Emergency Care for Children

Elizabeth M. Wertz, RN, BSN, MPM, PHRN, EMT-P, CMPE

Executive Director
Pediatric Alliance, PC

Chairperson, EMS for Children Advisory Committee
Pennsylvania Emergency Health Services Council

Immediate Past Chairperson
International Prehospital Trauma Life Support Committee
National Association of Emergency Medical Technicians

Pittsburgh, Pennsylvania

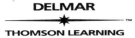
DELMAR
THOMSON LEARNING ™

Australia   Canada   Mexico   Singapore   Spain   United Kingdom   United States

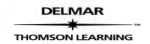

DELMAR
THOMSON LEARNING

Emergency Care For Children

Elizabeth Wertz

Business Unit Director:
William Brottmiller

Executive Marketing Manager:
Dawn Gerrain

Art/Design Coordinator:
Jay Purcell

Acquisitions Editor:
Doris Smith

Channel Manager:
Tara Carter

Cover Design:
Jay Purcell

Development Editor:
Darcy M. Scelsi

Project Editor:
Mary Ellen Cox

Editorial Assistant:
Jill Korznat

Production Coordinator:
Nina Lontrato

For permission to use material from this text or product, contact us by
Tel   (800) 730-2214
Fax   (800) 730-2215
www.thomsonrights.com

Library of Congress Cataloging-in-Publication Data

Emergency care for children
         p.   cm.
    ISBN 0-7668-1986-8 (alk. paper)
    1. Pediatric emergencies.   2. Pediatric intensive care.   3. Children—Wounds and injuries—Treatment.
    RJ370 .E417   2002
618.92′0025—dc21

                                      00-052284

NOTICE TO THE READER

Publisher does not warrant or guarantee any of the products described herein or perform any independent analysis in connection with any of the product information contained herein. Publisher does not assume, and expressly disclaims, any obligation to obtain and include information other than that provided to it by the manufacturer.

The reader is expressly warned to consider and adopt all safety precautions that might be indicated by the activities herein and to avoid all potential hazards. By following the instructions contained herein, the reader willingly assumes all risks in connection with such instructions.

The Publisher makes no representation or warranties of any kind, including but not limited to, the warranties of fitness for particular purpose or merchantability, nor are any such representations implied with respect to the material set forth herein, and the publisher takes no responsibility with respect to such material. The publisher shall not be liable for any special, consequential, or exemplary damages resulting, in whole or part, from the readers' use of, or reliance upon, this material.

Dedication

This book is dedicated to my beautiful children: Patrick, Amanda, and Ashley. I am blessed to have the opportunity to shape their lives.

To my son Patrick: You have grown into such a fine young man. Every day I watch you and am amazed at your knowledge, your positive attitude about life, and your sense of direction and purpose. You have made us so proud!

To my youngest daughter Ashley: You have given me more joy than you can possibly imagine. Experiencing life through your eyes and enjoying the "mother/daughter" relationship has been priceless. We appreciate every step you take, every task you learn to do, and, believe it or not, every word you speak—although sometimes, we need a small break!

My primary motivation for this book was my daugher, Amanda. Our unexpected journey with her began in her 10th week of life, and we have tackled many mountains and have withstood many disappointments over the last 13 years. I decided to turn my grief over all the things that we lost because of her seizures and subsequent disabilities into something positive—educating others about children with disabilities. She has taught our family so many things about life, and we are now advocates for all children with disabilities as well as their families.

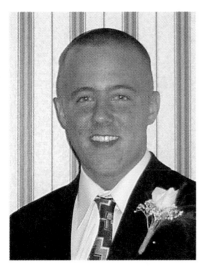 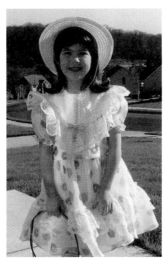 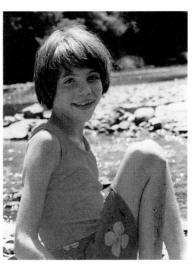

"I've learned that you can get beyond grief. Although it will always be a part of you, I learned that you can derive lessons from negative experiences . . . To heal yourself, you have to give to others. That is your responsibility."

Gianas, G. "Nurses who served in Vietnam: Silent heroes,"
Journal of Emergency Nursing, Vol. 20, No. 3, 247–249

I found ths quote several years after Amanda got sick. Those first few years were very difficult, and I was searching for somthing I could do to get past the frustration of not being able to change Amanda's diagnosis or prognosis. When I found this quote, I realized that what I could do was to give of myself to others. One avenue I chose was to write and teach others about children with special health care needs. If I could help one provider, one parent, or one family, I would be successful in my efforts.

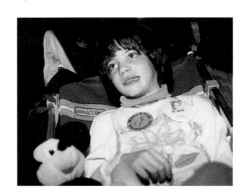

Over the last 11 years I have touched many lives and have dedicated myself to advocating for children with special health care needs and their families. To those of you who have been touched, thank you for listening. To others, please open your ears and your hearts. You may then be able to touch another person and keep the message alive.

Liz Wertz

Contents

Chapter 5   CARE AND RESUSCITATION OF THE NEONATE 67

Chapter 6   MEDICAL EMERGENCIES 77

Chapter 11   BURNS AND INHALATION INJURIES . 199

Contributing Authors

Susan A. Albrecht, PhD, MPM, RN
Associate Professor
University of Pittsburgh School of Nursing
Pittsburgh, Pennsylvania
Staff Nurse
Emergency Department
Jefferson Hospital
Pittsburgh, Pennsylvania

Lisa Marie Bernardo, PhD, MPH, RN
Assistant Professor
University of Pittsburgh School of Nursing
Pittsburgh, Pennsylvania
Staff Nurse
Emergency Department and Primary Care Center
Children's Hospital of Pittsburgh
Pittsburgh, Pennsylvania

John Chamberlin, NREMT-P, BS
EMS Specialist—Education
University of Pittsburgh Medical Center,
        Prehospital Care
Principal—Rock, Paper, Scissors & Chute, LLC

Kate Cronan, MD
Chief, Division of Emergency Medicine
Alfred I. duPont Hospital for Children
Wilmington, Delaware
Clinical Assistant Professor, Pediatrics
Thomas Jefferson Medical College
Philadelphia, Pennsylvania

Brian Gilchrist, MD
Assistant Professor of Surgery
State University of New York Health Science Center
Kings County Hospital Center
Brooklyn, New York

Judy Janing, PhD, RN, EMT-P
Emergency Program Specialist
IOCAD Emergency Services Group
Emmitsburg, Maryland
Former Program Director
Prehospital Education
Creighton University
Omaha, Nebraska

Susanne Kost, MD, FAAP
Clinical Assistant Professor
Pediatric Emergency Medicine
Jefferson Medical College
Alfred I. duPont Hospital for Children
Wilmington, Delaware

Max L. Ramenofsky, MD, FACS
Professor of Surgery
Chairman, Pediatric Surgery
Chief, Pediatric Trauma
State University of New York Health Science Center
Kings County Hospital Center
Brooklyn, New York

Richard Sobieray, MHA, MSEd, EMT-P
Senior Healthcare Consultant
Blue & Co., LLC
Columbus, Ohio

Illustrator:

Jill K. Gregory, MFA
Medical Illustrator
New York, New York

Special Assistants to the Author:

Ashley M. Wertz
Illustrator in Training
Student, Rowan Elementary School
Seven Fields, Pennsylvania

Patrick F. Wertz
Student, Seneca Valley High School
Seven Fields, Pennsylvania

Reviewers

Reg Allen, BS, NREMT-P
Monroe Community College
Rochester, New York

Rhonda Beck, NREMT-P
Macon Technical Institute
Macon, Georgia

Anne Clouatre, MHS, EMT-P
Porter and Littleton Adventist Prehospital Services
Denver, Colorado

Susan Fuchs, MD
Children's Memorial Hospital
Chicago, Illinois

Preface

This textbook represents several years of research to provide the reader with the most up-to-date information on prehospital pediatric emergency medicine. The text is written in a clear, easy-to-read style and is organized in such a way that the reader will naturally progress from usual growth and development to learning to care for critically ill or injured children. Objectives, Key Terms, a Case Study, and Review Questions are included with each chapter to address the competency-based level of achievement needed for success. Many photographs and illustrations are also included to enhance learning and reinforce didactic concepts.

The knowledge presented meets the objectives of the United States Department of Transportation 1998 National Standard Curriculum for Emergency Medical Technician (EMT)-Paramedics. It also includes recent changes to pediatric resuscitation as released by the American Heart Association in 2000. Some areas exceed the aforementioned objectives so as to provide a comprehensive educational tool for a variety of providers.

This textbook emphasizes "family-centered care" while many current products simply mention families. It discusses in-depth information about the prehospital providers' important relationship with the ill or injured child's family. Parents are an integral part of their children's lives and have not been traditionally involved in emergency medical services (EMS) publications. Many of the writers of this book are parents; and two are parents of children with special health care needs.

SPECIAL FEATURES

- Complete chapters on children with special health care needs (CSHCN), CSHCN assisted by technology, collaboration with other health care professionals and programs, child abuse, and ethical and legal issues.
- "Parent Perspectives" and "Sibling Sensitivities" are provided to give the reader a unique insight into the feelings of real parents and real siblings involved in pediatric emergencies. These "from-the-heart" comments emphasize the important roles played by the child's parents and siblings.
- "Exploring the Web" activities serve to acquaint the reader with the vast resources available on the web for dealing with pediatric emergencies.
- Detailed resource information is available for independent study in a stand-alone appendix. Addresses, telephone numbers, and Web addresses are included for those readers who want additional information.
- "Safety" boxes point out material that may pose a hazard to the patient or the prehospital professional and where special precautions must be taken.
- "Tricks of the Trade" provide the reader with tips from professionals in the field to provide insight into the real-life experiences of the prehospital professional.

Instructor's Guide

This supplement provides the instructor with valuable resources to simplify the planning and implementation of the instructional program. It includes student outline masters, motivational questions and activities, answers to questions in the text, and lesson plans to provide the instructor with a cohesive plan for presenting each topic. Additional material to assist the instructor in the preparation of lesson plans is included such as:

- Teaching Strategies comprised of suggestions for classroom activities such as role playing, small group discussion, research, simulations, and lab activities.
- Additional Case Studies with questions for student use.

- Skills Checklists that can serve as an evaluation tool for the instructor.
- Correlation Guide to the 1998 U.S. Department of Transportation (U.S. DOT) EMT-P National Standard Curriculum. For each objective in the pediatric portion of the curriculum page numbers are provided pointing to where specific matching content can be found in the text.
- Printed testbank will provide the instructor with five hundred new questions to create tests and exams.

Author Acknowledgments

Thank you to my dear husband. He has been "Mr. Mom" and our chef on so many occasions so that I could finish this project. In fact, he now *loves* to cook! His love and support continue to motivate me to take the time to "make a difference" in this life.

Thank you to my children. I know it was hard to understand why I had to stay focused on this book when you wanted to do other things. You inspire me every day.

Thank you to my parents for taking the time to raise me to fight for what I believe. My mother continues to be one of my dearest friends.

Thank you to my best friend Sharon and her family. You all have been there to celebrate the good things and to support us during the tough times.

Thank you to the physicians, Office Managers, and all staff at Pediatric Alliance throughout all of the offices in Pittsburgh, Pennsylvania. Your dedication to all children continues to impress me and empower me. I do not see my role with all of you as a job. I view each day as an opportunity to positively influence the lives of children and their families through your tireless efforts.

Thank you to all of the contributing authors for your time and expertise. It was great working with all of you.

Thank you to all of the children models: Kaitlin Beauseigneur, Rebecca Smith, Ashley Wertz, Amanda Wertz, Patrick Wertz, Pam Wills, and Lindsay Winkler. You were all so patient as I took picture after picture after picture. GO RAIDERS! We are . . . SV!!

Special thanks to Mark Lockhart and his beautiful family Suzanne, Tony, and Brandon for contributing pictures. You all were so helpful and look great on camera.

Thank you to Dr. Kate Cronan, husband Stephen, and their son Colin. I appreciate you sharing your personal experiences and pictures to teach others the wonders of raising a child with special health care needs.

Thank you to Cranberry Volunteer Ambulance Association and Shaler Area EMS. I appreciate the time and expertise you all contributed to the photo shoots! You are all stars in my book (literally!).

Thank you to Jill Gregory for her terrific illustrations. It was a long time coming but certainly worth the work. Thanks also to Jay Purcell at Delmar for his help in keeping all of the artwork and illustrations organized.

Thank you to Darcy Scelsi at Delmar. She has been such a great supporter of this project. Her "beacon of light" helped me get through the many revisions and multiple processes that come with writing a book.

And lastly, thanks to God for giving me the talent and perseverance to see this project through to completion. I am simply doing His work to make this world better for children.

About the Author

Liz Wertz has over 20 years of critical care, prehospital, flight, emergency nursing, and administrative experience. She has published numerous articles and textbook chapters and is a co-author of two editions of an EMT-Intermediate textbook. She was an editor for three editions of the Prehospital Trauma Life Support (PHTLS) textbook and developed the initial PHTLS-Basic course. She also developed an educational program for providing emergency care to children with special health care needs (CSHCN) and has presented it around the country.

Liz serves as Chairperson of the Pennsylvania Emergency Health Services Council's (PEHSC) EMS for Children Advisory Committee and the Children with Special Health Care Needs Subcommittee. She is also the Immediate Past Chairperson of the National Association of Emergency Medical Technicians' International PHTLS Division. She has served as Chairperson of PEHSC's Nursing Advisory Committee and School Nurse Subcommittee and was instrumental in developing and revising legislation in Pennsylvania to allow nurses to function in the prehospital setting.

She has been an Affiliate Faculty for Advanced Cardiac Life Support and PHTLS as well as an instructor for Pediatric Advanced Life Support, Basic Cardiac Life Support, Emergency Nursing Pediatric Course, and Assessment of Pediatric Emergencies in the School Setting developed by the Emergency Nurses Association and the National Association of School Nurses. She is also certified as a medical practice executive with the American College of Medical Practice Executives and is working toward fellowship.

Currently, Liz is the Executive Director of Pediatric Alliance, a physician practice with 24 pediatricians in nine offices throughout the Pittsburgh area. She has been married 18 years and is the parent of three children, one of whom is severely disabled with special health care needs.

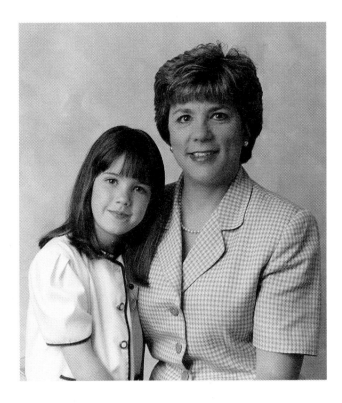

Chapter 1

Emergency Medical Services for Children

OBJECTIVES

Upon completion of this chapter, the student should be able to:

- Define *emergency medical services for children (EMSC)*.
- Identify the components of the EMSC system.
- Recall the first year that EMSC grants were awarded.
- List examples of pediatric equipment.
- Define *Emergency Department Approved for Pediatrics (EDAP)* and *Pediatric Critical Care Center (PCCC)*.
- List the seven issues to be included in EMSC data collection.
- Identify opportunities for pediatric injury prevention.
- Identify the components of the *Continuous Quality Improvement (CQI)* loop.
- Identify methods to contact the EMSC National Resource Center for additional information and materials.

KEY TERMS

Broselow system
Continuous Quality Improvement (CQI)
Emergency Department Approved for Pediatrics (EDAP)
Emergency Medical Services for Children (EMSC)
Isolette™

Pediatric Critical Care Center (PCCC)
primary transport
quality assurance (QA)
secondary transport

Case Scenario

You are dispatched to a motor vehicle accident on the main highway through town. Upon arrival, you discover a child was hit by a car while riding his bike. The child is lying on the side of the road on his back with a bystander holding his head still. The child is crying, and you are told his parents are coming up the road. He is not wearing a helmet. What would you do?

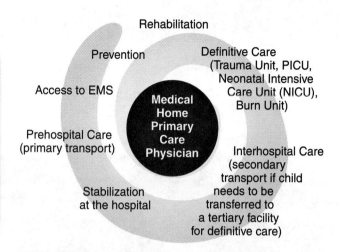

FIGURE 1-1 Components of the EMSC System. Seidel, J. S. & Henderson, D. P. (1991). *Emergency medical services for children: A report to the nation.* Washington, DC: National Center for Education in Maternal and Child Health.

INTRODUCTION

The **Emergency Medical Services for Children (EMSC)** program is a national program with the goal of ensuring that children receive the same high-quality emergency medical care that is provided to adults in the emergency medical services (EMS) system. The program was initiated in the mid-1980s with federal legislation and funding; and since that time, EMSC grants have been awarded to every state in the nation. Although prehospital and emergency department care are integral parts of the EMSC system, the program as a whole is geared toward the entire spectrum of caring for a child's unexpected accident or acute illness, from recognition of the problem by the parent to long-term rehabilitation (Figure 1-1).

The need for improving the existing EMS system by integrating a pediatric component is based on several well-recognized facts. First, children are not small adults. Health care providers need to recognize important pediatric differences in anatomy, physiology, and emotional responses to stress and spectrum of disease. Second, caring for ill or injured children may elicit stress responses in the health care provider, especially in the prehospital setting in which children account for a small proportion of the patient population. Finally, pediatric health care providers tend to focus more effort on prevention and rehabilitation than their adult counterparts; and the EMSC program has incorporated this philosophy.

This chapter presents a brief history of the EMSC program, as well as an overview of its components, including systems development, education, injury prevention, data analysis and research, and available resources for future program development. The objective of this chapter is to provide a contextual framework that identifies the role of the prehospital provider within the larger picture of EMSC and perhaps motivate the pre-

hospital provider to seek to expand that role for the sake of improving the health and lives of children.

HISTORY

The first organized EMS systems in the United States to provide rapid care and transportation for victims of heart attacks or trauma came about in the 1960s under the supervision of cardiologists and surgeons. While children have always used the EMS system, it was not recognized until the late 1970s that the system was not always meeting their needs. In the early 1980s, Senators Daniel Inouye, Orin Hatch, and Lowell Weicker in conjunction with Surgeon General Dr. C. Everett Koop (a pediatric surgeon) drafted legislation to provide organization and funding for the EMSC program. The program is operated jointly through the Maternal and Child Health Bureau (MCHB) of the Health Resources and Services Administration (HRSA) of the U.S. Department of Health and Human Services (DHHS), and the National Highway and Traffic Safety Association (NHTSA) of the U.S. Department of Transportation (DOT).

The organization and the goals of the program were established in the early 1980s with the help of Dr. Calvin Sia, president of the Hawaii Medical Association, along with the newly established Section on Pediatric Emergency Medicine of the American Academy of Pediatrics (AAP) (1981). The first grants were awarded to four states in 1985: Alabama, California, New York, and Oregon. By 1990, 20 states had received funding.

Exploring the Web

● Search the Web for EMSC grant projects in your state. What is available? How can you or your EMS organization get involved?

In order to assess the progress of the EMSC program and to provide unification and future direction for the program, HRSA commissioned a study from the Institute of Medicine (IOM) in 1990. As a result, a committee of experts from all aspects of pediatric emergency care met periodically over the course of two years. The publications produced by this committee, *EMSC: A report to the nation* (Seidel & Henderson, 1991) and *EMSC: Summary* (Durch & Lohr, 1993), provide a detailed analysis of the state of emergency medical care for children in this country and serve as the basis for the future of the EMSC program.

At present, all 50 states, four territories, and the District of Columbia have received some type of funding for improving emergency medical services for children. Grant projects have included a wide range of topics from prevention and education to systems issues and caring for children with special health care needs. However, the application of this information is by no means universal; and the ideal of an integrated, nationwide EMS/EMSC system remains to be achieved.

SYSTEMS DEVELOPMENT

Although the basic framework of an EMS system—personnel, communications, equipment, and record keeping—is the same for adults and children, optimal performance of the system from a pediatric standpoint requires special attention within many aspects of the system. Systems issues with a need for pediatric "extras" include access, protocols, medical control, transport, equipment, staffing, categorization, and rehabilitation.

Access

Access to the EMS system via the 911 and enhanced 911 systems is increasing throughout the country; however, rural areas and poor urban areas (i.e., areas where families lack telephones) remain underserved. The appropriate use of the 911 system also presents a problem. The

skills required for a parent or caretaker of an ill or injured child to recognize an emergency and to access EMS are neither taught nor assessed in any systematic manner in this country. Both overuse of the system for nonemergencies and failure to use the system for true emergencies are common mistakes. Goals of the EMSC program include universal 911 access and increasing education of the public about proper use of this system.

Protocols

Once the EMS system is accessed and help is on the way, the next step is ensuring that appropriate pediatric protocols are in place. Dispatchers can most effectively obtain triage information and assist parents in performing basic first aid or life support measures when protocols anticipate these circumstances.

In many states, pediatric field protocols are developed within a specific service area or region. Prehospital providers then have guidelines to use when initially treating the ill or injured child before contact with the medical control physician, ensuring that appropriate pediatric treatment is rendered.

Likewise, the medical control physician should have ready access to pediatric dosage cards, pediatric texts, and pediatric protocols. Utilization of these references again helps to assure that adequate pediatric care and pediatric medical oversight are provided.

In pediatric trauma cases, the trauma protocols or treatment guidelines should include appropriate pediatric adaptations. Disaster protocols should likewise prepare for events involving large numbers of children.

Medical Control

In complicated pediatric cases, the medical control physician and the child's pediatrician should communicate via a referral or consult call. While this communication is not always available during the emergency, an attempt at interaction with the child's primary care physician is recommended.

This discussion is particularly important in the instance of treating a child with special health care needs. The medical control physician may not be aware of specific pre-existing conditions that may affect the current emergency treatment (see Chapter 7—Children with Special Health Care Needs).

Transport

Fast, safe, and efficient transport of children depends on carefully coordinated services. In some cases, it may be prudent to bypass the closest facility in favor of a facility that is better equipped to handle pediatric cases.

Exploring the Web

● If one exists, search your state EMS Web site. Are state-wide protocols available for transporting a pediatric patient via ground, helicopter, or fixed-wing aircraft? Are regional protocols available? Research the guidelines that are used in your particular service area.

Interfacility transfer agreements should be in place before they are actually needed. In rural areas, the issue becomes one of what type of transport vehicle is most appropriate—ground, helicopter, or fixed-wing aircraft. Again, these problems should be addressed in advance through state- or region-wide policies.

Another issue of EMSC interest in the transport realm is that of ambulance design. Transport vehicles routinely used for complex pediatric emergencies (i.e., severe trauma or life-threatening medical illnesses), whether air or ground, need careful consideration and pre-planning. An **Isolette**™, for example, is a self-contained incubator unit that allows for the control of heat, humidity, and oxygen (Figure 1-2). It is used to transport high-risk neonates (e.g., premature and low-birth-weight neonates) and requires specific adaptations to properly secure the device within the ambulance, hel-

icopter, or fixed-wing aircraft. Proper planning, purchase, and installation of this adaptive structural equipment needs to occur before the transport is necessary.

Equipment

It is essential that the ambulance be appropriately stocked with pediatric treatment equipment such as child-sized cervical collars, masks, bag-valve devices, endotracheal tubes, blood pressure cuffs, and intravenous catheters. The types of equipment necessary depend on the capabilities of the ambulance (e.g., basic life support or advanced life support). As recently as 1997, only five states required EMSC-recommended advanced life support equipment on all ambulances (DHHS, HRSA, and MCHB, 1997).

Weight- or length-based charts for appropriate equipment and medication dosing are also essential. The **Broselow system** is an excellent example of a useful pediatric adjunct for resuscitation equipment. The system allows the prehospital provider to quickly identify the proper size of equipment to be used for that child. The color-coded, length-based tape correlates a rapid estimate of the weight of the child to appropriately sized equipment (Figure 1-3).

Staffing

All medical staff throughout the cycle of a pediatric illness or injury, from the prehospital phase to rehabilitation, should feel trained and adequately prepared to care for children. Local and state policymakers should set standards for pediatric education at all levels and desig-

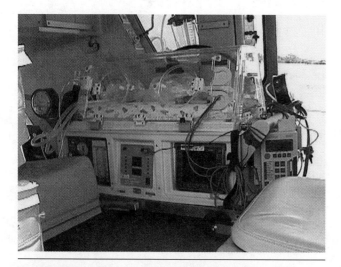

FIGURE 1-2 This Isolette is used in the helicopter for transport of a high-risk neonate to a tertiary facility with a Neonatal Intensive Care Unit (NICU).

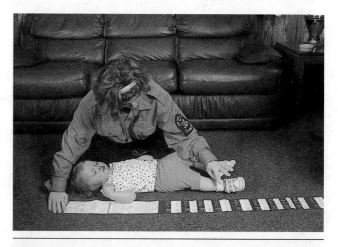

FIGURE 1-3 This child is being measured with a Broselow tape to determine what equipment and medications would be appropriate for her age and size.

nate facilities according to the training of the staff. The EMSC program is working to ensure that all health care professionals meet a minimum of training to provide pediatric standards of care and that pediatric referral centers are able to provide comprehensive care by pediatric specialists and pediatric surgeons.

Categorization

In much of the country, the transport of a critically ill child is based on geographical convenience rather than forethought as to the optimal location for pediatric care. A goal of the EMSC program is to have a system of pediatric-designated facilities, based on staffing and equipment standards, to allow a tiered or coordinated approach to care.

In rural settings, direct transport to a pediatric facility capable of meeting the child's complex trauma or medical needs may not be feasible. The tertiary facility may be more than 100 miles away so that the child is transported by EMS to the local facility for initial stabilization. This initial transport is known as **primary transport** (Figure 1-4). The child is then moved to a tertiary center by a second transfer or what is known as **secondary transport**.

In an urban setting, tertiary pediatric facilities may be readily accessible, and patients may be transported directly to those centers by the EMS system. In some instances, the patient may be transported initially to a suburban emergency department and then have secondary transport to the tertiary center.

California is a leader in tiered response with a system of **Emergency Departments Approved for Pediatrics (EDAPs)**. Children are initially stabilized at the EDAP where minimum pediatric staffing, equip-

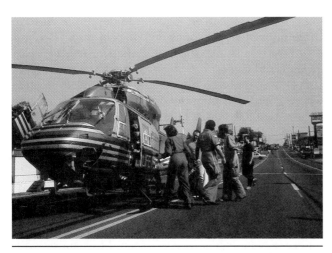

FIGURE 1-4 A helicopter is routinely used for primary transport.

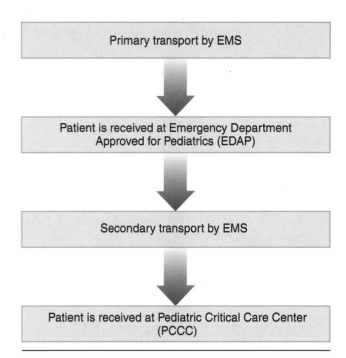

```
Primary transport by EMS
        ↓
Patient is received at Emergency Department
Approved for Pediatrics (EDAP)
        ↓
Secondary transport by EMS
        ↓
Patient is received at Pediatric Critical Care Center
(PCCC)
```

FIGURE 1-5 Tiered transport for a critically ill or injured pediatric patient.

ment, and supplies are available. The child is then taken to an appropriate **Pediatric Critical Care Center (PCCC)** which is designed to provide a higher level of care including a pediatric intensive care unit (PICU) as well as pediatric and trauma care specialists (Figure 1-5).

Rehabilitation

Although rehabilitation seems a long way from the ambulance and the emergency department, seriously ill or injured children often require some sort of physical or psychological rehabilitation. Another goal of EMSC is to integrate this phase into the care plan for the child as soon as possible. Ideally, data linkages will be established that will allow prehospital caretakers to know the long-term outcome of the child's illness or injury. Providers will learn what happened to the child throughout his or her hospitalization and rehabilitation and how the continuum of treatment affected the child's opportunity for return to the community, including the school setting. This knowledge will allow rational approaches to improving the initial steps of management so that the child's long-term functionality is positively affected.

Children in a rehabilitation situation may be temporarily or permanently dependent on technology, and they often require interfacility transport. Prehospital personnel should be familiar with the care of tracheostomies, vascular access devices, and feeding tubes (see

Chapter 8—Children with Special Health Care Needs Assisted by Technology).

Prehospital caretakers themselves may benefit from short-term psychological rehabilitation in the form of critical incident stress management (CISM), which is especially important when dealing with children. A well-planned EMS system will allow for the "care of the caretaker."

EDUCATION

A major focus of EMSC grants awarded to date has been education and training. The Institute of Medicine report recommended that education be directed toward both laypersons and health care professionals (Seidel & Henderson, 1991).

Training Laypersons

Recognizing that the most common cause of preventable morbidity and mortality in the pediatric population is trauma, EMSC programs directed education efforts for the public toward emphasis of injury prevention and safety. The EMSC program has supported dozens of excellent injury prevention projects, ranging from posters and coloring books to interactive videos.

An excellent example of a product supported in part by EMSC is Risk Watch™, developed by the National Fire Protection Association (NFPA) and Lowe's Home Safety Council. This curriculum is geared toward children in preschool through eighth grade and consists of five separate binders, one for each age range (i.e., preschool through kindergarten, grades 1 and 2, grades 3 and 4, grades 5 and 6, and grades 7 and 8). Schools or community groups may purchase one binder or the entire set with each binder containing reading materials and instructions for activities that promote developmentally appropriate topics (Figure 1-6).

In addition to injury prevention, EMSC supports public education in pediatric first aid, cardiopulmonary resuscitation (CPR), and appropriate access and use of the EMS system. Knowledge and skills of this nature are especially important for parents, but anyone responsible for the care of children (child care workers, teachers, and coaches) should have some background in basic emergency care.

Training Health Care Professionals

The EMSC program is active in the training of both prehospital and hospital personnel. The majority of the educational material produced to date has been directed

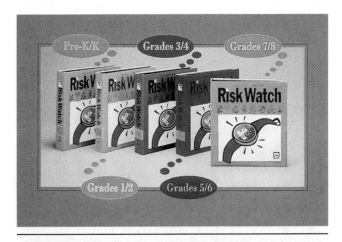

FIGURE 1-6 The *Risk Watch*™ document was developed by the National Fire Protection Association and Lowe's Home Safety Council to provide education regarding injury prevention for children from preschool through eighth grade. Photo courtesy of the National Fire Protection Association.

toward prehospital providers, in recognition of previous deficiencies in this area. Recent revisions to the emergency medical technician (EMT) curricula have increased the amount and quality of the pediatric education module. In the EMT-Basic National Standard Curriculum (NSC), the time devoted to pediatrics has increased from 2 to 6 hours of a 110-hour course, with an improved focus on pediatric airway management. The EMT-Intermediate and EMT-Paramedic National Standard Curricula have also increased the pediatric portion.

Many states have used EMSC grants to create supplemental prehospital educational materials, some geared especially toward rural areas. Idaho and Vermont grant recipients worked together to develop a series of three interactive programs on compact discs: *Respiratory Emergencies for Children, Pediatric Medical Emergencies*, and *Pediatric Trauma*. The discs allow a "flight simulation" approach to pediatric emergencies in areas where population is sparse and formal courses may be hundreds of miles away. Other supplemental prehospital educational products include printed materials, video tapes, and slides. These materials cover both broad topics, such as medical emergencies, and specific issues, such as intraosseous infusion.

EMSC has also devoted attention to the education of physicians and nurses in both office and hospital settings. Recent research has shown that pediatric offices may be inadequately prepared to stabilize critically ill children. An EMSC grant in North Carolina sponsored the development of a workshop, *Preparing*

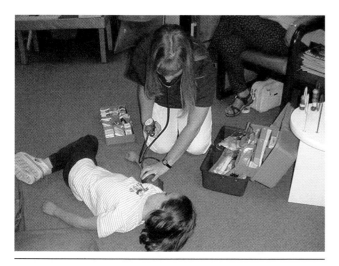

FIGURE 1-7 This pediatric office conducts mock codes in which all staff members participate.

the Office for Pediatric Emergencies, involving a didactic session and a "mock code" practical session, which has been presented to nearly every pediatric office in that state (Figure 1-7).

Another popular physician- and nurse-oriented course (though appropriate for paramedics also) is the Pediatric Advanced Life Support (PALS) course. PALS is sponsored by the American Heart Association, and the EMSC program encourages health care providers to take advantage of this resource.

In addition to providing and encouraging the voluntary use of pediatric emergency medicine educational materials, the EMSC program is active in attempting to set state and national standards for a minimum level of pediatric education, both for initial certification and for recertification in a health care field. As of 1997, fewer than 20 states had any formal pediatric requirements for EMT recertification. Likewise, in the public sector, fewer than 20 states require CPR training for licensed child care providers. From an EMSC standpoint, public policy has a long way to go regarding educational standards.

INJURY PREVENTION

Trauma remains the leading cause of death and disability in the pediatric population. Each year in the United States, approximately 120,000 children are permanently disabled as the result of a traumatic injury (National SAFEKIDS, 1999). Every day, over 39,000 children sustain injuries serious enough to require medical treatment for a total of 14 million children per year (National SAFEKIDS, 1999). Of children ages 14 and younger,

8.7 million are seen in an emergency department on a yearly basis (National SAFEKIDS, 1999). As Dr. C. Everett Koop testified to Congress in 1989, if an infectious disease affected this many children, the public would demand a cure quickly (Seidel & Henderson, 1991). However, as a nation we have become adapted to think of injuries as inevitable accidents, rather than preventable events.

Emergency service providers are uniquely suited to become involved in all aspects of injury prevention. Half of all pediatric EMS encounters are injury-related, providing plenty of first-hand experience with the problem. The EMSC program encourages prehospital and emergency care personnel to become involved in injury prevention in the areas of clinical practice, community education, policy making, and research.

Clinical Practice

In the area of clinical practice, health care providers can begin contributing to injury prevention by increasing their level of awareness as well as their "detective skills." Did the baby fall down the steps because the baby gate was improperly installed? *Was* there a baby gate? Was the child adequately supervised? Were the caretakers under the influence of alcohol or engaged in a domestic dispute? Prehospital personnel have a unique opportunity to assess the field situation directly and to offer advice when the parent may be most impressionable.

Community Education

Emergency service workers, whether EMTs, nurses, or physicians, are generally looked upon with respect by members of the community. First-hand experience will serve as a valuable resource when speaking to the media, schools, or community groups. By assisting at a school bicycle safety program or community car seat check, a health care worker may save more children in an afternoon than would be successfully resuscitated from major trauma in a career (Figure 1-8).

Policy Making

Medical professionals may also exert a profound influence on local and state policy. Lawmakers are human and are influenced by anecdotal stories as well as statistics. Dr. Barbara Barlow, a pediatrician in Harlem in New York City, developed an injury prevention group that, among other projects, encouraged enforcement of a window-guard law in high-rise apartments. The percentage of pediatric injury deaths in Harlem resulting from falls decreased from 12 to 0 percent in a five-year

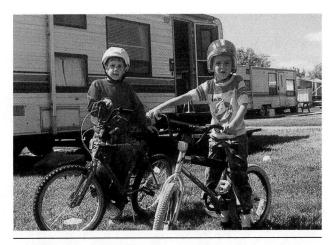

FIGURE 1-8 These children participated in a Bike Safety Day at a local campground.

period (Davidson, Durkin, O'Connor, Barlow, & Heagarty, 1994).

Prehospital and emergency care staff can also influence policy by complete documentation of the circumstances of an injury. National data sets that greatly influence public health, such as those maintained by the Consumer Product Safety Commission (CPSC), are dependent on accurate data from the scenes of the injuries.

Data Analysis and Research

Data collection and analysis are an essential part of any successful organization, and the EMS system is no exception. In order to know if children are receiving adequate emergency care, the EMSC program strongly advocates more extensive and uniform data collection through all phases of care, from the prehospital setting to the rehabilitation phase. Although there is certainly no shortage of information collection and paperwork in the health care system, the translation of these data into useful information for the purposes of large-scale com-

Exploring the Web

● Search the Consumer Product Safety Commission Web site. What children's resources are available? What resources are available for health care providers to report unsafe products?

parisons between systems or institutions is currently difficult or impossible. Patients are likely to be assigned separate identification numbers on the ambulance, at the hospital, in the trauma registry, and at the rehabilitation facility. Different ambulance companies and hospitals use different identification and coding systems. Patients with similar initial presentations may end up with very different diagnostic codes. Information about interventions and outcomes is likely to be entered into multiple computerized databases, few of which will be compatible, or worse, may not be entered into a computerized system at all. Finally, organizations may be averse to sharing data for reasons of patient confidentiality or competitive advantage.

The Institute of Medicine committee on EMSC suggests that data be obtained in a standardized manner to address the following seven issues:

1. Structure of the system—numbers and types of facilities, providers, and services available for children
2. Users of the system—demographics such as age, gender, race or minority group, address (rural, suburban, urban), and insurance status
3. Reasons that the system is used—types of illnesses and injuries that prompt parents or other caregivers to access the EMS system
4. Services that are provided to the patients—numbers and types of interventions and procedures
5. Timing of the services—down times, accident scene times, transport times, and hospital days
6. Outcomes of using the system—clinical outcomes, including survival-to-discharge and quality of life issues, as well as process outcomes such as admissions or referrals to specialty care facilities
7. Costs of the system—personnel, equipment, facility charges, and levels of reimbursement

The items on this list are important for determining the most efficient allocation of limited resources as well as in guiding injury prevention efforts and in maintaining financial stability in the EMS system.

While collection of data is vitally important, the data are useless unless they are employed in an organized effort to seek improvement. The terms **quality assurance (QA)** and **continuous quality improvement (CQI)** are becoming common in the health care workplace and should be an important part of the EMS system as well. QA refers to an organized system of tracking specific indicators to ensure that the quality of the system is maintained. The indicators are divided into structure (e.g., staff and equipment), process (e.g., protocols and procedures), and outcome (e.g., return of spontaneous circulation or return emergency depart-

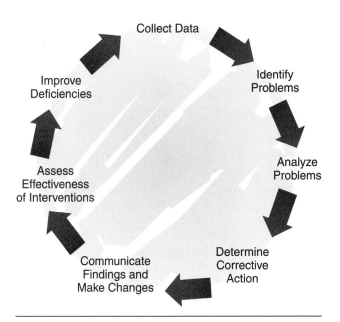

FIGURE 1-9 Continuous Quality Improvement (CQI) Loop. Seidel, J. S. & Henderson, D. P. (Eds.). (1991). *Emergency medical services for children: A report to the nation.* Washington, DC: National Center for Education in Maternal and Child Health.

ment visit in 48 hours). QA is taken one step further when it becomes CQI, in which data are used not only to maintain quality standards but also to enable health care providers to continually improve upon deficiencies via the CQI loop (Figure 1-9).

The founders of the EMSC program have taken large steps in these areas by adopting initial guidelines for structure and process of the system. Proposals for staffing, equipment, and supplies have been developed and published in the areas of prehospital, hospital, and posthospital care of pediatric emergencies. While these recommendations are not comprehensive, they serve as a basis for discussion and adaptation to the needs of individual communities.

RESOURCE NETWORK

The EMSC program supports a remarkable resource network, the EMSC National Resource Center (NRC).

Exploring the Web

● Become familiar with the Web site for the EMSC National Resource Center. What resources are available to help organize prevention programs in your area? What continuing education programs are available?

The purpose of the center is to provide assistance to the public, professional groups, and state or medical center grantees on issues of importance in developing and sustaining an EMSC system. Examples of resources provided by the center include a Web site, a quarterly newsletter (*EMSC News*), and multiple printed materials, including an annual catalogue of hundreds of EMSC products. Catalogue items include posters, pamphlets, stickers, books, videos, and compact discs aimed at all areas of EMSC interest. Many of these products are available free or for a minimal charge to cover cost of production.

For more information contact:
EMSC National Resource Center
111 Michigan Avenue, NW
Washington, DC 20010
(202) 884-4927; Fax: (301) 650-8045
e-mail: info@emscnrc.com

SUMMARY

In summary, the EMSC program is a federally funded program providing organizational and grant support for a variety of activities aimed at improving emergency medical care for children. While prehospital care is a vital component of EMSC, the program is designed to cover the spectrum of emergency care from prehospital to rehabilitative services. Prehospital care providers are encouraged to improve their professional pediatric skills and to become child advocates in the broader sense—by increasing public awareness of EMSC and by building coalitions within their communities with the goal of improving the health and safety of children.

Management of Case Scenario

Your partner gathers information as you examine the child. With the bystander continuing to hold the head, you find the airway patent as the child is softly crying. He cannot tell you his name or any other information. He has decreased breath sounds on the right side with a large abrasion on that side of his chest. A radial pulse is barely palpable, and the carotid pulse is rapid. Skin is cool, diaphoretic, and pale. Pupils are equal and sluggish to react to light. Abdomen is rigid to palpation. Abrasions are found on his arms and legs with minimal bleeding. The remainder of the exam is unremarkable.

Your partner comes over with the father and tells you the child is eight years old. He was wearing a helmet and was thrown about ten feet when the car hit him. He landed on the cement and stones at the side of the highway. He was initially unconscious when bystanders arrived. Another bystander finds the helmet and gives it to you. It has a large dent on the right side.

You speak with the medical control physician and request helicopter transport to the pediatric trauma center. You ask the father to talk with his son to reassure him. In the meantime, you apply oxygen at 15 liters per minute via a nonrebreather face mask. You then apply a pediatric cervical collar and immobilize the child to a long backboard. As you put the backboard in place, you quickly examine his back. No deformities are found. Multiple abrasions are present with minimal bleeding. You transfer the child on the backboard to the stretcher and into the ambulance. Vital signs are: pulse of 136, respirations of 24, and a blood pressure of 70/44.

You allow the father to stay with his son in the back of the ambulance and explain what will be happening. He rides restrained in the seat at the head of the stretcher. The father continues to talk to his son.

You meet the helicopter at the landing zone and provide report to the flight nurse and flight medic. The child is transferred into the helicopter and flown to the pediatric trauma center. The child's father is permitted to fly in the helicopter with his son.

At the trauma center, the child undergoes surgery for a grade II liver laceration. He also has a mild head injury and a pneumothorax on the right side for which he has a chest tube in for a few days. The child does well and is discharged home within two weeks.

All components of the EMS system worked well for this child as outlined in Table 1-1.

TABLE 1-1
Pediatric EMS System

EMSC Component	Result
Trauma prevention education	This child was wearing a helmet when he was riding his bike. He sustained a mild head injury instead of a catastrophic injury.
Bystander education	Bystanders assisted appropriately and maintained cervical immobilization until further help arrived.
Proper system development	• The ambulance and prehospital personnel responded within ten minutes. • Pediatric equipment was available on the ambulance. • Air transport was requested and properly coordinated. • The child was taken to a pediatric trauma center that was correctly staffed and equipped to treat his injuries.
EMS Pediatric Education	The child was properly treated and immobilized at the scene and in the air during transport.

REVIEW QUESTIONS

1. Define the following terms:
   a. Emergency Medical Services for Children (EMSC)
   b. Emergency Department Approved for Pediatrics (EDAP)
   c. Pediatric Critical Care Center (PCCC)
   d. Primary transport
   e. Secondary transport
2. List the components of the EMSC system.
3. The first EMSC grants were awarded in 1983. True or False?
4. Describe the concept of tiered transport and how it is accomplished.
5. Prehospital personnel have a unique opportunity to participate in injury prevention activities. True or False? Why?
6. The following issue(s) should be addressed in EMSC data collection:
   a. Structure and users of the system
   b. Timing of the services
   c. Costs of the system
   d. All of the above
7. List the components of the CQI loop.
8. The EMSC National Resource Center is located in Washington, DC. True or False? How do you contact them?

REFERENCES

Davidson, L. L., Durkin, M. S., Kuhn, L., O'Connor, P., Barlow, B., & Heagarty, M. C. (1994). The impact of the Safe Kids/Healthy Neighborhoods Injury Prevention Program in Harlem, 1988 through 1991. *American Journal of Public Health, 84(4)*: 580–586.

Durch, J. S., & Lohr, K. N. (Eds.). (1993). *Emergency medical services for children: Summary*. Washington, DC: National Academy Press.

National SAFEKIDS Campaign. Available e-mail: www.safekids.org

Seidel, J. S., & Henderson, D. P. (Eds.). (1991). *Emergency medical services for children: A report to the nation*. Washington, DC: National Center for Education in Maternal and Child Health.

U.S. Department of Health and Human Services, Health Resources and Services Administration, Maternal and Child Health Bureau. (1997). *5 Year plan: Midcourse review: Emergency medical services for children, 1995-2000*. Washington, DC: Emergency Medical Services for Children National Resource Center.

BIBLIOGRAPHY

Chameides, L., & Hazinski, M. F. (Eds.). (1999). *Pediatric advanced life support*. American Heart Association.

Henderson, D. P., & Seidel, J. S. (Eds.). (1997). *EMSC products catalogue*, National EMSC Resource Alliance.

Schafermeyer, R. W., & Frush, K. (1997). Emergency medical services for North Carolina's children. *North Carolina Medicine, 58(4)*, 293–295.

Widome, M. D. (Ed.). (1997). *Injury prevention and control for children and youth* (3rd ed.). Elk Grove Village, IL: American Academy of Pediatrics.

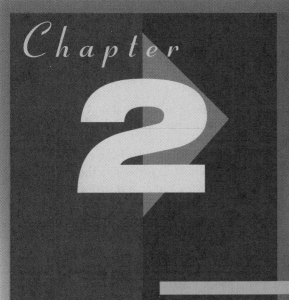

Chapter 2

Assessment of the Stable Child

OBJECTIVES

Upon completion of this chapter, the student should be able to:

- Identify and describe developmental characteristics and coping mechanisms of different age groups.
- Identify injuries and illnesses common to different age groups.
- Identify the major anatomical and physiological differences of various age groups as compared to adults.
- List the basic elements and parameters of assessment to include approach, history taking, and physical examination.
- Identify considerations for determining when to transport the stable child.

KEY TERMS

adolescent	fontanelle	sepsis
bronchiolitis	hypoperfusion	shock
cardiac output	infant	Starling's law
congenital	meningitis	startle reflex
croup	preschooler	stridor
dehydration	reactive airway disease (RAD)	stroke volume
diabetic ketoacidosis	respiratory syncytial virus (RSV)	sudden infant death syndrome (SIDS)
diaphoresis	retractions	tachypnea
epiglottitis	school aged	toddler
febrile seizure		

Case Scenario

You are dispatched at 10 a.m. to a private residence for an ill child. When you arrive, you find a four-year-old girl lying on the couch in the fetal position. She is awake and quiet. Her mother tells you she started complaining of abdominal pain this morning when she got up at 7 a.m. She ate a small breakfast and instead of going to play, she went immediately to the couch to lie down. When she checked on her a few minutes ago, she told her the pain was still there and she didn't want to move. The mother was concerned and called for an ambulance. How would you approach the assessment of this child?

INTRODUCTION

The prehospital provider needs to gain the cooperation of the stable child in order to conduct an adequate physical examination and gather a good history. Understanding normal developmental characteristics and coping mechanisms for the given age can help achieve this goal. To determine if a child's behavior or affect is atypical, the provider must first know what is typical for that age. There are also major anatomical and physiological differences in various age groups. Knowledge of these differences is necessary to recognize unusual and significant variances that may indicate a problem. In addition, a basic knowledge of common injuries and illnesses for various age groups can help focus assessment parameters for indicative signs and symptoms.

DEVELOPMENT, COPING, AND COMMON PROBLEMS

Stages of pediatric cognitive and emotional development can be approximated based on age. This section reviews mental development, including coping mechanisms and common medical problems, by age group.

The "Innocent"

The development of the **infant** from birth to one year is filled with "firsts." Infancy is a period of dramatic physical, motor, cognitive, emotional, and social growth. Infants progress rapidly from having little control over movement to becoming an almost "perpetual motion machine"—full of curiosity and adventure. The first year

of life is one of the most critical periods of growth and development.

Development

During the first three months, the infant has almost no ability to coordinate motor function. In the infant, sudden movements or loud noises are strong stimuli and may elicit the **startle reflex** (stiffening of the body and flexion of the extremities). Even though the startle reflex is appropriate for this age group, it is stressful; therefore, do *not* attempt to elicit this response deliberately during examination. Between three and six months, the infant begins to roll over independently. It is also common to see the infant with his or her hands or other objects in the mouth (Figure 2-1). From six months to a year, development progresses rapidly, from creeping and crawling to standing and walking. Table 2-1 summarizes the developmental skills of this age group.

Coping

Because infants are aware of familiar surroundings and are very attached to the parent/caregiver from approximately six months on, fear of the unknown and separation from the caregiver become significant. The major coping mechanisms for the infant up to one year is sucking (either a pacifier or the thumb) and close parental contact.

Common Problems

Problems are primarily medical in nature during the first six months of life. They include: **sudden infant death syndrome (SIDS)** (sudden and unexpected death), **dehydration** (excessive body fluid loss), **meningitis**

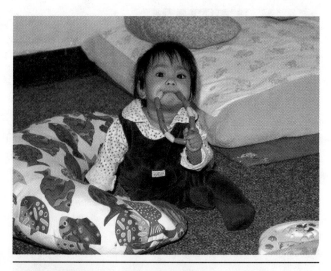

FIGURE 2-1 It is common to see infants three to six months of age with hands or other objects in the mouth.

TABLE 2-1
Growth and Development During Infancy

Age	Gross Motor	Fine Motor	Language	Sensory
Birth to 1 month	• Assumes tonic neck posture • When prone, lifts and turns head	• Holds hands in fist • Draws arms and legs to body	• Cries	• Comforts with holding and touch • Looks at faces • Follows objects when in line of vision • Alert to high-pitched voices • Smiles
2–4 months	• Can raise head and shoulders when prone to 45°–90°; supports self on forearms • Rolls from back to side	• Hands mostly open • Looks at and plays with fingers • Grasps and tries to reach objects	• Vocalizes when talked to; coos, babbles • Laughs aloud • Squeals	• Smiles • Follows objects 180° • Turns head when hears voices or sounds
4–6 months	• Turns from stomach to back and back to stomach • When pulled to sitting almost no head lag • By 6 months can sit on floor with hands forward for support	• Can hold feet and put in mouth • Can hold bottle • Can grasp rattle and other small objects • Put objects in mouth	• Squeals	• Watches a falling object • Responds to sounds
6–8 months	• Puts full weight on legs when held in standing position • Can sit without support • Bounces when held in standing position	• Transfers objects from one hand to the other • Can feed self a cookie • Can bang two objects together	• Babbles vowel-like sounds, "ooh" or "aah" • Imitation of speech sounds ("mama", "dada") beginning • Laughs aloud	• Responds by looking and smiling • Recognizes own name
8–10 months	• Crawls on all fours or uses arms to pull body along floor • Can pull self to sitting • Can pull self to standing	• Beginning to use thumb-finger grasp • Dominant hand use • Has good hand-mouth coordination	• Responds to verbal commands • May say one word in addition to "mama" and "dada"	• Recognizes sounds
10–12 months	• Can sit down from standing • Walks around room holding onto objects • Can stand alone	• Picks up and drops objects • Can put small objects into toys or containers through holes • Turns many pages in a book at one time • Picks up small objects	• Understands "no" and other simple commands • Learns one or two other words • Imitates speech sounds • Speaks gibberish	• Follows fast-moving objects • Indicates wants • Likes to play imitative games such as patty cake and peek-a-boo

Estes, M. E. Z. (1998). *Health assessment and physical examination.* Albany, NY: Delmar Thomson Learning. Copyright 1998 Delmar Thomson Learning.

(inflammation of the meninges), **sepsis** (systemic infection), and **congenital** (present at birth) diseases. See Chapter 6—Medical Emergencies for more information on these illnesses. Traumatic injuries, frequently the result of child abuse, are also seen in this age group. See Chapter 9—Head and Spinal Trauma, Chapter 10—Thoracic and Abdominal Trauma, and Chapter 12—Child Abuse for detailed information.

From six months to a year, the infant is prone to **febrile seizures** (seizures resulting from a rapid rise in temperature), **croup** (viral infection of the upper and lower respiratory tract), **bronchiolitis** (viral infection of the lower respiratory tract), **respiratory syncytial virus (RSV)** (virus causing bronchiolitis, bronchopneumonia, and the common cold in children), and **reactive airway disease (RAD)** (asthma) in addition to dehydration, sepsis, and meningitis. Again, refer to Chapter 6—Medical Emergencies for detailed discussions of these illnesses. Because the older infant is now mobile and curious, the incidence of ingestions of poisons and foreign body aspiration increases. Table 2-2 summarizes the common problems seen in this age group.

The "Creepers, Cruisers, and Climbers"

Children aged one to three (also known as toddlers) are busy learning about their new world. They test every aspect of their new reality through exploration, discovery, language, and intense activity. It is at this age that children develop very individual and independent personalities.

Development

Limited language develops by this age, although memory is short. The parents of a two-year-old child are likely to say that limited language consists primarily of the words "no" and "why." Motor skills increase making the toddler much more mobile. Toddlers are always on the go. Table 2-3 summarizes the developmental skills of the toddler.

Coping

This group remains very close to the parent/caregiver and fears separation, strangers, and loss of control. The primary coping mechanism continues to be parental contact. In addition, this age group often has a special object of affection such as a blanket, special toy, baby doll, or stuffed animal (Figure 2-2). Keep this in mind and, if at all possible, keep that object with the child.

Common Problems

Febrile seizures, croup, meningitis, and reactive airway disease continue to be common medical problems seen in this age group. Although the incidence of bronchiolitis is less frequent, the incidence of RAD increases. Incidence of foreign bodies and ingestions of poisons continue to be relatively common problems. Traumatic

---

TABLE 2-2
Common Problems of Infancy

Birth to Six Months	Six Months to One Year
• SIDS	• Febrile seizures
• Dehydration	• Dehydration
• Meningitis	• Meningitis
• Sepsis	• Sepsis
• Congenital diseases	• Croup
• Traumatic injuries from abuse/motor vehicle collision	• Bronchiolitis
	• Reactive airway disease/asthma
	• RSV
	• Ingestions
	• Foreign body aspiration

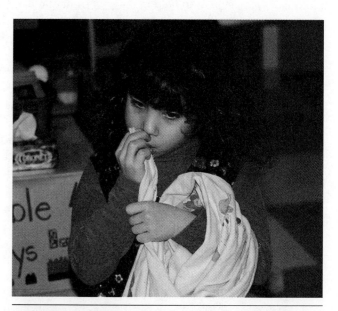

FIGURE 2-2 Toddlers often have a special object of affection such as a blanket, special toy, baby doll, or stuffed animal. If at all possible, keep that object with the child.

TABLE 2-3
Growth and Development of the Toddler

Age	Gross Motor	Fine Motor	Language	Sensory
12–15 months	• Can walk alone well • Can crawl up stairs	• Can feed self with cup and spoon • Puts raisins into a bottle • May hold crayon or pencil and scribble • Builds a tower of two cubes	• Says four to six words	• Binocular vision developed
18 months	• Runs, falling often • Can jump in place • Can walk up stairs holding on • Plays with push and pull toys	• Can build a tower of three to four cubes • Can use a spoon	• Says 10 or more words • Points to objects or body parts when asked	• Visual acuity 20/40
24 months	• Can walk up and down stairs • Can kick a ball • Can ride a tricycle	• Can draw a circle • Tries to dress self	• Talks a lot • Approximately 300-word vocabulary • Understands commands • Knows first name; refers to self • Verbalizes toilet needs	
30 months	• Throws a ball • Jumps with both feet • Can stand on one foot for a few minutes	• Can build a tower of eight blocks • Can use crayons • Learning to use scissors	• Knows first and last name • Knows the name of one color • Can sing • Expresses needs • Uses pronouns appropriately	

Estes, M. E. Z. (1998). *Health assessment and physical examination*. Albany, NY: Delmar Thomson Learning. Copyright 1998 by Delmar Thomson Learning.

injuries as the result of falls and auto/pedestrian collisions increase as the child becomes more active and expands the boundaries of his or her world past the confines of the home. Table 2-4 summarizes the common problems of toddlers.

The "Curious and Clever"

Curiosity and imagination abound in preschoolers from ages three to six. They often imitate adults during play (Figure 2-3). These children are openly loving of their parents and seem to be in constant motion.

TABLE 2-4
Common Problems of Toddlers

- Febrile seizures
- Croup
- Meningitis
- Reactive airway disease/asthma
- Foreign bodies
- Traumatic injuries from falls, auto/pedestrian collisions

Development

Verbal skills increase in this age group. The child often appears to talk constantly with a never-ending string of questions; however, comprehension is limited. Gross motor skills also increase, including the ability to ride tricycles, climb, and jump rope. This group is aware of a "private" zone. The concept of good touch versus bad touch appears to be understood. Table 2-5 summarizes the developmental skills of preschoolers.

Coping

Fears continue to include separation from parents and loss of control, as well as punishment and loss of body integrity. Coping mechanisms still include parental con-

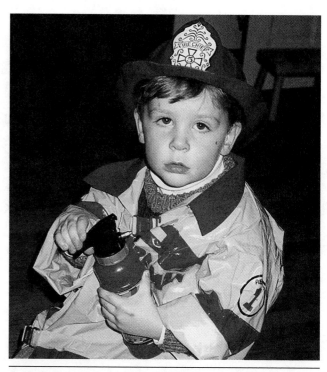

FIGURE 2-3 The active imagination of preschoolers often results in imitating adult roles.

tact but now expand to include talking, asking questions, and playing. This age group, as almost any parent can attest, also copes with minor injuries through the extensive use of Band-Aids!

TABLE 2-5
Growth and Development of Preschoolers

Age	Gross Motor	Fine Motor	Language	Sensory
3–6 years	• Can ride a bike with training wheels • Can throw a ball overhand • Skips and hops on one foot • Can climb well • Can jump rope	• Can draw a six-part person • Can use scissors • Can draw circle, square, or cross • Likes art projects, likes to paste and string beads • Can button • Learns to tie and buckle shoes • Can brush teeth	• Language skills are well developed with the child able to understand and speak clearly • Vocabulary grows to over 2,000 words • Talks endlessly and asks questions	• Visual acuity well developed • Focused on learning letters and numbers

.Estes, M. E. Z. (1998). *Health assessment and physical examination*. Albany, NY: Delmar Thomson Learning. Copyright 1998 by Delmar Thomson Learning.

Common Problems

Meningitis, febrile seizures, croup, and reactive airway disease continue to be some of the more common medical problems, as well as ingestions and foreign bodies. Although the incidence has decreased over the years due to vaccine, **epiglottitis** (bacterial infection resulting in swelling of the epiglottitis) surfaces as a problem. Traumatic injuries occur from falls with the addition of other mechanisms of injury that include tricycles and auto/pedestrian crashes. The incidence of drowning increases significantly in this age group. Table 2-6 summarizes the common problems of preschoolers.

The "Explorers"

With significantly improved communication skills, **school-aged** children (6 to 12) are very creative. They continue to test all limits that have been established. Their world expands beyond the family to include peers, neighbors, and teachers. It is at this age that children begin to be influenced by individuals other than the parent/caregiver.

Development

Motor skills, both gross and fine, continue to improve. Ability to concentrate increases to longer periods. Although peers gain considerable importance, parental attention is still highly desired. Modesty and privacy are very important to this group as they continue to realize their individuality and body integrity. Table 2-7 summarizes the developmental skills for school-aged children.

Coping

With increased awareness of self, this group fears pain and loss of body integrity and image. They also continue to fear separation and punishment. Primary coping mechanisms include parental contact, play, interaction with peers, and getting explanations for situations of concern (Figure 2-4).

Common Problems

Problems seen in this age group are primarily traumatic injuries such as fractures from falls, bicycles, rollerblades, and skateboards. The incidence of drowning or near drowning also continues to be significant. The frequency of febrile seizures, meningitis, sepsis, and epiglottitis decrease significantly as the child's temperature regulating mechanism and immune system mature. Although childhood RAD may resolve with age, its onset may occur between the ages of ten and thirty, with adult onset **reactive airway disease (RAD)** usually remaining a persistent condition. Table 2-8 summarizes the common problems encountered by school-aged children.

TABLE 2-6
Common Problems of Preschoolers

- Febrile seizures
- Meningitis
- Foreign bodies
- Drowning/near drowning
- Traumatic injuries from falls, tricycles, auto/pedestrian crashes
- Croup
- Ingestions of poisons
- Reactive airway disease (asthma)
- Epiglottitis (not common, but true emergency)

TABLE 2-7
Growth and Development During School-Age Years

Age	Gross Motor	Fine Motor	Language	Sensory
6–12 years	• Can use roller-blades or ice skates • Able to ride two-wheeler • Plays baseball	• Can put models together • Likes crafts • Enjoys board games, plays cards	• Vocabulary increases • Language abilities continue to develop	• Reading • Able to concentrate on activities for longer periods

---

Estes, M. E. Z. (1998). *Health assessment and physical examination.* Albany, NY: Delmar Thomson Learning. Copyright 1998 by Delmar Thomson Learning.

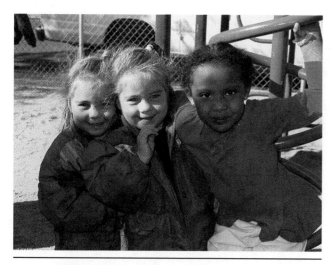

FIGURE 2-4 Play and interaction with peers are primary coping mechanisms for school-aged children.

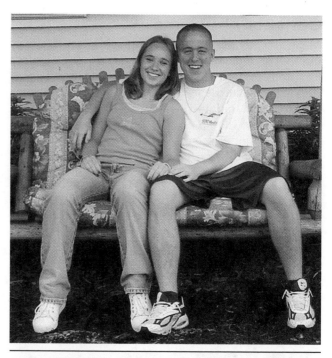

FIGURE 2-5 Teenagers develop strong relationships with their peers.

TABLE 2-8
Common Problems of
School-Aged Children

- Traumatic injuries such as fractures from falls, bicycles, rollerblades, and skateboards
- Drowning/near drowning
- Reactive airway disease/asthma

The "Dreamers"

Adolescents (12 to 18 years of age) are seeking independence and individuality. This time is an emotional period. Social relationships gain a prominent place as well as thoughts and plans for future adult life (Figure 2-5).

Development

This stage is the most complex developmental period of childhood. Puberty normally occurs earlier in girls than in boys and is accompanied by a growth spurt. Although fine motor skills are well developed, muscle development is still continuing and at times is accompanied by lack of coordination. Table 2-9 highlights the development of this age group.

Coping

Parents are still important; however, this group tends to respond more readily to peer pressure. It is not un-

common to see either dramatic over-reaction or under-reaction to situations based on peer pressure. Fear of separation from peers sometimes seems to be more significant than fear of separation from parents; however, parental contact is usually important even though this fact may not be obvious. Primary coping mechanisms are peer and parental contact and receiving accurate and honest information related to a given situation.

Common Problems

With increased independence, school activities, and peer contact, the focus of problems changes in this

Exploring the Web

- Search for Web sites that contain information on child development. Use the information you find to create flash cards for each age group that identify strategies that will help in assessment of each group.

TABLE 2-9
Growth and Development During Adolescence

Age	Gross Motor	Fine Motor	Language	Sensory
12–19 years	• Muscles continue to develop • At times awkward, with some lack of coordination	• Well-developed skills	• Vocabulary fully developed	• Development complete

Estes, M. E. Z. (1998). *Health assessment and physical examination.* Albany, NY: Delmar Thomson Learning. Copyright 1998 by Delmar Thomson Learning.

TABLE 2-10
Common Problems of Adolescents

- Traumatic injuries due to sports, motor vehicle collisions, violence
- Drug and alcohol abuse
- Suicide
- Pregnancy
- Sexual abuse

age group. There is a dramatic rise in the incidence of sports injuries, motor vehicle crashes, drug and alcohol abuse, suicide, pregnancy, and sexual abuse. There is also a significant increase in injury due to violence. Table 2-10 summarizes the common problems seen in adolescents.

ANATOMICAL AND PHYSIOLOGICAL CONSIDERATIONS

There are many anatomical and physiological differences between children and adults. These differences must be taken into account during both assessment and treatment interventions. These differences mature to adult anatomy and physiology at varying ages and stages of development.

Integumentary System

The body surface area of the child is larger in proportion to mass than the adult until approximately ten years of age. In infants and young children, the skin is thinner and there is less subcutaneous fat. Infants have poorly developed thermoregulatory mechanisms. All of these factors contribute to problems in maintaining body temperature and increase the risk of hypothermia. The prehospital provider must ensure that the child is kept warm during examination, treatment, and transport.

Neurological System

The head is larger and heavier in proportion to the rest of the body and remains so until approximately four years of age (Figure 2-6a). Because of this difference, the provider must take care to align the spine of children properly during immobilization by using padding under the shoulders. The anterior **fontanelle** (space between the bones of an infant's skull) does not close until 12 to 18 months (Figure 2-6b).

The brain is approximately 25 percent of its adult weight at birth. By two and one-half years, it is 75 percent of adult weight and by age six, it is 90 percent of adult weight.

In addition to increasing in mass, brain circuitry at birth is not the same as that of the adult. There are many "extra" pathways in infancy. The normal neonatal reflexes such as the startle reflex are the result of the extra pathways. These eventually disappear as the brain develops and forms. Rapid brain growth and circuitry development make it difficult to predict outcomes of neurological problems in children. The brain may develop and use some of the "extra" pathways to compensate for pathways lost due to injury or disease. Motor

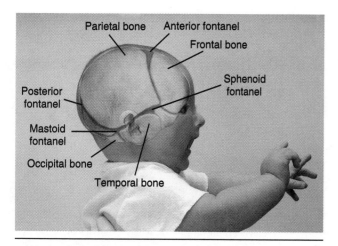

FIGURE 2-6 a. The infant's head is larger and heavier in relation to the rest of the body until approximately four years of age.

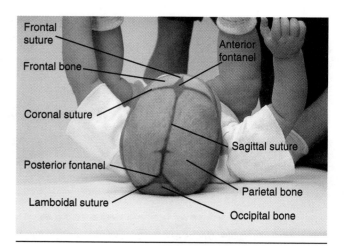

FIGURE 2-6 b. The fontanelles on the top of the infant's head can be palpated to assess for dehydration (i.e., sunken), or increased intracranial pressure (i.e., bulging). The anterior fontanelles do not close until approximately 18 months of age.

control develops from head to trunk to extremities as the nerve connections develop. This results in the infant developing head control before sitting or walking.

Respiratory System

The nasal bridge is flat and flexible. Nasal passages are small, allowing for easy obstruction. Remember that infants are obligate nose breathers up to the age of approximately one month; therefore, any obstruction of the nasal passages may result in respiratory compromise.

The diameter of the trachea in an adult is approximately 20 mm, while that of the infant is approximately 4 mm (Figure 2-7). The smallest diameter of the trachea in the child is at the cricoid ring. Because of the small diameter in this area, cuffed endotracheal tubes should not be used on children younger than the age of eight years. The tracheal rings are more elastic, allowing for tracheal collapse if the head is hyperextended.

The vocal cords of the adult are located at approximately C-5 to C-6. The vocal cords of the infant are located at approximately C-3 to C-4. Besides being higher, the vocal cords are also more anterior in the child than in the adult.

The rib cage in young children is very compliant. This difference allows the ribs to be compressed significantly without resulting in fracture. Although fractures are uncommon, severe compression of the ribs may affect the underlying lung tissue, resulting in pulmonary contusion and compromised ventilation.

The intercostal muscles are not well developed. Infants primarily use the diaphragm for breathing. The diaphragm increases the vertical diameter of the chest

✚ Tricks of the Trade

Severe compression of the ribs in infants and young children may cause underlying injury to the lungs *without* any rib fractures. Monitor the patient carefully for respiratory distress and the need for assisted ventilation.

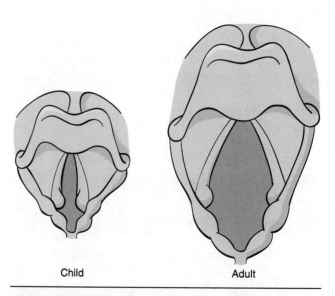

Child   Adult

FIGURE 2-7 The diameter of the infant's trachea is approximately 4 mm while the adult's trachea is approximately 20 mm!

by pulling the thoracic cavity down. The intercostal muscles increase the horizontal diameter and lift the thoracic cavity out. Therefore, only minimal chest expansion occurs with respirations, while the abdomen rises with inspiration and falls with expiration.

A secondary result of poorly developed respiratory muscles is the inability to sustain a rapid respiratory rate for a prolonged period of time. The child who is attempting to compensate for a respiratory problem by increasing rate and effort will fatigue and decompensate easily, sometimes in a matter of minutes.

In infants and young children, there are fewer and smaller alveoli. Collateral pathways of ventilation are not completely developed resulting in less surface area for gas exchange to occur. Thus, any airway obstruction can compromise gas exchange to a greater extent in children. Due to an increased metabolic rate, infants and young children have one and a half to two times the oxygen consumption of the adult. Meeting this increased need for oxygen is evidenced by the normally faster respiratory and heart rates of the child. The child's respiratory anatomy and physiology approximates that of the adult's anatomy and physiology by eight to ten years of age.

Cardiovascular System

Cardiac output (blood pumped by the heart in one minute) is determined by **stroke volume** (blood pumped by the heart with each contraction) and heart rate. Stroke volume is affected by the degree to which the heart muscle stretches as it fills. **Starling's law** states that the more the heart muscle stretches, the greater the force of contraction (to a point) and thus, the greater the stroke volume. The myocardium of the newborn is less compliant with less contractile mass than that of the adult. In the infant and young child, the stroke volume (1.5 cc/kg/beat) is considerably less than that of the adult. The 20-kg child has a stroke volume of approximately 30 cc per beat compared to the normal adult stroke volume of 70 to 80 cc per beat.

Cardiac output (CO) is the result of stroke volume (SV) times heart rate (HR) (CO = SV × HR). Since stroke volume in the child is limited, the primary compensatory mechanism for maintaining cardiac output is to increase heart rate. Stimulation of the sympathetic nervous system results in the release of adrenaline and norepinephrine. Adrenaline results in increased force or contraction and increased heart rate. It is important to remember that the sympathetic nervous system innervation of the heart is incomplete in the newborn; therefore, the newborn tends to respond to decreased cardiac output with bradycardia. Older children respond to decreased cardiac output by increasing the heart rate. However, cardiac output will continue to decrease if the

heart rate reaches 180 to 200 beats/minute. This rate does not allow adequate ventricular filling time, thus stroke volume decreases.

Although circulating volume by weight is greater in children (90 cc/kg in infants and 80 cc/kg in children) compared to the adult (70 cc/kg), the absolute circulating volume amount is significantly less in the child. The 20-kg child has 1,600 cc of circulating volume compared to the 70-kg adult with approximately 5,000 to 6,000 cc of circulating volume.

Abdomen

The liver and spleen in children up to the age of puberty are larger in proportion to those in the adult body. The abdominal muscles are immature, offering less protection to the organs. Both the liver and spleen are susceptible to injury. However, due to its increased size, the liver is more often injured since it is less protected by the ribs. Young children often rely on abdominal muscles to assist in breathing; therefore, any child suffering from an abdominal injury or abdominal pain may exhibit an altered respiratory pattern.

 Tricks of the Trade

Young children suffering from an abdominal injury or abdominal pain may exhibit an altered respiratory pattern due to their reliance on the abdominal muscles to assist in breathing.

Musculoskeletal

Long bone growth in the extremities occurs from the epiphyseal (growth) plates near the end of the bones. Bones begin as cartilage and harden only as minerals are deposited. This process is not complete until puberty. As a result, the bones in children are softer than in adults and more easily fractured. Because of bone composition, fractures can be incomplete, resulting in the classic "greenstick" type of fracture associated with children.

All muscle fibers are present at birth. They lengthen and stretch as the bones grow. The mandibular muscles are immature and the tongue is large relative to the size of the oropharynx. These differences can lead to potential problems when ventilating a child with a bag-valve mask and are addressed in Chapter 4—Respiratory Emergencies.

Neck muscles are not well developed in infants, resulting in minimal control of the head. Head control is

Exploring the Web

● Search for Web sites that identify anatomical and physiological differences between children and adults.

not attained until approximately six months of age. Remember to support the head of the infant to prevent "flopping" which may result in flexion, hyperextension, or exaggerated lateral movement.

ELEMENTS OF ASSESSMENT

The assessment of a stable child involves gathering the appropriate history and conducting the physical examination in a manner that may need to be tailored to the age group. This section discusses the elements of assessment as they apply to a stable child.

Environment

Conduct a "from-the-door" evaluation. How "bad" or "good" does the child look? What is the mental status? Is the child alert and aware of his or her surroundings? What does the child's respiratory status look like? Is breathing easy or labored? What is the child's general appearance? Is skin color normal, pale, or cyanotic? Does he or she appear slow to respond or unresponsive?

Observe the child's environment (e.g., cleanliness and temperature of the house, condition of the child's clothing, or condition of any animals). Are there pill bottles sitting in the open or any clues to the nature of the problem? Pay attention to the child's interactions with the parent or caregiver. Does the relationship appear appropriately loving or is the child hesitant to be with the adult? Is the child aware of the parents' presence, and does the child recognize the parents? Lack of awareness and recognition of parents by any child over two months is an ominous sign and indicative of severe cerebral **hypoperfusion** (decreased blood flow).

History

The tendency of most prehospital providers is to gather all of the history from the parent or caregiver. This technique is important since the parent or caregiver may tell of subtle differences or changes in the child that are not noticeable to the provider.

Children over the age of two, however, may be able to appropriately answer questions and relay a history. When communicating with the child, the provider should be positioned at the child's eye level and use terms the child understands. All the components of the history should be ascertained in the stable child. Adolescents' histories regarding sexual activity or potential drug use should be conducted in private. Table 2-11 summarizes the components of the history and includes suggested questions to ask.

Vital Signs

In order to recognize abnormal vital signs in children, the prehospital provider must have a knowledge of normal vital signs. Normal vital signs in the pediatric patient vary considerably from normal adult vital signs. Table 2-12 presents the estimated normal vital signs for children by age. Children over the age of 12 have vital signs very similar to those of the adult.

Enhancing Cooperation

Conducting a physical examination on a child is dependent on that child's cooperation. Gaining the cooperation of a sick or injured child often presents challenges to the prehospital provider. Following are some general strategies as well as some specific strategies for each age group that will help the provider in the ability to gain the necessary information from the history and physical examination.

General Strategies

When the child is stable, the provider should allow for a "transition" phase by talking calmly and in a soft, gentle voice. Let the child hold a favorite toy if there is one. Allow the child to touch any equipment to be used in the physical assessment. Encourage the parent or caregiver to get involved in touching the equipment with the child. If time permits, demonstrate on the parent how the equipment will be used such as placing the stethoscope against the chest to listen.

Examine the stable child starting at the toes and working toward the head. By giving the child an opportunity to accept the provider's presence for a few minutes, he or she may feel less threatened. Rushing up to the child and touching the head may be quite intimidating, resulting in an uncooperative child.

Most children will cooperate if they understand what is going to happen and feel they retain some control. Explain what is going to happen throughout the

TABLE 2-11
Components of the History

Parameter	Description
S—Signs/symptoms	• Pain—What is the quality, severity, or radiation? Does anything make it better or worse? • Dyspnea—How severe is it? Does anything make it better or worse? • Time—When did the problem begin? Have there been any changes in signs/symptoms since onset? • What treatments have already been attempted? • Has the child seen a physician for this problem? When? What did the physician say it was? • Is the child's behavior usual for that child? (Parents notice subtle changes that may not be apparent to the provider.)
A—Allergies	• Does the child have any allergies? • To what? (food/medication) • What type of reaction occurred?
M—Medications	• Is the child on any prescription medication for other illnesses? • Has any medication been given for the current problem (over the counter, aspirin, Tylenol®)? • When was the last dose?
P—Past medical history	• Does the child have any significant health problems/chronic diseases? • Is there a history of congenital problems? • Has the child had any major injuries? • Has the child had surgery for anything? • When was the last time the child saw a physician?
L—Last oral intake	• When did the child eat or drink last? • Has the child been eating and drinking normally? • Has the child had any vomiting/diarrhea? • Has the urine output been normal? • Do you see tears when the child cries? • If diapers are used, how long has it been since the last diaper change?
E—Events leading to current problem	• What was the child doing when and before the problem began? • Did the problem begin suddenly or occur over time?
Weight	• How much does the child weigh? • What is the best estimate or weight from the last checkup? • Has the child had a recent weight gain or loss?

TABLE 2-12
Normal Pediatric Vital Signs

Age	Weight	Respirations	Heart Rate	Systolic BP
Newborn	4–5 kg	30–50/min.	120–160 bpm	60–90
Infant	4–11 kg	20–30/min.	80–140 bpm	87–105
1–3 years	11–14 kg	20–30/min.	80–130 bpm	95–105
3–6 years	14–25 kg	20–30/min.	80–120 bpm	95–105
6–13 years	25–63 kg	(12–20)–30/min.	(60–80)–100 bpm	97–112
13–16 years	62–80 kg	12–20/min.	60–100 bpm	112–128

American Heart Association (1997). *Pediatric advanced life support.* Dallas, TX: American Heart Association; & Wertz, E. (1997). *Pediatric emergencies.* In B. Shade, M. Rothenberg, E. Wertz, & S. Jones, (Eds.), *Mosby's EMT—intermediate textbook.* St. Louis, MO: Mosby-Year Book.

Wertz, E. (1997a). Infants and children. In N. McSwain, R. White, J. Paturas, & W. Metcalf, (Eds.), *The basic EMT—comprehensive prehospital patient care.* St. Louis, MO: Mosby-Year Book.

entire assessment as it progresses. Touching before talking or not explaining what is about to occur may result in the relatively quiet, cooperative child becoming a kicking, screaming child simply out of fear of the unknown.

Never lie to a child. Once a child recognizes a lie, all trust is gone and cooperation may cease to exist. If a procedure is going to be painful, tell the child it will hurt. Set parameters for acceptable behavior. For example, as the IV is started, tell the child it is okay to cry; but he or she must not move the arm.

Strategies by Age Group

There are specific strategies that will help the prehospital provider gain the cooperation of the stable child. These strategies depend on the age group of the child and are based on the coping mechanisms common for that group.

Infants—The infant is extremely attached to the parent. Allow the parent to be present and take part in the assessment process as much as possible. The infant senses anxiety in the parent, so efforts must be made to reduce that anxiety. Finally, attempt to have one provider conduct the entire assessment and remain with the infant and parent throughout. This approach will help decrease the fear the infant has of strangers.

 Tricks of the Trade

Whenever possible, have one provider interact with the child. Having more than one person asking questions and touching is confusing and overwhelming and may change a cooperative child into an uncooperative child.

Toddlers—Toddlers fear separation from parents and loss of control. In addition to allowing this age group a "transition phase" and time to touch and play with equipment, allow the parent to be present and part of the assessment process as much as possible. Remember, choose words carefully and keep explanations to the child simple.

Preschool—Preschoolers have a very literal interpretation of words. Choose words carefully and keep explanations brief and simple. Always be honest.

School Age—This age group may listen attentively to what is said, may not comprehend the information, and is reluctant to ask questions. Ask the child to explain what he or she understands. This age group is beginning to assert independence and is often faced with some form of punishment. Assure the child that whatever procedures are necessary as part of the treatment, they are not a form of punishment.

Adolescents—This age group values independence. Allow them as many decisions about their care as appropriate. Explain the importance of any assessment step or treatment to their well being. Be honest about consequences and help them control emotional responses by gentle speech and encouraging relaxation techniques such as deep breathing.

Regardless of effort, cooperation may never be gained in some children. Do not waste a great deal of time attempting to get a detailed physical assessment on an extremely uncooperative child. Complete the initial assessment to the degree possible and then begin transport. If the child is screaming and crying, there is probably no life-threatening cardiopulmonary compromise. Table 2-13 summarizes methods to enhance cooperation in a stable child.

Physical Examination

The initial assessment should always be focused on finding and treating life-threatening problems. Following the immediate general evaluation of mental status, overall respiratory effort, and general appearance (skin color), the examination should follow a format that allows rapid identification of life-threatening injuries to the critical body systems. There are several models for the primary assessment. One of the most recognized by prehospital providers is the ABCDES model.

TABLE 2-13
Enhancing Cooperation in the Stable Child

- Talk calmly using a soft voice.
- Look and talk BEFORE touching.
- Let the child hold a favorite toy.
- Allow the child to touch equipment before using it.
- Demonstrate equipment on the parent or caregiver.
- Allow the parent to hold the child.
- Move slowly and deliberately.
- Conduct the assessment from toe to head.
- NEVER lie!

- A—Airway
- B—Breathing
- C—Circulation
- D—Disability
- E—Expose to determine other injuries
- S—Status—determine if rapid transport is indicated

Airway

Check the airway for foreign bodies, blood, or secretions that might compromise air entry. Observe the airway by having the alert child open the mouth. Even in stable, alert children, there may be gum or candy present that presents the potential for airway compromise. Have the child remove these objects if they are present.

If respiratory status is compromised, check to make sure the airway is open and clear following basic life support guidelines. Suction may be needed. It must be remembered that the epiglottis is higher in the child and the trachea collapses easily. The location of the epiglottis increases the risk of aspiration if the neck is hyperextended. Hyperextension may also lead to tracheal collapse. Therefore, the child should be placed in the neutral or "sniffing" position to open the airway.

Breathing

Once the airway is open and clear, assessment of respiratory rate and effort should take priority. ***Most children who deteriorate to the point of cardiac arrest have an underlying respiratory problem.*** **Tachypnea** (rapid respiratory rate) may be due to respiratory distress, or it may be an attempt to compensate for an existing metabolic acidosis (e.g., **diabetic ketoacidosis** resulting from by-product of fat metabolism) or **shock** (inadequate tissue perfusion). A slow respiratory rate in the acutely ill child is ominous and usually leads to respiratory failure and arrest.

Assessment of respiratory status should include observation of breathing effort, auscultation of breath sounds, and palpation of the thorax if trauma is suspected. Observe and evaluate the child for signs of

 Tricks of the Trade

Most children who deteriorate to the point of cardiac arrest have an underlying respiratory problem. Slow respiratory rates in the acutely ill child are ominous and usually lead to respiratory failure and arrest.

respiratory distress. The signs of respiratory distress include:

- nasal flaring
- **retractions** (drawing inward)
- **stridor** (high-pitched sound indicating upper airway obstruction)
- prolonged expiration
- grunting
- "see-saw" movement
- head bobbing
- circumoral (around the mouth) cyanosis.

See Chapter 4—Respiratory Emergencies for a detailed description and explanation of the significance of these signs and symptoms.

Auscultate the lungs of a stable child by having the parent hold the child over his or her shoulder whenever possible. Auscultate the midaxillary region or on the back if the child resists listening on the front. Breath sounds are easily transmitted from side to side in young children due to small size and lack of muscle development. Have the child try to "blow out the candle" if breath sounds are difficult to hear. In order to obtain the most accurate breath sounds, it is important to use a pediatric-size stethoscope (see Figure 2-8).

Circulation

Observe the overall appearance of the child to gauge the adequacy of cardiac output. Specific assessment of the cardiovascular status should begin with the pulse. Assess

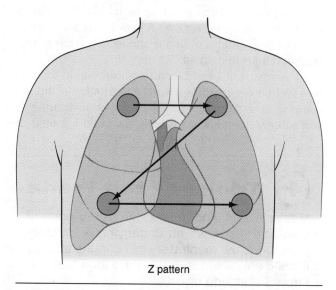

Z pattern

FIGURE 2-8 Auscultation of a child's lungs should be done using the "z" pattern.

the pulse for rate, rhythm, and quality. In the older child, assess the radial pulse. Assess the brachial pulse on an infant since a radial pulse is extremely difficult to obtain. An infant's rate can also be checked by taking an apical pulse for one minute; however, it is important to palpate the brachial pulse even if the rate is obtained apically. An apical pulse does not provide any information as to peripheral perfusion. If the peripheral pulses are weak or unobtainable, check the central carotid pulse. It is not uncommon to note some irregularity in pulse rate due to sinus arrhythmia. This increase in rate on expiration and decrease in rate on inspiration is normal in children.

Assess the skin for color, temperature, moisture, and capillary refill. Peripheral vasoconstriction results in pallor. Pallor may indicate shock or exposure to cold. The presence of cyanosis is unreliable by itself. Peripheral cyanosis may be the result of cold or may be indicative of shock. Peripheral cyanosis with central cyanosis is more indicative of respiratory failure.

Skin that appears flushed may be indicative of fever, infection, or allergic reaction. The temperature may be taken orally on the older child, rectally or tympanically on the infant and young child. If one of these methods of measuring temperature is not available, estimate skin temperature by placing the back of the hand or wrist on the child's forehead or extremities.

Cool or cold skin indicates peripheral vasoconstriction. This condition, like pallor, may be the result of shock or cold exposure. Skin that is warm or hot to the touch may indicate infection, fever, or heat exposure. Skin that is warm, hot, and dry should be assessed for turgor that may indicate the presence of dehydration. **Diaphoresis** (profuse sweating) may indicate either a response to heat exposure (either external or internal as the result of a breaking fever) or uncompensated shock.

Assess capillary refill on the nail beds. Normal capillary refill is two seconds or less. Delayed capillary refill may be an early indicator of inadequate cardiac output, but it may also indicate cold exposure. It is unreliable by itself and should be evaluated in the context of other assessment findings.

In very young children and infants, accurate blood pressure measurement may not be possible in the field setting. If measurement is to be accurate, the appropriate size cuff must be used. The array needed for all age groups may not be available. The appropriate cuff should be two-thirds the length of the upper arm, and the bladder should encircle the arm. If the cuff is too wide or loose, it will give a false low reading. A cuff that is too narrow or tight results in a false high reading.

Strong cardiovascular compensatory mechanisms in children will maintain a normal blood pressure for a prolonged time. When hypotension occurs as the result of inadequate cardiac output, it is often sudden and late in the shock cycle. It is far more important to assess the parameters of pulse rate and quality, skin temperature and color, and neurological status to determine the adequacy of cardiac output.

Disability

Assessment of the neurological status involves evaluating level of consciousness, pupillary response, and sensory/motor capability. Determining mental status can be more difficult in children. The traditional "oriented to time, place, and person" does not work when assessing the infant or young child. The AVPU method should be utilized in the context of the child's age (Figure 2-9). It is here that a knowledge of appropriate behaviors and developmental characteristics for age is extremely helpful.

Observe the child's response to his or her surroundings. The parent or caregiver can be very helpful in determining mental status. They know the child's usual behavior and response and can identify subtle changes that are not apparent to the prehospital provider.

Look at the face for expressions or grimacing that may indicate pain in the child too young to communicate. The quality of the cry in an infant can also help assess the neurological status. A weak, irritable cry may indicate compromise of the central nervous system and decreased cerebral perfusion.

Assess the child's muscle tone. Movement should be symmetrical and purposeful for the child's age. If the child is limp and floppy, the central nervous system is severely compromised.

Palpate the anterior fontanelle on any child less than 18 months. Gently stroke the index and middle finger over the fontanelle to determine if it is level, sunken, or bulging. A sunken fontanelle may indicate dehydration. A bulging fontanelle may indicate increased intracranial pressure. In order for the findings to be accurate, assess the child with the head elevated slightly

and when the child is quiet. Often the fontanelle will bulge when the child is crying.

Exposure

In unstable children, exposing is crucial to finding life-threatening problems; however, exposure for assessing the stable child should be limited to relevant areas of the body. Children have a strong sense of modesty that must be respected. Always consider the alert child's sense of "private" areas and good touch/bad touch when conducting the physical examination. Respecting the sense of modesty will go a long way in enhancing cooperation in a child. Once the assessment is complete, all efforts should be made to cover the child with a blanket to maintain body heat. Keep the child covered when not directly reassessing specific areas.

Status

When to begin transport is based on the child's condition and cooperation. If the child is unstable or presents with a critical illness or injury, transport should never be delayed to complete a thorough examination. Life systems should be supported and transport begun immediately.

If the child is stable and cooperative, take time to allow the "transition phase" discussed earlier and to complete a thorough history and physical examination. If all attempts to gain the child's cooperation fail, complete the initial assessment to the degree possible and then begin transport.

Exploring the Web

● Search for Web sites that identify common pediatric emergencies. Do they provide tips for assessment and treatment for the prehospital provider? Are there any professional journals that provide information on pediatric assessment?

Tricks of the Trade

Fear of the unknown crosses all age groups. Don't forget to talk to the child enroute! With stable children, talk about things of interest to them. Prepare them as much as possible, in general terms, for what is to come at the hospital.

Neurological Assessment — AVPU

A → **A**lert

V → responds to **V**erbal stimuli

P → responds to **P**ainful stimuli

U → **U**nresponsive

FIGURE 2-9 AVPU is used for the neurological assessment.

SUMMARY

Proficiency in treatment and intervention skills is necessary to administer adequate care to the pediatric patient. However, the most important knowledge base is an understanding of normal pediatric anatomy, physiology, and behavioral characteristics. An understanding of what are usual assessment findings increases the ability to recognize significant deviations. Without that understanding, problems may be missed or findings misinterpreted when in reality they are appropriate for the child's developmental age. A sound, basic knowledge of normal development and anatomical differences will increase the confidence of the provider to relate to children, recognize significant problems, and intervene appropriately.

Management of Case Scenario

Your "from-the-door" assessment should include the child's apparent mental status, color, and respiratory effort. Approach the child slowly and speak with a gentle, calm voice. Kneel down beside the couch so you can make contact at the child's eye level. Since the child is alert, begin by telling her that you are going to feel her wrist to count how fast her heart is beating. You can also ascertain the respiratory rate and skin condition at this time. Be sure to ask her mother about any allergies and medications (prescription or over-the-counter) that the child has taken and if this type of problem has occurred before.

Because this child is in the school-age group, she can give you a great deal of information regarding the history. Specifically ask her to tell you what the pain feels like and does anything make it better or worse. Ask her what she was doing when the pain began. Have her point to the area that hurts. Choose your words carefully and make sure you are using terms the child can understand.

Check her blood pressure while asking questions related to the history, but be sure to tell the child exactly what that involves. Show her the cuff and stethoscope. Tell her that you are going to wrap the cuff around the upper part of her arm and pump it up. It may feel tight but does not hurt. Then you will let it down while you listen with the stethoscope on her arm. Use the same type of explanation before listening to breath sounds.

The last area you want to assess is the abdomen, since that involves palpation and may increase the pain. Be sure to tell the child what you are going to do. Tell her that it may hurt a little more when you touch her, but it is important to do it to help find out what is wrong. Palpate gently.

Remember that this age group is very sensitive about privacy and modesty. Do not expose any more than necessary. Explain why you must look. Asking the child's permission after explaining often increases cooperation by giving the child some sense of control.

Allow the mother to remain close to the child. Allowing the mother to hold the child's hand while you conduct the physical examination can do a great deal to diminish fear in the child. Be sure to answer any questions the mother might have and make sure she understands what and why you are doing the steps of the assessment. The child will assume the position of comfort. Make every attempt to let the child remain in that position during assessment, treatment, and transport.

▶ REVIEW QUESTIONS

1. Identify the primary coping mechanism for children ages one to three.

2. Identify the age group in which health problems tend to shift from medical in nature to trauma.

3. Identify the more common injuries/illnesses seen in the infant.

4. Identify and compare the anatomical and physiological differences in the respiratory system between children and adults.

5. Describe the conditions that indicate transporting a stable child before a *complete* physical examination is accomplished.

6. Describe the appropriate approach and parameters for assessing the neurological status of a one-year-old child. Include rationale.

▶ REFERENCES

American Heart Association. (1997). *Pediatric advanced life support*. Dallas, TX: American Heart Association.

Estes, M. E. Z. (1998). *Health assessment and physical examination*. Albany, NY: Delmar Thomson Learning.

Wertz, E. (1997a). Infants and children. In N. McSwain, R. White, J. Paturas, & W. Metcalf, (Eds.), *The basic EMT—comprehensive prehospital patient care*. St. Louis, MO: Mosby-Year Book.

Wertz, E. (1997b). Pediatric emergencies. In B. Shade, M. Rothenberg, E. Wertz, & S. Jones, (Eds.), *Mosby's EMT—intermediate textbook*. St. Louis, MO: Mosby-Year Book.

▶ BIBLIOGRAPHY

National Association of Emergency Medical Technicians (1999). *Basic and advanced prehospital trauma life support* (4th ed.). St. Louis, MO: Mosby-Year Book.

Sanders, M. (2000). *Mosby's paramedic textbook* (2nd ed.). St. Louis, MO: Mosby-Year Book.

Wong, D. (1999). *Whaley & Wong's nursing care of infants and children* (6th ed.). St. Louis, MO: Mosby-Year Book.

Chapter 3

The Critically Ill Child

OBJECTIVES

Upon completion of this chapter, the student should be able to:

● Identify the two major causes of cardiac arrest in the pediatric patient.

● Describe the signs of respiratory distress and their significance.

● Explain appropriate pediatric airway management during resuscitation.

● Compare and contrast the major causes of shock.

● Explain the pathophysiology of the shock cycle.

● Given a scenario, explain the resuscitative measures for shock in the pediatric patient, including rationale.

● Describe the major rhythm disturbances and underlying causes in the pediatric patient.

● List the indications, dosages, and special considerations for drugs used during pediatric resuscitation.

● Explain the considerations involved in determining initiation of transport.

KEY TERMS

adenosine
amiodarone
anaphylactic shock
asystole
atropine
bradycardia
bradydysrhythmia
capnograph
cardiogenic shock
diazepam

distributive shock
epinephrine
hypercarbia
hypovolemic shock
hypoxemia
intraosseous
lidocaine
midazolam
neurogenic shock

pulse pressure
pulseless electrical activity
  (PEA)
respiratory failure
salicylism
septic shock
shock
sinus tachycardia
stridor

stroke volume
supraventricular
  tachycardia (SVT)
tachydysrhythmia
tachypnea
temperature demarcation
ventricular fibrillation (VF)
ventricular tachycardia (VT)
verapamil

Case Scenario

You are dispatched for an unresponsive three-year-old child, who may have a possible overdose. As you arrive, an elderly woman runs out of the house carrying a limp boy. He appears pale and his face is cyanotic. His grandmother tells you that she put him down for his nap after lunch. When she went to check on him an hour and a half later, she found him lying on the floor with an open bottle of her Elavil® lying beside him. She could not wake him and called 911 immediately. His respirations are irregular at approximately six breaths/minute. He has no detectable radial pulse or blood pressure but has a weak, slow carotid pulse. He is unresponsive to all stimuli and flaccid. How would you manage this child?

INTRODUCTION

The most common causes of cardiac arrest in the pediatric patient are respiratory failure and shock. Respiratory failure or shock, regardless of the underlying cause, rarely occurs as a sudden event. These states often result from a progressive deterioration of either the respiratory or circulatory system and ultimately end in arrest. Once the state of cardiac arrest occurs, the resuscitation rate is extremely poor. Therefore, the key to managing the critically ill child is early recognition and intervention to correct the underlying problem(s).

RESPIRATORY FAILURE

Respiratory failure is a clinical state of either **hypercarbia** (inadequate carbon dioxide elimination) or **hypoxemia** (inadequate oxygen in the blood). It may result from inadequate respiratory effort, airway obstruction, or an intrinsic lung or airway disease such as reactive airway disease (RAD) or asthma. Hypoxemia in children may develop rapidly due to high metabolic rates and increased oxygen consumption. Infants have one and a half to two times the oxygen consumption of an adult. This rate can rapidly deplete reserves. For more information, see Chapter 4—Respiratory Emergencies.

TYPES OF SHOCK

Shock is a clinical state of inadequate tissue perfusion. Adequate perfusion maintains normal metabolism by delivering enough oxygen and nutrients to the tissues and by removing the waste products. It is important to understand that the clinical state of shock may exist even when cardiac output is normal or increased as well as when cardiac output is decreased. If metabolic demands are significantly increased, even with normal cardiac output, some organs or tissues may be inadequately perfused. The shock state may also exist when the patient exhibits a normal blood pressure. Regardless of cause, shock follows a predictable cycle. This cycle is illustrated in Figure 3-1.

Field classification of the stages of shock is based on blood pressure. This method is convenient since estimating blood loss in the field is usually unreliable and other shocks such as cardiogenic and distributive do not involve blood loss. If the blood pressure is normal in the presence of other signs and symptoms of shock, the patient is considered to be in the *compensated* stage. The compensatory mechanisms are able to shunt blood from the nonvital organs to maintain blood pressure and perfusion of vital organs. When hypotension exists, the patient is considered to be in the *uncompensated* stage. In the uncompensated state, perfusion to vital organs is compromised.

Hypovolemic Shock

Hypovolemic shock is the most common type of shock seen in children. It is the result of a decrease in circulating blood volume. Severe dehydration and blood loss are the most common causes of volume depletion in children. Children have less total circulating volume than an adult. Therefore, a small actual volume loss may be a large circulating volume. For instance, a 55-pound (25-kg) child has a circulating volume of 2,000 cc while a 154-pound (70-kg) adult has approximately 5,000 cc of

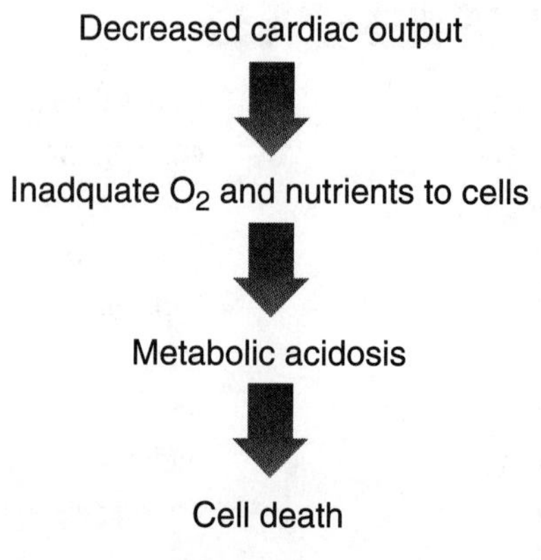

Decreased cardiac output

⬇

Inadaquate O_2 and nutrients to cells

⬇

Metabolic acidosis

⬇

Cell death

FIGURE 3-1 The shock cycle.

circulating volume. If the child were to lose 300 cc of fluid, that would be 15 percent of the circulating volume versus only 6 percent of the adult's circulating volume.

Distributive Shock

Distributive shock is the result of massive vasodilatation. There is no actual volume loss outside of the body. There are three types of distributive shock: septic shock, neurogenic shock, and anaphylactic shock.

Septic Shock

One of the most common causes of distributive shock in children is **septic shock**, which results from an overwhelming infection. In the initial stage of septic shock cardiac output increases, blood pressure remains normal, and vascular resistance decreases. The patient appears well perfused, may be warm to the touch, and often presents with a bounding pulse. However, in this stage, some tissues receive excessive blood flow while other tissues are inadequately perfused. This process leads to the development of metabolic acidosis. The presentation of septic shock is subtle and requires a high index of suspicion. Because newborns have an immature temperature-regulating mechanism, fever may be absent, making this form of shock even more difficult to detect.

Neurogenic Shock

Another type of distributive shock is **neurogenic shock**. This form of shock produces massive vasodilatation resulting from the loss of sympathetic innervation after an injury to the spinal cord. Although neurogenic shock can occur in children, it is rare since spinal cord injuries in children are rare.

Anaphylactic Shock

Anaphylactic shock is the result of a profound allergic reaction. The release of histamine in response to the allergen causes vasodilation and increased capillary permeability. Fluid leaks out into the interstitial space and reduces the overall blood volume returning to the heart. It does occur in children but is not as common as hypovolemic or septic shock.

Cardiogenic Shock

Cardiogenic shock is the inability of the heart to maintain adequate cardiac output (pump failure) and is usually the result of myocardial ischemia. Cardiogenic shock is rare in children but may occur in those who have a congenital heart defect, prolonged supraventricular tachycardia, severe electrolyte imbalance, advanced septic shock, or hypoglycemia.

GENERAL SIGNS AND SYMPTOMS

Timely intervention depends on early recognition of the signs and symptoms of respiratory distress and/or shock. Signs and symptoms include changes in respiratory rate and effort, alteration of normal air movement as noted by lung auscultation, changes in heart rate, and changes in organ perfusion as assessed by quality of pulses, skin, vital signs, and level of consciousness. These system parameters should be assessed in the primary examination and reassessed frequently. Table 3-1 summarizes the signs and symptoms and possible causes for respiratory failure and shock.

Exploring the Web

- Search for each type of shock discussed in the chapter. What information can you find on each of these? Is there information specific to children?

ASSESSMENT

A thorough assessment is necessary to determine the level of shock and how treatment should be prioritized. Attention is directed toward evaluation of airway, breathing, and circulation.

Respiratory Rate

Tachypnea (rapid breathing) is often the first indication that a child is suffering from respiratory distress. However, tachypnea may also occur as a compensatory mechanism for an underlying medical problem ("quiet tachypnea"). Quiet tachypnea is an increased respiratory rate that is initiated as a compensatory mechanism for an underlying metabolic acidosis. Conditions that may cause compensatory tachypnea include: shock, diabetic ketoacidosis (DKA), dehydration, sepsis, and **salicylism** (aspirin overdose). The chemical composition of aspirin is acetylsalicylic acid. An overdose of aspirin releases the acid, resulting in metabolic acidosis.

The respiratory muscles of children are less developed than those of an adult and tire easily. Rapid respiratory rates for a prolonged period of time will result in fatigue. Children with respiratory rates above 40 breaths/minute require rapid assessment and intervention since fatigue will develop rapidly leading to a slowing of the

TABLE 3-1
Signs/Symptoms of Respiratory Failure and Shock

Signs/Symptoms	Possible Causes
Respiratory Failure	
Nasal flaring	Inadequate respiratory effort
Stridor	Intrinsic lung disease (RAD)
Retractions	Airway obstruction
Prolonged expiration	Infection
Grunting	
"See-saw" respirations	
Head bobbing	
Circumoral cyanosis	

Shock

Hypovolemic

Pale, cool, clammy skin	Hemorrhage
Line of temperature demarcation on extremities, moving up toward the trunk as shock progresses	Dehydration
	Burns
Tachycardia	
Tachypnea	
Altered to decreasing level of consciousness	
Hypotension (late)	

Septic

Early	Systemic infection
Skin warm and pink	
Bounding pulse	
Fever (except in infants)	
Normal blood pressure	
Late	
Pale, cool, clammy skin	
Tachycardia (except infants)	
Tachypnea	
Altered to decreasing level of consciousness	
Hypotension	

Cardiogenic

Pale, cool, clammy skin	Congenital heart defect
Tachycardia → bradycardia	Prolonged SVT
Tachypnea	Severe electrolyte imbalance
Wet lung sounds	Advanced septic shock
Altered to decreasing level of consciousness	Hypoglycemia

Neurogenic (also called spinal shock)

Rare in children	Spinal cord injury
Warm and dry skin below level of the injury	Vasodilatation from loss of sympathetic tone
Pale, cool, clammy skin above level of injury	

Signs/Symptoms	Possible Causes
Hypotension	Vasodilation below the level of injury → blood pools in extremities
Normal heart rate or bradycardia	Compensatory mechanism lost due to loss of sympathetic nervous system function

Anaphylactic

Early signs:	
Headache	After exposure to an antigen, the sooner the reaction occurs, the more serious it can become.
Flushed skin; urticaria (hives)	
Feeling of impending doom	
Later signs:	
Change in level of consciousness	
Laryngeal edema; stridor	
Bronchospasm	
Hypotension	Tracheal swelling
Tachycardia	Bronchiolar constriction
	Vasodilation

American Heart Association. (2000). Guidelines 2000 for cardiopulmonary resuscitation and emergency cardiovascular care. *Journal of the American Heart Association, 102(8)*. I-307-319.

Wong, D. (1999). *Whaley & Wong's nursing care of infants and children* (6th ed.). St. Louis: Mosby-Year Book.

respiratory rate. This slowing does not indicate the child is improving, rather that the child is deteriorating. In addition to fatigue, slow respiratory rates may result from hypothermia, central nervous system (CNS) depression, or overdoses. Slow respiratory rates in the acutely ill child are ominous and often signal impending respiratory arrest.

Respiratory Effort

Normal respiratory effort should be quiet and require minimal work. Anatomical differences in children can contribute to the development of increased respiratory effort. The child's airway diameter is much smaller than the diameter of the adult airway. This smaller diameter increases the resistance to air flow. Obstruction from

 Tricks of the Trade

Slow respiratory rates in the acutely ill child are ominous and often signal impending respiratory arrest.

mucus or edema increases resistance and thus, significantly increases the work of breathing. As the work of breathing increases, so does the oxygen demand of the respiratory tissues and muscles necessary to produce adequate air exchange. Increased oxygen demand results in shunting of blood to perfuse these tissues and an increase in carbon dioxide production.

Multiple signs may manifest increased respiratory effort. Nasal flaring may be obvious. Head bobbing with each inspiration is often a sign of increased respiratory effort. Retractions may be noted on inspiration in the intercostal, subcostal, and suprasternal areas. Retractions are usually obvious in children since the ribs are pliable and fail to support the lungs as they do in the adult. The pliable ribs result in retraction rather than expansion of the lung. Figure 3-2 illustrates a child with retractions.

Inspiratory **stridor** (crowing sound heard on inspiration) indicates an upper airway problem. Causes of stridor include infections (e.g., croup, epiglottitis), edema (e.g., allergic reaction) and congenital abnormalities (e.g., large tongue). A prolonged expiratory phase indicates a lower airway problem; usually located in the bronchi or bronchioles. It is often accompanied by wheezing. Causes of prolonged expiration include RAD, bronchiolitis, and foreign body aspiration. Grunting at

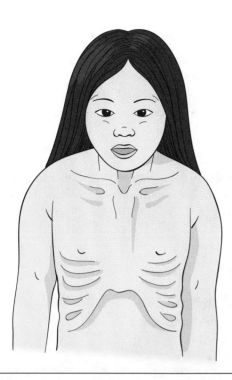

FIGURE 3-2 Inspiratory retractions are indicative of increased respiratory effort and may be seen in the intercostal, subcostal, and suprasternal areas.

the end of expiration is an attempt to keep the alveoli open by increasing the end expiratory pressure. It is the result of premature closure of the glottis. Grunting is often heard in children with underlying alveolar problems such as atelectasis or pneumonia.

"See-saw" respirations, sometimes called abdominal respirations, usually indicate an upper airway obstruction. They are evidenced by obvious chest retraction accompanied by abdominal distention. Children are dependent on the diaphragm for air movement to the lungs. When the diaphragm contracts, the chest wall retracts and the abdomen expands. The actions result in the characteristic paradoxical movement of the chest and abdomen. This breathing pattern results in inadequate air exchange due to decreased tidal volume and energy consumption, and leads to early fatigue.

 Tricks of the Trade

Head bobbing with each respiration is often a sign of increased respiratory effort.

Air Movement

If tidal volume and respiratory effort are normal, the chest should expand and breath sounds should be easily heard bilaterally. Children have a thin chest wall, resulting in breath sounds being easily transmitted. Sound may be transmitted from one area of the lung and heard in another area; therefore, it is possible to hear breath sounds even when the child has atelectasis or a pneumothorax. When auscultating air movement, it is important to listen for equality of sounds on both the anterior and posterior chest wall as well as under the axillae.

Pulse oximetry may be a useful assessment tool to determine oxygen saturation. However, adequacy of ventilation cannot be determined by the oximeter. It must be determined by other assessment methods.

Heart Rate

Cardiac output in children is more affected by heart rate than by stroke volume. In other words, an increased heart rate increases cardiac output. The neonate is the exception, in that response to hypoxemia is often **bradycardia** (heart rate of less than 60 beats per minute).

The tachycardic (heart rate greater than 100 beats) response may fail to maintain adequate oxygenation. Inadequate oxygenation results in hypoxia and hypercarbia, which leads to acidosis and resultant bradycardia. Bradycardia in an acutely ill child is considered an ominous sign and may indicate impending cardiac arrest. Guidelines established by the American Heart Association for heart rates indicating the need for rapid assessment and possible intervention for children are:

- Less than five years of age—rate below 80/minute or above 180/minute
- Over the age of five—rate below 60/minute or above 160/minute

Quality of Pulses

Peripheral pulses that can be easily palpated in infants and children are the radial, brachial, dorsalis pedis, and posterior tibial. Central pulses that are easily palpated are the carotid and femoral. The quality of the pulse is dependent on the **pulse pressure** (difference between the systolic and diastolic pressures). As cardiac output decreases, peripheral vasoconstriction begins and the pulse pressure narrows. This change results in a weak, thready pulse that ultimately disappears. Differences in the quality of the peripheral pulse and the central pulse may be an early indicator of decreased cardiac output (shock). However, it must be remembered that a cold environment will also induce peripheral vasoconstriction

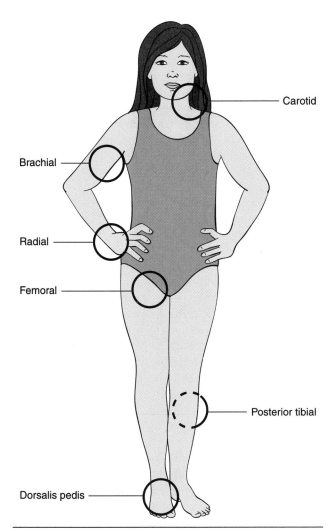

Carotid

Brachial

Radial

Femoral

Posterior tibial

Dorsalis pedis

FIGURE 3-3 The radial, brachial, dorsalis pedis, and posterior tibial pulses are peripheral pulses that can be palpated on a child. The carotid and femoral pulses are the central pulses that are easily palpated.

and may alter pulse quality. Figure 3-3 illustrates the pulse points on a child.

Blood Pressure

Cardiac output and systemic vascular resistance determine blood pressure. Increasing systemic vascular resistance (vasoconstriction) can maintain blood pressure when cardiac output falls. Tachycardia also helps increase and maintain cardiac output. A tachycardic rate will continue until all cardiac reserve is spent. Most children have extremely good vascular tone and will maintain a normal supine blood pressure in hypovolemic shock up

to a 20 to 25 percent volume loss. Because children often maintain normal blood pressures until all compensatory mechanisms are exhausted, hypotension is usually late and sudden. The prehospital provider should not rely on the presence or absence of hypotension to determine the potential for shock in the pediatric patient.

Skin

In a normal warm environment, the skin temperature and color should be the same over the trunk and extremities. Mucous membranes, nail beds, palms of the hands, and soles of the feet should be pink. Capillary refill should be normal. Environmental temperature is a major factor in skin color and temperature. If the environment is cold, peripheral vasoconstriction may result in cool, mottled skin and delayed capillary refill.

If the environment is warm, the signs associated with peripheral vasoconstriction indicate shunting of blood and oxygen to vital organs. Vasoconstriction begins in the periphery (fingers and toes) and proceeds toward the trunk. Assessing the extremities for a line of **temperature demarcation** (where cool skin ends and warm skin begins) on a frequent basis may serve as an indicator of the progression of shock or success of resuscitation efforts.

Vasoconstriction results in changes in skin color. In newly borns, the skin takes on a gray or ashen color; in older children the skin becomes pale. Peripheral cyanosis resulting from vasoconstriction is another indicator of poor skin perfusion. Central cyanosis may be present with hypoxemia. However, cyanosis may not be present in anemic conditions despite severe hypoxemia. Cyanosis alone should not be considered a reliable sign of poor perfusion. It must be considered in conjunction with other presenting signs.

Level of Consciousness

The signs of cerebral ischemia depend on the severity and duration of the episode. If inadequate perfusion is sudden and significant, loss of consciousness is rapid, with few preceding signs. If ischemia develops gradually, altering levels of consciousness may occur. Altered levels of consciousness include confusion, irritability, or alternating states of agitation and lethargy.

Normally, an infant can recognize and focus on the parents by the age of two months. Failure to focus or recognize and respond to the parents is an ominous sign and usually indicates severe hypoperfusion of the brain. The parents may recognize changes in the child's neurological behavior but may not be able to describe those changes other than saying something is wrong. The prehospital provider should take this assessment by the parents seriously. They are usually aware of subtle differences in behavior that may not be apparent to the provider.

MANAGEMENT OF THE RESPIRATORY SYSTEM

The goal of prehospital management should be to support the respiratory system because it may not be possible to determine the underlying cause of the respiratory distress. Any child who exhibits signs of respiratory distress should receive high concentration oxygen. The method of delivery is dependent on the severity of the distress. The oxygen administration device for children with effective ventilation should be determined by the oxygen concentration desired. Nasal cannulas are not indicated for children exhibiting signs of significant respiratory distress. Simple masks deliver 35 to 60 percent concentration when the flow rate is set at 6 to 10 liters/minute. The nonrebreather mask can deliver a concentration of 95 percent when the flow rate is set at 12 to 15 liters/minute. These delivery concentrations are based on the mask being placed on the child's face. If the oxygen is administered using the blow-by method (holding the mask to the side of the face), inspired concentrations will decrease due to dilution with room air. Figures 3-4a and b show the oxygen delivery devices needed for pediatric resuscitation.

Suctioning may be required to provide a patent airway. Flexible suction catheters are appropriate for aspirating thin secretions from the oropharynx or endotracheal tube. A variety of catheter sizes (8 to 12 French) should be available to accommodate different age groups.

The procedure of suctioning the endotracheal tube should be carried out under sterile conditions. A rigid (tonsil tip) catheter may be required to remove thick, particulate matter from the oropharynx. A force of 80 to 120 mm Hg is normally required to provide enough suction to clear the airway. Stimulation of the posterior pharynx or trachea with the suction catheter may induce vagal stimulation and a resultant bradycardia. Therefore, it is important that the heart rate be monitored while suctioning. Suctioning should not exceed five seconds and should be preceded and followed by ventilation with 100 percent oxygen to prevent hypoxia.

Children that exhibit signs of severe respiratory distress or impending respiratory failure should receive assisted ventilation. If ventilation is initiated with the bag-valve mask, it is important that the mask be the appropriate size for the child. The mask should fit from the bridge of the nose to the cleft of the chin in order to provide an airtight seal and to decrease the amount of dead air space (Figure 3-5). This position helps prevent rebreathing exhaled air that is trapped in the bottom of the mask

The tongue of a child is larger in relationship to the oropharynx than in the adult. Therefore, if the ventilator's fingers are placed below the jaw, the tongue may be forced upward and result in a partial or complete obstruction of the airway. The fingers should rest no lower than the mandible or may be curled around the bottom of the mask.

The cartilaginous rings of a child's trachea are not as developed as those of the adult. This difference results in the trachea being soft and prone to collapse if the child's head is hyperextended for ventilation. The head should be maintained in a neutral, "sniffing" position to prevent this complication. It may be necessary to reposition the head and neck to find the best position for effective ventilation. In the absence of trauma, placing a folded towel under the head and neck may be helpful in

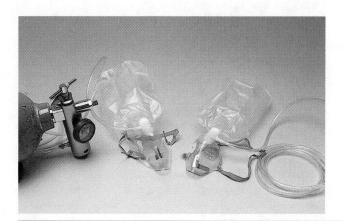
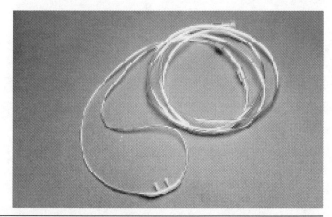

FIGURE 3-4a and b A variety of oxygen delivery devices must be available to manage the pediatric patient with respiratory distress, simple and nonrebreather masks as well as nasal cannulas are available.

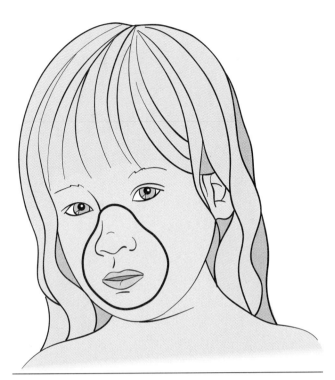

FIGURE 3-5 To achieve an adequate seal and decrease dead air space, the mask should fit from the bridge of the nose to the cleft of the chin.

achieving the anterior displacement of the cervical spine required for the best positioning of the child over the age of two years.

The bag itself should have a minimum volume of 450 cc. The neonatal bag, which has a volume of 250 cc, is usually inadequate to achieve effective ventilation in the infant. The amount of volume delivered should be based on chest rise and fall. Care must also be taken to squeeze the bag slowly. Squeezing the bag too quickly will force air into the stomach instead of the lungs.

Bags used to ventilate the pediatric patient should not have pop-off valves or the valve should be easy to occlude. Occluding the valve may be accomplished by holding it down with a finger or twisting it into a closed position. Pop-off valves are normally set with a pressure limit of 35 to 45 cm of water. Children with respiratory distress or underlying lung problems that result in increased airway resistance or poor lung compliance may require higher pressures for effective ventilation.

Even with attention to technique, children are prone to developing gastric distention from air being forced into the stomach during ventilation using a mask. This gastric air may result in vomiting and aspiration. Cricoid pressure (Sellick maneuver) to occlude the esophagus against the cervical spine may help control

this distention. Care must be taken to prevent too much pressure, which could result in tracheal compression and obstruction. If local protocols allow, insertion of a nasogastric tube should be considered as a more definitive method of minimizing distention along with endotracheal intubation.

The procedure of endotracheal intubation of the pediatric patient must take into consideration certain anatomical differences between children and adults. The larynx is located higher and more anterior. The narrowest portion of the trachea in the child up to eight years of age is the cricoid ring. Uncuffed tubes should be used in children eight years of age or under since the cricoid ring serves the same function as the cuff.

Appropriate endotracheal tube size (in mm) for children can be determined by a variety of methods. For children over the age of one, the American Heart Association suggests calculating the size using the formula of age in years divided by four plus four ([age in years/4] + 4). Another formula that may be used when cuffed tubes are indicated is age in years divided by four plus three ([age in years/4] + 3). Endotracheal tube size for newborns can be determined by weight. Finally, commercially available resuscitation tapes use the length of the child to determine endotracheal tube size. Be aware that estimating endotracheal tube size with an outside diameter that is approximately the same as that of the child's little finger has been shown to be difficult and unreliable (American Heart Association, 2000).

Ideally, three endotracheal tubes should be available—one at the estimated size, one 0.5 mm smaller, and one 0.5 mm larger. These extra tubes allow for individual variance in the child's trachea.

Laryngoscope blades come in a variety of sizes. A straight blade should be used for infants and toddlers since it provides better visualization of the more anterior cords. A curved blade for the older child may provide better tongue displacement than the straight blade. A guide to tube and blade size is provided in Table 3-2.

It is important that the heart rate be monitored during intubation for the development of bradycardia due to vagal stimulation. If the heart rate drops below 60 beats/minute or the attempt takes longer than 30 seconds, the procedure should be stopped and the child ventilated with 100 percent oxygen until the rate increases.

The pulse oximeter, if available, should be used to monitor oxygen saturation while the child is being intubated. The pulse oximeter reading should always be confirmed with an assessment of the patient. Since displacement and extubation can occur easily, it is critical that the effectiveness of ventilation be continually assessed following intubation. If a **capnograph** is available, in-line monitoring of end-tidal carbon dioxide provides better evidence of proper ventilation than does the pulse oximeter.

TABLE 3-2
Guidelines for Pediatric Endotracheal Tube and Laryngoscope Blade 2.5–3.5 Size

Age	Endotracheal Tube Size	Laryngoscope Blade Size
Premature Infant 0 month–1 year/infant	3.5–4.0 mm	0–1
1 year/small child (10–13 kg)	4.0 mm	1
3 years/child (14–16 kg)	4.5 mm	2
5 years/child (16–20 kg)	5.0 mm	2
6 years/child (18–25 kg)	5.5 mm	2
8 years/child to small adult (24–32 kg)	6.0 mm cuffed	2
12 years/adolescent (32–54 kg)	6.5 mm cuffed	2
16 years/adult (50+ kg)	7.0 mm cuffed	3

American Heart Association. (2000). Guidelines 2000 for cardiopulmonary resuscitation and emergency cardiovascular care. *Journal of the American Heart Association, 102(8)*. I-307-319.

Chricothyroidotomy is rarely required in children, but may allow oxygen administration and ventilation in the child with complete upper airway obstruction when all other methods fail. This procedure is discussed in depth in Chapter 4—Respiratory Emergencies.

MANAGEMENT OF THE CIRCULATORY SYSTEM

Vascular access is necessary for fluid administration and preferred for drug administration. The feasibility of peripheral venous access should be assessed first. Although scalp veins are acceptable venous access sites in infants, they should not be used for resuscitation. These vessels are extremely small, and rapid administration of drugs or fluid will result in infiltration. Due to location, attempts to use these veins can also result in interference of airway management. Peripheral veins that may be utilized include the medial cubital, basilic, or cephalic vein in the upper extremities and the saphenous or dorsal venous arch in the lower extremities (Figures 3-6 and 3-7).

Since exposure to critically ill children in the field is limited, proficiency in establishing a peripheral line may be less than desired. If venous access cannot be established within the first 90 seconds of resuscitation or within the allowed attempts by local protocol, the provider should consider using the **intraosseous** route (insertion of a needle into the marrow cavity of the tibia) in children six years of age or less. The intraosseous route has been used successfully in children over the age of six; however, at that age, the bone marrow becomes smaller and more difficult to successfully cannulate.

The intraosseous route may be used for all resuscitation medications and fluid administration. It results in drug uptake and fluid resuscitation equivalent to that of peripheral venous access. Complications following intraosseous cannulation include growth disturbances (if the epiphyseal plate is entered), tibial fracture, osteomyelitis, and compartment syndrome as the result of infiltration. Although rare, because these complications are severe, intraosseous cannulation should be used only in the critically ill or injured child. See Appendix C for a skills review of intraosseous infusions.

Fluid resuscitation for the child who is volume depleted should be initiated with an isotonic crystalloid

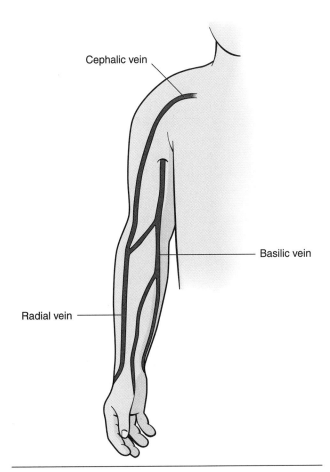

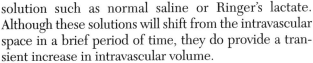

FIGURE 3-6 Peripheral veins in the upper extremities.

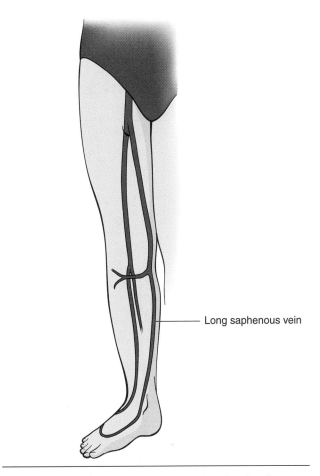

FIGURE 3-7 Peripheral veins in the lower extremities.

solution such as normal saline or Ringer's lactate. Although these solutions will shift from the intravascular space in a brief period of time, they do provide a transient increase in intravascular volume.

Fluid resuscitation is indicated for the child demonstrating clinical signs of shock, regardless of the normality of the blood pressure. Because rapid infusion of unmonitored amounts of fluid may result in pulmonary edema in the critically ill child with underlying cardiac or pulmonary disease, infusion should be initiated using a fluid bolus of 20 cc/kg. Rapid fluid administration may not be possible if minidrip tubing is used to establish the intravenous drip. Rapid infusion may be accomplished if the fluid is drawn into a 35 or 50 cc syringe and pushed.

Fluid resuscitation of children requires ongoing reassessment of the parameters of heart rate, skin, vital signs, and mental status to determine the effectiveness of treatment and the need for additional boluses. Although some children may require large amounts of fluid replacement (i.e., over 100 cc/kg), the number of

boluses recommended in the field is limited to three (60 cc/kg). The number of boluses should be determined by the service program protocols and be adhered to by the provider.

MANAGEMENT OF RHYTHM DISTURBANCES

Classifying rhythm disturbances that affect cardiac output in children can be done by looking at the rhythm in terms of being too fast (**tachydysrhythmias**), too slow (**bradydysrhythmias**), or pulseless (asystole, ventricular fibrillation, and pulseless ventricular tachycardia). Cardiac output is determined by **stroke volume** (the amount of blood pumped out with each beat) times the heart rate. Tachycardic rates can compromise cardiac output by decreasing filling time, thus decreasing stroke volume. Although stroke volume may be adequate, bradydysrhythmias decrease cardiac output due to inadequate heart rate.

Tachydysrhythmias

Tachydysrhythmias are abnormally rapid heart rates that are accompanied by an irregular heart rhythm. Several forms are outlined below.

Sinus Tachycardia

Sinus tachycardia is not usually considered a true dysrhythmia. It usually occurs in response to fever, anxiety, or as a compensatory mechanism for a decrease in cardiac output. Sinus tachycardia usually occurs with a rate of less than 200 beats/minute in children. There is no specific therapy for sinus tachycardia. Assessment and treatment should be directed at determining and correcting the underlying cause, which may include anxiety, shock, or respiratory distress.

Supraventricular Tachycardia

Supraventricular tachycardia (SVT) is usually caused by a re-entry mechanism involving an accessory pathway or the AV conduction system. The rate of SVT is usually above 240 beats/minute in infants and above 180 beats/minute in children but can vary with age. **Adenosine** (Adenocard®) is the drug of choice for symptomatic SVT. Adenosine is an endogenous nucleoside that causes a transient AV block that interrupts the re-entry circuit. Adenosine has a very short half-life (10 seconds) and produces minimal side effects. The dose is 0.1 mg/kg and should be injected as a rapid IV or IO bolus, as close to the hub of the catheter as possible. No more than 6 mg should be given in the initial bolus. It should be followed immediately by a 2 to 3 cc saline flush. If the initial dose has no effect, it may be doubled (0.2 mg/kg) and repeated once. The maximum single dose should not exceed 12 mg.

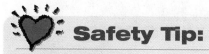

Safety Tip:

Adenosine

- Always follow adenosine administration with 2–3 cc saline flush.
- Never administer more than 12 mg in a single dose.
- Monitor patient for transient bradycardia or ventricular ectopy during conversion.

Verapamil (Calan®, Isoptin®) is a calcium-channel blocker that acts to slow conduction in the atrioventricular junction. Although used in adult SVT, its use is contraindicated in infants due to reports of profound bradycardia, hypotension, and asystole. It should not be used in children who are taking beta-adrenergic blocking drugs or those with signs of congestive failure or myocardial depression.

The treatment of choice for the child exhibiting signs of unstable SVT (poor perfusion, congestive heart failure, or hypotension) is synchronized cardioversion at an initial setting of 0.5 to 1.0 joules/kg. If the initial attempt at cardioversion is unsuccessful, it should be repeated at double the setting with a maximum of 360 joules. If the second attempt is unsuccessful, it is possible that the rhythm is not SVT.

If IV access has been established, adenosine may be administered before cardioversion. However, in the unstable patient, cardioversion should never be withheld to establish IV access.

If the child is conscious, sedation should be considered after consultation with medical control. **Midazolam** (Versed®) may be given intravenously at 0.1 mg/kg (maximum individual dose of 2.0 mg.). **Diazepam** (Valium®) may also be administered intravenously at 0.2 mg/kg with a maximum individual dose of 5.0 mg.

SVT may also present with aberrant conduction, creating the appearance of ventricular tachycardia. In the field setting, if the rhythm appears to be ventricular tachycardia, it should be treated as such.

Ventricular Tachycardia with a Pulse

Ventricular tachycardia is at least three consecutive ventricular complexes at a rate of more than 100 beats/minute. It is rare in pediatrics and is normally associated with underlying heart disease. However, hypoxemia, acidosis, electrolyte imbalance, and drug toxicity (particularly tricyclic antidepressants) can also cause ventricular tachycardia. If the child presents with signs of shock but still has a palpable pulse, the treatment of choice is synchronized cardioversion beginning at 0.5 joules/kg. A history of potential underlying causes should be sought, and treatment to correct those problems should be initiated.

Lidocaine (Xylocaine®) raises the threshold for ventricular fibrillation and suppresses ventricular ectopy. If IV access is established, a loading dose of 1.0 mg/kg should be administered IV push or intraosseous. The dose may be repeated twice as necessary with a maximum dose of 3.0 mg/kg. A lidocaine drip at 20 to 50 micrograms/kg/minute should follow the bolus if the rhythm is converted successfully. Lidocaine may also be given down the endotracheal tube if the child is intubated.

Amiodarone (Cordarone®) is being used more often for a wide range of atrial and ventricular dysrhythmias in children. It is an antidysrhythmic that prolongs the QT interval by inhibiting the outward potassium current. It also slows conduction in the ventricular myocardium and prolongs QRS duration by inhibiting sodium channels.

A loading infusion of 5 mg/kg given over 20–60 minutes is recommended for both supraventricular and ventricular dysrhythmias. The rate of the infusion depends on the need to have a rapid drug effect.

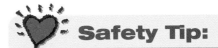

Safety Tip:

Atropine

- Always administer a minimum of 0.1 mg to avoid paradoxical bradycardia.
- Never administer more than 0.5 mg in a single dose or 1.0 mg total dose to a child.
- Never administer more than 1.0 mg in a single dose or 2.0 mg total dose to an adolescent.

Bradydysrhythmias

Bradydysrhythmias are the most common terminal rhythms seen in children. It is not critical to determine the specific dysrhythmia in the child who exhibits signs of poor perfusion. Any child with a heart rate less than 60 beats/minute with signs of poor perfusion (regardless of blood pressure) should be treated. Since the underlying cause of most cardiopulmonary failure and arrest is respiratory in nature, the initial intervention is aimed at correcting hypoxia and hypoxemia by providing effective ventilation with 100 percent oxygen. If ventilation does not rapidly increase the heart rate, chest compressions should be initiated, endotracheal intubation considered, and IV access obtained.

Epinephrine is the first-line drug for children in hypoxia-ischemia induced bradycardia. Epinephrine has both alpha- and beta-adrenergic effects. The beta-adrenergic effects increase myocardial contractility and heart rate. Alpha-adrenergic effects induce vasoconstriction, which elevates the perfusing pressure during chest compressions and enhances oxygen delivery to the heart muscle and brain. The initial dose for bradycardia is 0.01 mg/kg of a 1:10,000 solution via intravenous or intraosseous route with a maximum of 1.0 mg. If the child is intubated, 0.1 mg/kg of a 1:1,000 solution may be given through the endotracheal tube. If administering epinephrine via the endotracheal tube, it should be diluted in 3 to 5 cc of saline. Epinephrine can be repeated every 3 to 5 minutes until the bradycardia or the severe compromise of the cardiopulmonary system resolves.

Epinephrine should ideally be given through a central line. When given through a peripheral vascular line, local ischemia, tissue injury, and ulceration may occur if the drug infiltrates into the tissue. Remember also not to give sodium bicarbonate through the same line as epinephrine because the epinephrine will be inactivated by the alkaline solution.

Atropine is a parasympathetic blocker that accelerates the sinus or atrial pacemaker and increases AV conduction. Atropine is indicated in bradycardias with

AV block or those that are vagally induced. However, most bradycardias in children result from hypoxemia; therefore, oxygen and ventilation should be the initial treatment, rather than atropine. Dosage is 0.02 mg/kg IV or intraosseous. This dose should be doubled or tripled and diluted in at least 3 to 5 cc of saline for administration via the endotracheal tube. A minimum dose of 0.1 mg should be given, since lesser doses may result in a paradoxical bradycardia. Atropine may be repeated every five minutes. The maximum single dose for a child is 0.5 mg with a total maximum dose of 1.0 mg. The maximum single dose for an adolescent is 1.0 mg with a maximum dose of 2.0 mg.

Pulseless Dysrhythmias

Rhythms without pulses demand immediate attention. Rapid treatment is required as soon as it is determined that the patient is pulseless.

Pulseless Ventricular Tachycardia/ Ventricular Fibrillation

Ventricular fibrillation (VF) is a dysrhythmia characterized by rapid, disorganized depolarization of the ventricles of the myocardium. It is a rare occurrence in children and is seen in only about 10 percent of pediatric patients. It is associated with electrolyte imbalance, glucose imbalance, hypothermia, and drug toxicity (especially tricyclic antidepressants). The definitive treatment for VF and pulseless ventricular tachycardia (VT) is defibrillation. However, ventilation with 100 percent oxygen and chest compressions should be initiated immediately and continued until the defibrillator is prepared and ready for use.

Defibrillation depolarizes a critical mass of myocardial cells. This depolarization allows the potential for spontaneous normal depolarization (contractions) to resume. If normal contractions do not resume, the fibrillating heart will progress to asystole. Defibrillation should be administered as quickly as possible with an initial setting of 2 joules/kg. If this is unsuccessful, defibrillation should be repeated at 4 joules/kg and again at 4 joules/kg if the second attempt is unsuccessful. If conversion is not achieved with the third defibrillation, ventilation and compressions should be resumed and epinephrine administered. If there is a recurrence of VF following a successful conversion, defibrillation should be repeated at the same energy level (joules/kg) that resulted in the previous successful conversion.

The initial dose of epinephrine is 0.01 mg/kg (1:10,000) if given by IV or intraosseous route and 0.1 mg/kg (1:1,000) diluted in 3 to 5 cc of normal saline if given via the endotracheal tube. Epinephrine may be repeated every three to five minutes at a dose of 0.1 mg/kg (1:1,000) by all routes (IV, intraosseous, and endotracheal). Defibrillation at 4 joules/kg should follow 30 to 60 seconds after each medication administration.

Lidocaine may be administered in an attempt to decrease automaticity and raise the VF threshold. Lidocaine should be administered as a loading dose of 1.0 mg/kg by IV or intraosseous route and repeated once at the same dose.

There are no data on the effectiveness of **bretylium** in pediatrics. However, it may be administered if defibrillation and lidocaine fail to convert the VF. The initial dose of bretylium is 5.0 mg/kg IV push. It may be repeated one time at 10 mg/kg. The American Heart Association only recommends magnesium sulfate administration in the pediatric patient with torsades de pointes VT.

Pulseless Electrical Activity/Asystole

In **pulseless electrical activity (PEA)**, the electrical activity of the heart remains organized; but there is lack of, or severely compromised, cardiac output resulting in the loss of central pulses. **Asystole** is the lack of both cardiac output and electrical activity. Asystole must be confirmed by clinical assessment rather than just the cardiac monitor, since loose electrodes can result in a flat line tracing.

 Tricks of the Trade

Confirm asystole by an examination of the patient in addition to seeing a flat line on the cardiac monitor. If the electrocardiogram (EKG) electrodes are loose, a flat line will appear even though the patient is not in asystole.

 Exploring the Web

● What information can you find on dysrhythmias in children? Does the American Heart Association Web site provide any information? Are there links to other sites with information on dysrhythmias in children?

Causes of PEA include hypovolemia, tension pneumothorax, cardiac tamponade, hypoxemia, and severe acidosis. PEA may also result from drug overdoses including tricyclic antidepressants, beta-blockers, and calcium-channel blockers. Effective treatment of PEA depends on identification of the underlying cause. However, intubation and ventilation with 100 percent oxygen, chest compressions, and epinephrine should be administered while attempting to determine the underlying cause.

Resuscitation rates in asystole are dismal. Treatment should be aimed at oxygenating and stimulating the heart with epinephrine while performing chest compressions. Treatment for both PEA and asystole include cardiopulmonary resuscitation (CPR), intubation, ventilation with 100 percent oxygen, and the administration of epinephrine as previously described.

See Table 3-3 for a summary of pediatric dysrhythmias.

Additional Drug Therapy

In addition to the first-line drugs already discussed, several other pharmaceutical agents may be used. These drugs may not always be given depending on local protocols, the patient's response to the initial round of drugs, the length of the cardiac arrest, and the transport time.

Sodium Bicarbonate

During cardiac arrest, hypoxia leads to the development of metabolic acidosis, and hypercarbia leads to the development of respiratory acidosis. Although sodium bicarbonate is an alkalizing agent, it may result in a transient increase in cellular acidosis, which can depress cardiac function. If too much bicarbonate is administered, metabolic alkalosis may result. An alkalotic state alters the oxyhemoglobin dissociation curve, resulting in decreased oxygen delivery to the tissues. The standard adult sodium bicarbonate (8.4% solution) is hyperosmolar and has been associated with cerebral bleeds in premature infants. Thus, if the commercial 4.2 percent

TABLE 3-3
Pediatric Dysrhythmias

Cause, Signs, and Symptoms	Treatment
TACHYDYSRHYTHMIAS	
Sinus tachycardia	
• HR between 100 and 200 beats/minute • Not usually considered a true dysrhythmia • Usually in response to fever, anxiety, or compensatory mechanism for decrease in CO • Rapid pulse (usually less than 200/min) • Other signs dependent on underlying cause	• Determine and treat underlying cause
Supraventricular tachycardia	
• Caused by re-entry mechanism via accessory pathway or AV conduction system • HR > 240 beats/minute in infants • HR > 180 beats/minute in children • Stable—rapid pulse (usually greater than 200/min) • Unstable—signs of poor perfusion, congestive heart failure, hypotension	• Adenosine 0.1 mg/kg rapid IV or IO bolus (MAX DOSE: 6 mg) • Repeat once at 0.2 mg/kg (MAX DOSE: 12 mg) • Synchronized cardioversion at 0.5 to 1.0 joules/kg • Repeat at double the setting with max of 360 joules • Consider sedation before cardioversion
Ventricular tachycardia with a pulse	
• More than three ventricular complexes with HR > 100 beats/minute • Rare in pediatrics; associated with underlying heart disease • May be caused by hypoxemia, acidosis, electrolyte imbalance, and drug toxicity • Signs of poor perfusion and hypotension	• Synchronized cardioversion at 0.5 to 1.0 joules/kg • Lidocaine 1.0 mg/kg IV or IO (MAX DOSE: 3.0 mg/kg) • Follow with a lidocaine drip at 20–50 mcg/kg/minute • Treat underlying causes (e.g., tricyclic overdose with sodium bicarbonate 1.0 mEq/kg) • Consider amidarone at 5 mg/kg IV over 20 to 60 minutes • Consider procainamide at 15 mg/kg IV over 30 to 60 minutes
BRADYDYSRHYTHMIAS	
• Pulse rate < 60 beats/minute • Signs of poor perfusion	• Correct hypoxia with 100 percent oxygen and effective ventilation • Epinephrine 0.01 mg/kg (1:10,000) IV or IO (MAX DOSE: 1.0 mg) • OR epinephrine 0.1 mg/kg (1:1000) diluted with 3–5 cc of NSS via ET tube • Repeat same dose every 3–5 minutes

(continues)

TABLE 3-3
Continued

Cause, Signs, and Symptoms	Treatment
• Bradycardias with AV block or vagally induced	• Atropine 0.02 mg/kg IV or IO • OR Atropine 0.04–0.06 mg/kg in 3–5 cc of NSS via ET tube • Initial dose must be at least 0.1 mg to prevent paradoxical bradycardia • Repeat every 5 minutes to total dose of 1.0 mg for child or 2.0 mg for adolescent

PULSELESS DYSRHYTHMIAS

Pulseless ventricular tachycardia/ventricular fibrillation

• No vital signs • Unconscious	• Ventilate with 100 percent oxygen • Cardiac compressions • Defibrillate ASAP at 2 joules/kg followed by 4 joules/kg and then 4 joules/kg • Continue ventilations and compressions • Epinephrine 0.01 mg/kg (1:10,000) IV or IO or 0.1 mg/kg (1:1000) in 3–5 cc of NSS via ET tube • Repeat every 3–5 minutes at 0.1 mg/kg (1:1000) by all routes. Follow with defibrillation at 4 joules/kg 30–60 seconds after each dose of medication • Lidocaine 1.0 mg/kg IV or IO • Repeat lidocaine once at same dose • Consider amiodarone at 5 mg/kg IV over 20 to 60 minutes

Pulseless electrical activity/asystole

• No vital signs • Unconscious	• Ventilate with 100 percent oxygen • Cardiac compressions • Epinephrine 0.01 mg/kg (1:10,000) IV or IO or 0.1 mg/kg (1:1000) in 3–5 cc of NSS via ET tube • Repeat every 3–5 minutes at 0.1 mg/kg (1:1,000) by all routes

Abbreviations: ASAP, as soon as possible; AV, atrioventricular; CO, cardiac output; ET, endotracheal; HR, heart rate; IO, intraosseous; IV, intravenous; NSS, normal saline solution.

solution is not carried by the service, the adult solution should be diluted 1:1 (4.2 percent) if administered to infants younger than three months. Because actual blood gas analysis of acidosis is not possible in the field, sodium bicarbonate is rarely used before hospitalization.

The primary method of managing acidosis associated with cardiac arrest in the field is effective ventilation. Sodium bicarbonate is indicated in tricyclic antidepressant toxicity and should be administered in a dose of 1.0 mEq/kg.

Dextrose

Children have high glucose needs and limited glycogen stores. The increased demands of cardiopulmonary distress can rapidly deplete the glycogen stores and lead to hypoglycemia. Clinical signs of hypoglycemia can mimic those of hypoxemia. Therefore, blood sugars should be monitored in all critically ill, unstable children. If hypoglycemia is documented by the field glucose test, dextrose should be administered. The dose of dextrose for children is 2 to 4 mL/kg of a maximum concentration of 25 percent ($D_{25}W$) glucose (250 mg/mL) which provides 0.5 to 1.0 g/kg. $D_{25}W$ is available commercially. If the 25 percent concentration is not carried by the service, the 50 percent concentration must be diluted 1:1 before administration. This dilution is necessary since 50 percent dextrose is very hyperosmolar. Even 25 percent dextrose is hyperosmolar; therefore, it is preferable to dilute the dextrose to a 10 percent concentration (1:4) and run a 5 to 10 cc/kg infusion over 20 minutes. IV boluses of dextrose may result in periods of hyperglycemia. Hyperglycemia has been associated with worsened outcomes of children with head injury and shock.

TRANSPORT GUIDELINES

Children suffering from respiratory failure or shock require rapid transport to an appropriate facility for definitive care. Efforts should immediately be directed at maintaining the airway and providing necessary oxygenation and ventilation. Transport should never be delayed to gain venous access. Protocol treatment of shock or dysrhythmias should be carried out enroute.

SUMMARY

The majority of children arrest from either respiratory failure or shock. Once arrest has occurred, resuscitation rates are extremely poor. Children who are resuscitated often suffer neurological compromise. The key to dealing with these problems is early recognition and intervention with emphasis on ventilation for respiratory failure and fluid resuscitation for shock.

Rapid transport to the hospital is of prime importance in the care of the critically ill child. Definitive treatment by health care professionals with specific pediatric skills offers the best chance for a positive outcome.

Management of Case Scenario

This child is suffering from profound respiratory failure and circulatory collapse. Immediate intervention to gain airway control and ventilation are crucial. This child has both respiratory and metabolic acidosis as the result of inadequate ventilation and perfusion. Positive pressure ventilation with 100 percent oxygen must be initiated. Compressions should also be initiated since the heart rate is below 60 with signs of inadequate perfusion. Although intravenous sodium bicarbonate is indicated for tricyclic overdoses, no time should be wasted attempting venous access on this child. Definitive treatment for specific problems associated with tricyclic overdose is complex. This child should be managed with aggressive airway maintenance and ventilation, compressions, and rapid transport.

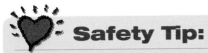

REVIEW QUESTIONS

1. List the two major causes of cardiac arrest in the pediatric patient.
2. Slow respirations in the critically ill child may be the result of which of the following:
   a. Hypothermia
   b. CNS depression
   c. Fatigue
   d. All of the above
3. Compare the cause of the following types of shock.
   a. Hypovolemic
   b. Cardiogenic
   c. Septic
4. What are the three principles of field management that will provide the critically ill child the best chance for a positive outcome?

Safety Tip:

Sodium Bicarbonate and Dextrose

• Both sodium bicarbonate and dextrose, as packaged for adult use, are hyperosmolar. If commercially diluted packages are not carried by the ambulance service, these drugs should be diluted 1:1 before administering to children.

Questions 5, 6, and 7 apply to the following scenario.

You are managing a five-year-old child suffering from blunt abdominal trauma. Her skin is pale and cool from the elbows down. She is agitated and complaining of abdominal pain. Her respiratory rate is 24, shallow, and somewhat labored. Her heart rate is 120 and regular and blood pressure is 96/72.

5. Is this child in compensated or uncompensated shock? What criteria did you use for your decision?

6. How would you manage this child's respiratory system? Explain your rationale.

7. How would you manage this child's circulatory system? Explain your rationale.

▶ REFERENCES

American Heart Association (2000). Guidelines 2000 for cardiopulmonary resuscitation and emergency cardiovascular care. *Journal of the American Heart Association, 102(8).* I-307-19.

Wong, D. (1999). *Whaley & Wong's nursing care of infants and children.* St. Louis, MO: Mosby-Year Book.

▶ BIBLIOGRAPHY

National Association of Emergency Medical Technicians. (1999). *Basic and advanced prehospital trauma life support* (4th ed.). St. Louis, MO: Mosby-Year Book.

National Association of EMS Physicians (1999). *Model pediatric protocols.*

Sanders, M. (2000). *Mosby's paramedic textbook.* St. Louis, MO: Mosby-Year Book.

Wertz, E. (1997a). Infants and children. In N. McSwain, R. White, J. Paturas, & W. Metcalf. (Eds.), *The basic EMT—comprehensive prehospital patient care.* St. Louis, MO: Mosby-Year Book.

Wertz, E. (1997b). Pediatric emergencies. In B. Shade, M. Rothenberg, E. Wertz, & S. Jones. (Eds.), *Mosby's EMT—intermediate textbook.* St. Louis, MO: Mosby-Year Book. 482–517.

Chapter 4

Respiratory Emergencies

OBJECTIVES

Upon completion of this chapter, the student should be able to:

- Describe pathophysiology, signs/symptoms, and appropriate field management of the following diseases:
  a. Croup
  b. Epiglottitis
  c. Bronchiolitis
  d. Reactive airway disease (RAD)
  e. Foreign body aspiration (not related to trauma)
- Define drowning and near-drowning.
- Explain pathophysiology and differences between:
  a. Wet and dry drowning
  b. Salt water and fresh water drowning
  c. Cold water drowning
- Identify factors affecting survivability, management principles, and transport criteria for near drowning

KEY TERMS

atelectasis	dysphagia	hypotonic	status asthmaticus
bronchiolitis	epiglottitis	hypoxia	subglottic
bronchoconstriction	foreign body aspiration	hypoxemia	surfactant
circumoral cyanosis	hemoptysis	laryngospasm	transtracheal jet insufflation
cricothyroidotomy	hypercarbia	mammalian diving reflex	tripod position
croup	hyperkalemia	reactive airway disease	ventilation-perfusion mismatch
drowning	hypertonic	(RAD) or asthma	wet drowning
dry drowning	hypothermia		

Case Scenario

You are dispatched at 2 p.m. for a child having difficulty breathing. You are met at the door by a frantic mother who leads you to a two-year-old girl in the kitchen. The child is sitting very still on the kitchen chair. You notice she is leaning forward in the tripod position. Her mother tells you she was playing loudly with her older sister and friends. There were dolls and accessories strewn about the room. The mother states the child was making a funny noise when she breathed and refused to eat or drink anything for lunch. The child continued to make "that funny noise," and so the mother called for help. How would you manage this child and why?

INTRODUCTION

Respiratory distress in children may rapidly lead to failure due to immature development of respiratory muscles and fatigue. Managing respiratory distress requires rapid assessment and intervention. A knowledge of the signs of respiratory distress or failure and respiratory problems frequently encountered in children gives the prehospital provider a sound basis for interpreting assessment findings and implementing appropriate interventions.

SIGNS OF RESPIRATORY DISTRESS

Signs of respiratory distress are often more noticeable in children than in adults. Table 4-1 provides the description and significance of the common signs of respiratory distress in children. In addition to the signs listed in the table, the inability to speak or to speak only in one- to two-word sentences is indicative of severe respiratory distress.

Exploring the Web

- What Web sites can you find related to respiratory problems?

UPPER AIRWAY PROBLEMS

There are several respiratory problems that are specifically caused by upper airway infection. Initial signs and symptoms are caused by partial airway obstruction which may progress to respiratory distress or failure if not adequately treated.

Croup

Croup is a self-limiting viral infection that results in **subglottic** (below the glottis) edema and edema of the vocal cords. History often includes a low-grade fever and upper respiratory tract symptoms, such as a runny nose for one to three days prior to onset.

Incidence

Croup occurs more often in boys than girls and increases in the late fall through the early winter months. It primarily affects children from ages six months to three years, especially those children two years of age. About 1 to 15 percent of all children affected require hospitalization; and of that group, 1 to 5 percent are intubated (Wong, 1999).

Etiology

A viral infection develops around the larynx. The area below the glottis and the larynx itself become swollen and produce the characteristic "seal bark" cough. The child actually sounds worse than he or she looks.

Assessment

Signs and symptoms include inspiratory and expiratory stridor and a classic "seal bark" cough. The cough results from the narrowing produced by edema. Edema of the vocal cords usually results in hoarseness. Most children can be treated at home with humidified air. However, signs and symptoms may worsen at night due to the dry, warm air of a bedroom and lying in the supine position. These changes will result in more pronounced respiratory distress.

Management and Transport

Allow the child to assume a position of comfort. If available, administer humidified oxygen. If humidified oxygen is not available, do not withhold dry oxygen if the child is in respiratory distress. Allowing the parent to hold the mask for blow-by oxygen administration will often help decrease the child's agitation. Improvement of signs and symptoms may occur as the result of moving to cooler, outside air when the child is moved from

TABLE 4.1
Signs of Respiratory Distress

Sign	Description	Significance
Nasal flaring	• Nares flare out on inspiration	• Some respiratory distress
Retractions	• Skin appears to pull in between ribs during inspiration • May be seen supraclavicular, substernal, or intercostal	• Due to immature respiratory muscles • Indicative of moderate to severe respiratory distress
Stridor	• High pitched, harsh sound heard during inspiration	• Partial upper airway obstruction
Wheezes	• High pitched, whistling sound • Usually heard first on expiration, but may be heard on both expiration and inspiration	• Partial lower airway obstruction
Prolonged expiration	• Expiratory phase is extended	• Bronchoconstriction
Grunting	• Grunting sound heard at the end of expiration • Most common in infants	• Premature closure of glottis during early expiration • Increases airway pressure
"See-saw" movements	• Tidal volume in young children much more dependent on diaphragm • Extreme respiratory effort causes chest to draw in and pushes abdomen out	• Severe respiratory distress
Head bobbing	• Head moves up and down with inspiration and expiration	• Often indicative of impending respiratory failure
Circumoral cyanosis	• Bluish discoloration around the mouth	• Hypoxia/hypoxemia

Wertz, E. (1997a). Infants and children. In N. McSwain, R. White, J. Paturas, & W. Metcalf, (Eds.). *The basic EMT—comprehensive pre-hospital patient care*. St. Louis, MO: Mosby-Year Book. pp. 643–682.

the house to the ambulance for transport. Inspiration of cooler air contributes to decreasing the existing edema.

 Tricks of the Trade

Always move slowly and speak calmly when dealing with a child in respiratory distress to prevent further agitation and increased distress.

Epiglottitis

Epiglottitis is an acute bacterial infection resulting in inflammation and swelling of the epiglottis. It is a life-threatening problem and results from serious obstructive inflammatory processes.

Incidence

Epiglottitis occurs most frequently between the ages of two and five years (Wong, 1999). It can, however, occur at any time between infancy and adulthood. Many infants now receive vaccination against the bacteria that causes epiglottis. This widespread vaccination has significantly reduced the incidence of this infection.

Etiology

Epiglottitis is most commonly caused by type B *Hemophilus influenzae* bacteria. It is characterized by a rapid onset that may progress from initial signs and symptoms to complete obstruction in a few hours. The child may go to bed without any symptoms and wake up later with a sore throat and pain on swallowing.

Assessment

The child with epiglottitis presents with anxiety and looks acutely ill. The child is usually found in the classic **"tripod" position**, sitting upright and leaning forward with the arms down and extended. This position causes the epiglottis to fall slightly forward and allows air to pass. Inspiratory stridor may be present due to partial obstruction by edema. **Dysphagia** (difficulty swallowing) due to edema is often exhibited as the classic drooling associated with the disease. High fever (102° F to 103° F) is also characteristic.

Management

Make every effort to prevent increasing the anxiety of the child. Slow movements, a calm voice, and involving the parents in the interaction whenever possible will contribute to keeping the child calm. Under no circumstances should an attempt be made to visualize the oropharynx. Provide high-concentration supplemental oxygen if the child will tolerate it. If possible, have the parent hold the mask to prevent further anxiety in the child.

If loss of consciousness or obstruction occurs, immediately ventilate the child with a bag-valve mask device. It is usually possible to provide ventilation with the bag and mask. Remember that the ventilation must be done slowly and requires high inspiratory pressures. Bags with pop-off valves are set to release at 30 to 35 cm of water pressure. To effectively achieve the needed higher pressures, use a bag without a pop-off valve. Although the American Heart Association's Pediatric Advanced Life Support guidelines recommend that pop-off valves are inappropriate in any setting, some prehospital services may still carry equipment with them. If the only bag available is one with a pop-off valve, seal the valve with a finger or tape.

Cricothyroidotomy (emergency opening between the thyroid and cricoid membrane) is rarely required but should be considered if all other means of ventilation fail. Cricothyroidotomy is performed with a large-bore (14- or 16-gauge) intravenous catheter through the cricothyroid membrane. Be aware that there is significant risk of injury to the carotid arteries or jugular veins if performing this procedure on an infant or child. See Appendix C for a skills review of cricothyroidotomy.

Due to the diameter of the intravenous catheter, high resistance to air flow, and the need for high inspiratory inflation pressures, effective ventilation using the bag is not usually possible. Oxygenation may be possible only if pop-off valves are disabled. A transtracheal jet insufflator is required to provide enough pressure to ventilate through the catheter. This method may buy some time, but it will eventually result in **hypercarbia** (increased carbon dioxide in the blood) and hyperinflation of the lungs that can lead to pneumothorax. Subcutaneous emphysema may also result if the catheter tip is not in the lumen of the trachea.

Pediatric Advanced Life Support (PALS) guidelines of the American Heart Association discuss needle cricothyroidotomy and point out that there is no published experience with this procedure in infants and small children. Needle cricothyroidotomy and **transtracheal jet insufflation** (ventilation through the catheter used for the cricothyroidotomy) should be considered only if they are part of system protocols and the prehospital provider has adequate training and practice. See Appendix C for a skills review of transtracheal jet insufflation.

Transport

The child should be left in the sitting position for transport. Attempting to place the child in the recumbent or supine position may result in complete obstruction of the airway.

Epiglottitis is a true emergency. Transport should not be delayed for a prolonged assessment.

 Tricks of the Trade

Epiglottitis is a true emergency! Do not do anything to upset the child or delay transport for a detailed assessment.

LOWER AIRWAY PROBLEMS

Lower airway problems are caused by changes in the lungs and not the airway leading to the lungs. Commonly, the bronchioles and alveoli are affected.

Bronchiolitis

Bronchiolitis is an acute viral infection that primarily affects the bronchioles. Even though few children require a stay at the hospital, it can be a serious disease.

Incidence

Bronchiolitis occurs in infants and children under two years of age and usually has a gradual onset. It tends to be a seasonal disease, with higher incidence in winter and spring, since the responsible viruses are most abundant at those times. It usually reaches its peak in the winter (Wong, 1999).

Etiology

Bronchiolitis is most commonly caused by the respiratory syncytial virus (RSV). It causes inflammation and edema of the bronchioles that produces a thin, watery fluid that collects in the alveoli. It also results in **bronchoconstriction** (narrowing of the bronchioles).

Assessment

The infant may present with a cough or signs of respiratory distress such as tachypnea, nasal flaring, or retractions. Lung auscultation often reveals wheezes and fine rales at the end of expiration. The infant may have a history of a runny nose or cough. Bronchiolitis is most often confused with reactive airway disease in its presentation.

Management and Transport

If the infant is in respiratory distress, administer high-concentration oxygen. Nebulized beta-adrenergic agents such as albuterol sulfate may also help. Since infants cannot use a mouthpiece, administer the treatment by holding the nebulizer close to the face to allow the medication to be taken in using the blow-by method or administer it through a loosely applied facemask. Subcutaneous epinephrine is not effective in the treatment of bronchiolitis, but racemic epinephrine may provide some relief. Transport the infant in a position of comfort.

Reactive Airway Disease (RAD/Asthma)

Reactive airway disease (RAD) or **asthma** is a chronic inflammatory disorder of the airways and includes three components:

1. Airway obstruction that can be reversed
2. Airway inflammation
3. Increased (hyperreactivity) airway responsiveness to stimuli (Jackson & Vessey, 1996)

Incidence

Asthma is the most common chronic disease of childhood and is the primary cause of children being absent from school (Wong, 1999). In addition, the majority of pediatric admissions to the Emergency Department and hospital are because of asthma and its complications. Overall, about $1 billion is spent each year treating children with asthma (Wong, 1999).

Asthma may occur at any age yet 80 to 90 percent of children have their first asthma symptoms before four or five years of age (Wong, 1999). In young children, boys are affected more often than girls. Once adolescence occurs, girls are affected more often than boys.

Etiology

Various stimuli or events can trigger an asthma exacerbation or attack (Table 4-2). Bronchospasm, inflammation and edema of the mucosa, and production of thick mucus leading to plugging narrow the child's lower airways. Air then becomes trapped behind narrowed or blocked airways. This process leads to retention of carbon dioxide and air trapping. The child tries to breathe harder, and hyperinflation of the lungs allows gas to be exchanged and the airways to be kept open. Hypoxemia eventually occurs as ventilation and perfusion decrease, leading to the development of acidosis and dehydration (Figure 4-1).

Mortality from asthma is on the rise in all age groups with the highest mortality occurring in blacks (Jackson & Vessey, 1996). Factors that may contribute to the increased rate of reported mortality include:

- Increase in the severity of the disease
- Pharmacological treatment is misused or underutilized
- The severity of symptoms is not recognized
- Treatment is delayed
- Psychosocial issues (Jackson & Vessey, 1996)

Assessment

When assessing the child with an asthma exacerbation, the following signs and symptoms may be present:

- Shortness of breath that progressively worsens
- Wheezing
- Cough
- Chest tightness
- Change in level of consciousness. Infants and young children become irritable, restless, and unable to be comforted while older children become restless, apprehensive, lethargic, and may lose consciousness.

TABLE 4-2
Asthma Triggers

Type of Trigger	Examples	Type of Trigger	Examples
Allergens	Outdoor • Air pollution • Trees and shrubs • Weeds • Grass • Molds and pollens Indoor • Mold • Dust • Dust mites	Animals	• Cats • Dogs • Horses • Rodents
		Medications	• Aspirin • Antibiotics • Beta-blockers • Nonsteroidal anti-inflammatory drugs (NSAIDs)
Irritants	• Tobacco smoke • Sprays • Odors • Wood smoke	Strong emotions	• Fear • Anger • Laughing • Crying
Exercise	• School sports	Conditions	• Gastroesophageal reflux • Tracheoesophageal fistula
Cold air	• Winter		
Changes in weather or temperature	• Very warm day in the winter • Very cool day in the summer	Food additives	• Sulfite preservatives
		Foods	• Milk and dairy products • Nuts
Environmental change	• Starting new school • Moving to new house	Endocrine factors	• Menses • Pregnancy • Thyroid disease
Colds and infections	• Upper respiratory infection • Flu		

Wong, D. (1999). *Whaley and Wong's nursing care of infants and children* (6th ed.). St. Louis, MO: Mosby-Year Book.

• Pale skin leading to cyanosis

• Older child speaks in broken, short, panting phrases

• Upright position. Young children will use a tripod position while older children will sit upright with shoulders hunched over and hands on bed or chair (Figure 4-2).

Early in the attack, the patient may present with coughing since expiration requires more effort than inspiration. Respiratory rate and effort increase as the attack worsens. The expiratory phase becomes prolonged, and wheezing may be heard. Expiratory wheezes are most common, but inspiratory wheezes may also be present. The dyspnea caused by the attack

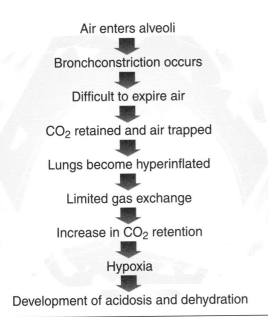

Air enters alveoli

↓

Bronchconstriction occurs

↓

Difficult to expire air

↓

CO_2 retained and air trapped

↓

Lungs become hyperinflated

↓

Limited gas exchange

↓

Increase in CO_2 retention

↓

Hypoxia

↓

Development of acidosis and dehydration

FIGURE 4-1 Pathophysiology of reactive airway disease (asthma).

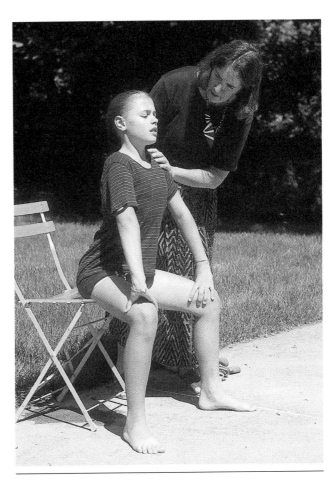

FIGURE 4-2 This position in an older child is a classic sign of an asthma attack.

results in the child breathing through the mouth. Since intake of air through the mouth is not humidified, this dry air contributes to dehydration of the airway resulting in thicker mucus and increased respiratory distress.

In some situations, no breath sounds or wheezing may be audible. DO NOT be fooled that the child is improving. In fact, this finding represents a severe spasm or obstruction and can be fatal! Immediate intervention is needed! *A silent chest is an ominous sign.*

The increased rate and effort of breathing over time may result in respiratory arrest from exhaustion. The child suffering from a reactive airway disease attack who appears sleepy is in trouble and requires immediate assistance. In severe cases, wheezing may be absent with only minimal air movement heard on auscultation.

Management

If the child is alert, administer a nebulized beta-adrenergic agent such as albuterol (Proventil®; Ventolin®) metaproterenol (Alupent®), or terbutaline (Brethine®). If the

child is not able to use the inhaler, the hands-free mask should be used for the nebulizer treatment.

Epinephrine may be indicated to reduce bronchoconstriction. Administer epinephrine at a total dosage of 0.01 mg/kg of a 1:1,000 solution (maximum dose: 0.35 cc) via subcutaneous injection. These dosages are usually divided into 3 doses at 20-minute intervals. Beware that epinephrine may increase an already tachycardic heart rate.

Tricks of the Trade

A silent chest is an ominous sign! If wheezing is absent but only minimal air movement is heard on auscultation, the child needs *immediate* assistance.

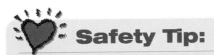

Safety Tip:

Epinephrine

- Never administer more than 0.35 cc of epinephrine
- Monitor pulse rate. Epinephrine may increase an already tachycardic rate

If the child presents with severe respiratory distress, administer high-concentration oxygen. Depending on the child's condition, intubation and ventilation with in-line nebulizer of a beta-adrenergic agent should be considered. Because of hyperinflation and air trapping, significant resistance is often encountered when attempting to ventilate with a bag-valve mask device.

Terbutaline (Brethine®) may also be given to those children who do not respond to beta-agonists or epinephrine. Give up to 3 doses at 0.25 mg subcutaneously over 30 minutes.

Transport

Transport should not be delayed to wait for treatment effects. Allow the child to assume a position of comfort if he or she is alert. Continue to monitor and support the child's respiratory status. Talk calmly to the child in order to prevent further agitation and increased distress. Try to involve the child as much as possible in his or her treatment depending on the child's age. Allow the parents to participate as well.

Table 4-3 presents a summary comparison of the signs and symptoms of croup, epiglottitis, bronchiolitis, and RAD/asthma.

Status Asthmaticus

Status asthmaticus is an acute, severe, and prolonged asthma attack. The ongoing bronchospasm, edema, and mucus plugging critically reduce the diameter of the airway. The child continues to struggle to breathe without any improvement.

TABLE 4-3
Comparison of Common Respiratory Problems

	Croup	Epiglottitis	Bronchiolitis	RAD/Asthma
Age	6 months–3 years	2–5 years (may occur at any age)	6–18 months	Any age
Cause	Viral	Bacterial	Viral	Allergies Infection Weather change Emotions Exercise
Onset	Slow	Rapid May progress in matter of hours	Slow	Relatively rapid
Precipitating Events	History of upper respiratory infection	Usually none	History of upper respiratory infection	Exercise Allergy Inhaled irritant Weather change
Signs and Symptoms	• Low-grade fever • Inspiratory and expiratory stridor • "Seal bark" cough • Hoarseness	• High fever • Anxious • Drooling • Inspiratory stridor • Tripod position	• No fever • Cough • Tachypnea • Nasal flaring • Rales and wheezes	• No fever • Tachypnea • Nasal flaring • Retractions • Expiratory wheezes

Wertz, E. (1997a). Infants and children. In N. McSwain, R. White, J. Paturas, & W. Metcalf, (Eds.). *The basic EMT—comprehensive prehospital patient care*. St. Louis, MO: Mosby-Year Book.

Wong, D. (1999). *Whaley & Wong's nursing care of infants and children* (6th ed.). St. Louis, MO: Mosby-Year Book.

Tricks of the Trade

Status asthmaticus is a medical emergency! If left untreated, respiratory failure and death will occur. DO NOT waste any time in the field.

Status asthmaticus is a medical emergency! If untreated, respiratory failure and death will occur. Continue to provide high-concentration oxygen, and rapidly transport the child to the closest facility. DO NOT waste any time in the field.

Exploring the Web

- Search for specific key terms such as croup, epiglottitis, reactive airway disease/asthma, and bronchiolitis. What information can you find? Create a fact sheet for each disorder based upon your findings.

OTHER CONDITIONS AFFECTING THE RESPIRATORY SYSTEM

In addition to upper and lower airway problems, children may have other conditions that may cause respiratory emergencies. These situations also require prompt assessment, treatment, and transport.

Foreign Body Aspiration

Children are prone to putting everything into the mouth as a way of exploring and learning about new things in their world. If they have access to items that are small, aspiration may occur once those items are in the oral cavity. **Foreign body aspiration (FBA)** is the inhalation of a foreign body into either the upper or lower airway.

Incidence

FBA is most common in older infants as well as children from ages one to three (Wong, 1999). Aspiration of a for-

eign body can, however, occur at any age. Of the number of deaths that occur each year from FBA, 20 percent occur in children under four years (Wong, 1999).

Etiology

About 75 percent of all items get caught in the mainstem or lobar bronchus. The site of the obstruction is dependent upon the object aspirated. Heavier items such as nails or coins go to the most dependent portions of the tracheobronchial tree. Some objects stay in one place while others move around in the airway.

Common causes of foreign body obstruction include food (peanuts, hot dogs, and hard candy), small toys (Lego® blocks and marbles), coins, buttons from stuffed animals, and balloons. The most common objects aspirated in order of frequency are:

- Hot dog
- Round candy
- Peanut or other nut
- Grape
- Cookie or biscuit
- Other meat
- Carrot
- Apple
- Peanut butter (Wong, 1999)

Hot dogs, round candy, peanuts (or other nuts), and grapes are responsible for more than 40 percent of all items aspirated. Another serious offender is latex balloons whether they are inflated, not inflated, or broken into small pieces. Items that swell when wet (e.g., popcorn) or items that do not dissolve (e.g., seeds) are also dangerous.

Assessment

FBA may present as either an upper or lower airway problem. Signs and symptoms of foreign body obstruction may range from a mild cough to life-threatening, complete obstruction. The child may be choking, drooling, or unable to swallow. Marked inspiratory stridor and frantic efforts to breathe may be present. Maximal effort to breathe may suck the foreign body into the trachea or beyond. Therefore, lung sounds may be decreased or completely absent on the side of the aspiration. Wheezing may be noted with partial obstruction of the bronchus. If wheezing occurs as the result of FBA (versus reactive airway disease), it will be on one side only.

History can be extremely helpful in determining the possibility of an FBA. The onset of symptoms is sudden and usually occurs right after eating or playing with small toys. The child's caregiver may tell you the child has been gagging or vomiting.

Management

Initial management of children with upper airway obstruction, either partial or complete, should follow basic life support (BLS) guidelines. If the obstruction is partial and the child is awake, attempt to calm the child and encourage slow, deep breathing. No attempt should be made at this point to forcefully dislodge the object. Supplemental oxygen may be necessary and should be administered in a way that prevents further agitating the child. Holding the mask to the side and away from the face to provide blow-by oxygen is one way to decrease apprehension and agitation. Punching the oxygen tubing through the bottom of a paper cup can allow the child to "drink" the oxygen (Figure 4-3). Do not use a Styrofoam cup since there is a risk the child might bite the cup, breaking off and aspirating bits of Styrofoam. Oxygen "bears" can also help calm fears of oxygen administration and are available commercially.

If the obstruction is complete, the child is unresponsive, and basic life support maneuvers are unsuccessful, try to visualize the object with a laryngoscope. If the object is visible, attempt to remove it with Magill forceps. If the removal attempt is unsuccessful, intubation may push the object into the right mainstem bronchus and allow for ventilation of the left lung.

Transport

All children with suspected foreign body aspiration should be transported to the hospital, even if there are no obvious signs or symptoms. If an aspiration has occurred, the object must be removed. If the object is not removed, secondary respiratory problems such as pneumonia, bronchitis, or **hemoptysis** (coughing up blood) may develop.

SUBMERSION

Drowning is now recognized as a death due to submersion events in which the child dies at the scene, in the Emergency Department, or in the hospital. If the child dies after 24 hours of the episode, the death is referred to as a "drowning-related" death (American Heart Association, 2000). Drowning can occur with or without inhalation of surrounding medium.

The American Heart Association recommends that the term "near-drowning" not be used any longer. Water rescue should be used to describe someone who is alert but has some difficulty while swimming. Submersion is now used to describe someone who has distress related to swimming and who requires treatment in the field as well as transportation to an emergency facility for additional treatment and observation (American Heart Association, 2000).

Dry drowning or drowning without aspiration is death caused from respiratory obstruction and asphyxia when submerged. The usual cause is prolonged laryngospasm. This form of drowning accounts for approximately ten percent of all deaths (Wong, 1999).

Wet drowning or drowning with aspiration is death from asphyxia as well as changes caused by fluid aspiration while submerged. The lungs fill with water or whatever medium in which the child has been submerged.

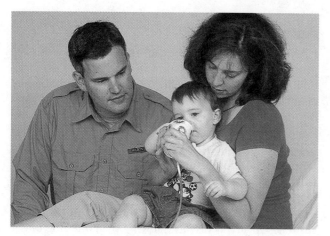

a.

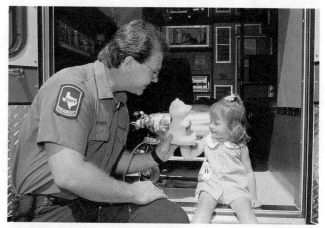

b.

FIGURE 4-3   a. This child is able to pretend to drink the oxygen from the cup, thus making administration of the oxygen more tolerable. **b.** Oxygen bears provide a child-friendly way of providing necessary oxygenation. Courtesy of Laerdal Medical Corporation, Wappingers Falls, NY.

Incidence

Drowning is the second leading cause of accidental death in children (Wong, 1999). Four times more males than females are victims of accidental drowning. Most instances are related to the age of the child (Table 4-4). For every child who drowns, another four are hospitalized for near drowning. For every hospital admission, approximately four more children are treated in hospital emergency departments (National SAFEKIDS Campaign, 1998).

The peak ages of drowning/drowning-related episodes occur in children ages one to four and in teenagers. The most common location is a private or residential swimming pool. The incidence of drowning/drowning-related in younger children is often associated with bathtubs or pools when the child is unsupervised. Of the 320 children that have drowned in buckets since 1984, 88 percent were between the ages of 7 and 15 months (National SAFEKIDS Campaign, 1998). The child at that age may not be strong enough to lift the head out. In teenagers, drowning is often associated with alcohol

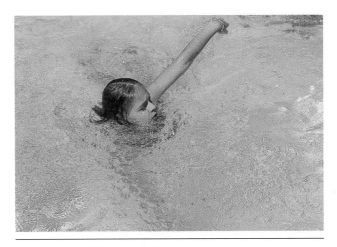

FIGURE 4-4 Drowning occurs when children become exhausted while swimming.

use, boating accidents, or exhaustion while swimming (Figure 4-4). The majority of drowning/drowning-related episodes involve those who do not know how to swim and occur less than ten feet from safety. In 1997, more than 200 children ages 14 and under were injured while riding a personal watercraft device.

Factors Affecting Survivability

Those children discovered within two minutes of submersion represent the majority of children who survive (92 percent). Children found after 10 minutes of submersion usually die (86 percent). Any child who requires cardiopulmonary resuscitation has a greater likelihood of dying or sustaining severe brain injury (National SAFEKIDS Campaign, 1998).

Several factors affect survivability. These include:

- Age
- Submersion time
- Past medical history/head or spine trauma related to diving
- Water temperature
- Water contaminants
- Effectiveness of resuscitative efforts

Age

The younger the child, the greater the chance of survival. The extra pathways that are still present in the brain of young children allow for recovery with less neurological deficits. In addition, children rarely have underlying medical conditions that complicate recovery.

TABLE 4-4
Drowning Risks

Age Group	Activity
Infants	• Bathtub
Preschool	• Private swimming pools (highest rate: two–three years of age) • Bathtub • Wading pool • Bucket • Diaper pail • Toilet • Hot tub • Spa
School age	• Private swimming pools • Open water sites such as lakes, rivers, and oceans
Adolescents	• Open water sites

1998 National SAFEKIDS Campaign.

Wong, D. (1999). *Whaley & Wong's nursing care of infants and children* (6th ed.). St. Louis, MO: Mosby-Year Book.

Submersion Time

As submersion time increases, chance of survival decreases. Prolonged hypoxia and asphyxia decrease the chance of survival.

Past Medical History

Past medical history such as seizures or respiratory problems can complicate both the submersion and after effects of drowning and lessen the chance of survival.

Water Temperature

The temperature of the water has a major effect on survivability. Cold water submersion rapidly induces hypothermia as the result of both water temperature and the child's large body surface area. Generalized hypothermia lowers metabolic rate and oxygen demands which may preserve brain function. In addition, the **mammalian diving reflex** (apnea, bradycardia, and shunting of blood to the heart and brain) initiated by cold water on the face and forehead results in lowering metabolic needs and maintaining perfusion of vital organs. These mechanisms no doubt contribute to neurologic recovery following prolonged cold water submersion. As of this writing, the longest documented submersion with survival is 88 minutes (Schmidt, Fritz, Kasperczyk, & Tscherne, 1995). All children suffering from cold water submersion should be transported despite presentation or submersion time. Death should not be assumed until rewarming has been initiated and the determination made by hospital personnel.

Water Contaminants

Water contaminants such as silt, salt, sand, bacteria in fresh or sea water, chlorine in swimming pools, and cleaning products in buckets or toilets irritate the respiratory system and can lead to bronchoconstriction or chemical pneumonia that complicates and lessens the chance of survival.

Effectiveness of Resuscitative Efforts

Initiation and effectiveness of resuscitative efforts following submersion have a major effect on survivability, especially following cold water submersion. An unconscious child who is apneic and pulseless requires immediate initiation of basic life support upon removal from the submersion and rapid transport to the hospital.

Etiology

Regardless of the type of submersion, the underlying problems are the same: hypoxia and acidosis. A drowning episode follows a predictable sequence of events that begins with gasping and breath-holding at the onset of submersion. Once the involuntary stimulus to breathe occurs, the victim panics and struggles. This action results in water being swallowed and aspirated. Swallowing of water leads to gastric distention that may result in vomiting. Aspirating water triggers **laryngospasm** (spasm of the larynx). This laryngospasm and aspiration lead to profound hypoxia with resultant **hypoxemia** (decreased oxygen in the blood) and acidosis.

As hypoxia increases and cerebral perfusion decreases, loss of consciousness ensues. In 85 to 90 percent of occurrences, the laryngospasm subsides, allowing water to freely enter the respiratory tract (i.e., wet drowning). In 10 to 15 percent of occurrences, the laryngospasm is so severe that very little water is aspirated (i.e., dry drowning). Because there is no aspiration of material and resultant complications, dry drowning accounts for the majority of survivors of near drowning episodes.

Salt Water versus Fresh Water

Salt water is **hypertonic** (causes cells to shrink) in comparison to plasma. As salt water is inhaled, it osmotically pulls plasma and water into the alveoli in an attempt to equalize the salt concentration. This process results in pulmonary edema with **ventilation-perfusion mismatch** (inability to exchange gases) and subsequent severe hypoxia that leads to hypoxemia and acidosis.

Fresh water is **hypotonic** (causes cells to swell) in comparison to plasma. As fresh water is inhaled, it chemically alters the alveolar-capillary membranes and "washes out" **surfactant**. Surfactant is the protein in the lungs that reduces the surface tension of pulmonary fluids and allows the exchange of gases in the alveoli. It maintains alveolar stability. When alveolar stability is altered, **atelectasis** (alveolar collapse) and ability to exchange gases is diminished resulting in a ventilation-perfusion mismatch. These changes result in the same underlying problems as salt water aspiration: severe hypoxia, hypoxemia, and acidosis.

Fresh water is osmotically pulled into the blood. If enough fresh water is aspirated (approximately 20 cc/kg), the water dilutes the electrolytes to a dangerous level and diffuses into the red blood cells. The red blood cells then rupture and release potassium into the extracellular spaces resulting in **hyperkalemia** (elevated potassium) that may contribute to cardiac rhythm disturbances.

Both salt water and fresh water contain contaminants and particulate matter. These contaminants can obstruct the alveoli and alter chemical balances, leading to initial respiratory tract irritation and bronchoconstriction and later to pulmonary infection.

Management

The prehospital management of the child who has suffered a submersion episode is the same regardless of whether the submersion occurred in salt water or fresh water. Provider safety is the number one priority. Attempts by untrained and unprepared personnel to provide water rescue are dangerous and may well result in additional submersion victims. Because survivability following a submersion episode cannot always be correlated to the time of submersion, the prehospital provider should follow local protocol or seek advice from the local medical control physician as to when a "rescue operation" becomes a "recovery operation."

If it is necessary to wait for water rescue personnel, use the time to gather information from witnesses to assist in the rescue effort.

- **Who** is involved? Include information on the age and sex of the child. If possible, find out the type of clothing the victim was wearing.
- **What** happened? Were any other victims involved?
- **When** did the incident occur, and when was the child last seen?
- **Where** did the incident occur and where is the "last seen" point?
- **Why** did the incident occur? Did it involve a boating or water sport accident, alcohol, diving, etc.?

Water rescue personnel should initiate spinal precautions as soon as access to the child is gained. Full immobilization can actually begin in the water and be completed once the child is out of the water.

The child involved in a drowning may present from asymptomatic to complete respiratory and cardiac arrest. Prehospital management should focus on the initial assessment findings. If trauma is suspected, open the airway using the jaw-thrust method. Make sure suction is available since patients who drown are prone to vomiting swallowed water. Initiate cardiopulmonary resuscitation (CPR) if indicated. If necessary, intubate the child and hyperventilate with high-concentration oxygen to reduce acidosis. Reassess lung sounds frequently.

Use caution with fluid resuscitation. Since hypoxia, hypoxemia, and acidosis can cause severe cardiac ischemia, fluid overload may lead to cardiogenic shock. If the child's condition allows, check the blood glucose. Hypoglycemia is common following a drowning/drowning-related episode.

Hypothermia (body temperature below 95° F) is a major factor in cold water submersion episodes. It may also be a factor in warm water submersions due to evaporation following rescue. Remove wet clothing. Dry and warm the child with blankets as soon as possible. Handle the child gently. Rough handling or stimulation of the hypothermic patient may induce ventricular fibrillation. There is some disagreement over whether the hypothermic child with apnea should be intubated. The provider should follow the local system's protocols.

It is well established that drug therapy is ineffective with hypothermia and should be withheld until rewarming occurs. Since drug therapy is not indicated in this situation and stimulation may induce ventricular fibrillation, many prehospital system protocols also withhold initiation of intravenous access on the victims of cold water submersion who present in cardiac arrest. Again, follow local protocols.

Transport

Any child who meets any of the guidelines listed below should be transported to the hospital for examination:

- All cold water submersions, regardless of how the patient appears
- Submersion time of one minute or longer
- Any period of apnea
- Any history of cyanosis following submersion
- Any resuscitation required following submersion

Most children meeting any of the above criteria will be observed for complications in the Emergency Department.

 Exploring the Web

● What Web sites can you find related to drowning? Can you find information related to prehospital care? Are there any sites that provide help or chat rooms for families?

SUMMARY

Respiratory emergencies in children require early recognition of respiratory distress and rapid intervention with appropriate management to prevent respiratory failure. Because a child in respiratory distress may progress to failure quickly, constantly reassess the respiratory status for indications that would require more aggressive management. Be aware of potential secondary complications such as spinal injuries that may be present and require management.

Exploring the Web

● What professional journals cover topics that are discussed in this chapter?

Management of Case Scenario

Based on history and presentation, you should suspect a foreign body obstruction. After your "a foreign body obstruction" evaluation, you would approach the child slowly and speak calmly. Get down to the eye level of the child. Explain what you are going to do before you touch the child. You do not want to increase the child's anxiety and fear with any sudden or unexpected moves. Increasing anxiety in the child could lead to agitation and crying resulting in further obstruction. Keep the mother with you at all times to decrease the anxiety and fear of the child.

Allow the child to remain in the sitting position or another position of comfort to assist the respiratory effort. Do not attempt to look in the child's mouth. Having the child lie down or looking in the mouth could cause the foreign body to fall back and completely obstruct the airway.

Administer high-concentration oxygen by nonrebreather face mask. If the child does not want the mask on her face, administer it blow-by. Allowing the mother to hold the mask may go a long way in decreasing the child's fear and accomplishing oxygen administration that the child may not accept from you.

Transport the child immediately. Advanced providers should attempt no additional care beyond basic level. Do not attempt to insert an IV. This activity will simply increase the child's fear and agitation and serves no useful purpose in the prehospital environment. Be prepared to ventilate the child enroute if necessary.

▌ REVIEW QUESTIONS

1. List four signs of respiratory distress, describe how the signs present, and explain the significance of each.

2. Compare and contrast the upper airway problems of croup and epiglottitis in terms of:
   a. Age group
   b. Cause (viral/bacterial)
   c. Onset
   d. Precipitating events
   e. Signs/symptoms

3. Compare and contrast the lower airway problems of bronchiolitis and asthma/RAD in terms of:
   a. Age group
   b. Cause (viral/bacterial)
   c. Onset
   d. Precipitating events
   e. Signs/symptoms

4. Describe the prehospital management of epiglottitis and asthma/RAD and explain the rationale.

5. List four of the most common objects aspirated.

6. Explain the difference between drowning and drowning-related episodes.

7. List at least three factors that affect survivability from a submersion episode.

8. Compare and contrast the pathological differences between salt water and fresh water drowning.

9. Identify the transport criteria for submersion episodes.

▌ REFERENCES

Jackson, P., & Vessey, J. (1996). *Primary care of the child with a chronic condition*. St. Louis, MO: Mosby-Year Book.

National SAFEKIDS Campaign. (1998). Drowning fact sheet.

Schmidt, U., Fritz, K., Kasperczyk, W., & Tscherne, H. (1995). Successful resuscitation of a child with severe hypothermia after cardiac arrest of 88 minutes. *Prehospital and Disaster Medicine, 10(1),* 60–62.

Wertz, E. (1997). Infants and children. In N. McSwain, R. White, J. Patuaras, & W. Metcalf (Eds.), *The basic EMT—comprehensive prehospital patient care*. St. Louis, MO: Mosby-Year Book.

Wong. D. (1999) *Whaley & Wong's nursing care of infants and children* (6th ed.). St. Louis, MO: Mosby-Year Book.

▌ BIBLIOGRAPHY

American Heart Association (2000). Guidelines 2000 for cardiopulmonary resuscitation and emergency cardiovascular care. *Journal of the American Heart Association, 102(8).* I-307-19.

Emergency Nurses Association (1997). *Emergency nursing pediatric course.* Chicago, IL: Kay Graphics.

National Association of EMTs. (1998). *Prehospital trauma life support—basic and advanced* (4th ed.). St. Louis, MO: Mosby-Year Book.

Sanders, M. (2000). *Mosby's paramedic textbook* (2nd ed.). St. Louis, MO: Mosby-Year Book.

Wertz, E. (1993) Pediatric and infant intubation. *Emergency, 25(12),* 53–56.

Wertz, E. (1997b). Pediatric emergencies. In B. Shade, M. Rothenberg, E. Wertz, & S. Jones, (Eds.), *Mosby's EMT—intermediate textbook.* St. Louis, MO: Mosby-Year Book.

Chapter 5

Care and Resuscitation of the Neonate

OBJECTIVES

Upon completion of this chapter, the student should be able to:

- List and describe the major differences in fetal circulation and its effects.

- Discuss the assessment and routine care required for the neonate.

- Explain the sequence and rationale of resuscitative efforts for the depressed neonate.

- Describe the pathophysiology, signs/symptoms, and management of the neonate suffering from meconium staining/aspiration.

KEY TERMS

acrocyanosis
air leak syndrome
Apgar scoring
central cyanosis
conduction
convection
ductus arteriosus
evaporation

foramen ovale
intraosseous
meconium
persistent pulmonary hypertension
premature newborn
radiation
retrolental fibroplasia

Case Scenario

You are dispatched to a possible delivery in progress. On arrival you find a 27-year-old female, gravida 2, para 1, who is crowning. The patient tells you she is seven months pregnant. Following delivery, you note the newborn is pale with central cyanosis. Brachial pulse is 100. Respirations are irregular at a rate of 20. The newborn has little movement. The newborn appears to weigh approximately 5 pounds. How will you manage this newborn and why?

INTRODUCTION

Assisting in the delivery of a healthy newborn is an exciting and rewarding experience; however, when the newborn is distressed, it can become a stressful experience. Understanding the changes that occur in the newborn at the time of birth, learning the appropriate interventions, and practicing those interventions on a regular basis help prepare the prehospital provider to deal effectively with both healthy and distressed newborns.

FETAL CIRCULATION AND RESPIRATORY PHYSIOLOGY

Because the placenta supplies the fetus with oxygen during intrauterine life, the lungs serve no ventilatory purpose. Fetal lungs are filled with fluid, so blood passing through the lungs cannot pick up oxygen. Blood flow through the lungs while in the uterus is greatly decreased compared to the blood flow necessary after birth due to the partial closing of the arterioles in the lungs. This partial closing results in the majority of the blood being diverted away from the lungs through the **foramen ovale** (the opening in the septum between the right and left atria in the fetal heart) and **ductus arteriosus** (the vascular channel in the fetus that joins the pulmonary artery directly to the descending aorta) (Figure 5-1).

Several changes occur at birth that allow the lungs to take over supplying the body with oxygen. About one-third of the fetal lung fluid is removed through the newborn's nose and mouth when the chest is compressed while moving through the birth canal. As the newborn takes the first few breaths, several changes occur. The lungs expand with air. The arterioles in the lungs begin to open, and the blood previously shunted by the ductus

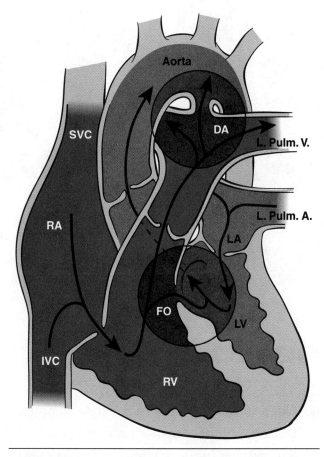

FIGURE 5-1 Blood is diverted away from the lungs through the foramen ovale and ductus arteriosus while the fetus is in the uterus.

arteriosus flows through the lungs to pick up oxygen. It takes a great deal of pressure to overcome the force of the fluid and open the alveoli for the first time. The first several breaths by the newborn may require two to three times the pressure of succeeding breaths. As pulmonary circulation is established, there is no need for the foramen ovale and ductus arteriosus and they eventually close.

There must be both air entering and adequate blood flow to the lungs for normal respirations to occur. If the newborn is suffering from asphyxia, hypoxemia, and accompanying acidosis, the pulmonary arterioles remain constricted and the ductus arteriosus remains open.

ROUTINE CARE

The majority of newborns require no resuscitation beyond maintenance of body temperature, suctioning, tactile stimulation, and proper positioning. This care is reflected in the inverted pyramid developed by the

Assess and Support: Temperature (warm and dry)
Airway (position and suction)
Breathing (stimulate to cry)
Circulation (heart rate and color)

Frequently Needed: Dry, Warm, Position, Suction, Stimulate

Oxygen

Establish Effective Ventilation
Bag-valve mask
Endotracheal intubation

Chest
Compressions

Infrequently Needed: Medications

FIGURE 5-2 Method of neonatal resuscitation per Pediatric Advanced Life Support (PALS). © Reproduced with permission Pediatric Advanced Life Support, 1997. Copyright American Heart Association

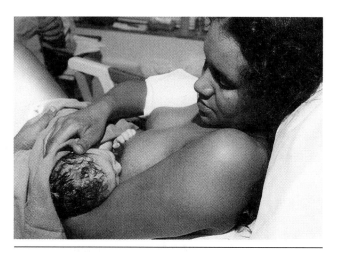

FIGURE 5-3 Place the stable newborn against the mother's bare skin and cover with blankets to decrease heat loss.

American Heart Association (Figure 5-2). It is important to remember that body substance isolation should be observed when handling the neonate. There is a high risk of exposure to blood and/or body fluids during delivery, and the infectious state of the patient is often unknown.

Maintenance of Body Temperature

A cold environment is difficult for all newborns to tolerate. Hypothermia is a special problem for newborns born in the prehospital environment. Loss of heat in newborns occurs from both external causes and the decreased ability to produce heat. Newborns have a proportionally larger body surface area compared to weight. The head accounts for a large part of the body surface area.

External heat loss can occur through a variety of mechanisms. **Convection** involves the transfer of heat away from the body by air movement; therefore, preventing drafts is important. **Radiation** involves electromagnetic waves. Warmer surfaces radiate heat to cooler areas with no physical contact occurring. The body can emit or absorb heat. **Evaporation** occurs as low humidity in the air converts water to vapor, thereby drawing heat from the core. Internal factors contributing to heat loss are the result of the newborn's minimal shivering response. Newborns produce heat primarily by increasing metabolic rate. This increased metabolic rate leads to increased oxygen demands and can worsen hypoxia,

acidosis, and hypoglycemia. **Conduction** is the transfer of heat from a warmer to cooler surface.

Heat loss can be controlled by rapidly and thoroughly drying off the amniotic fluid covering the newborn. Remove all wet towels used during the drying process, and wrap the newborn in warm blankets or towels. Cover the newborn's head since it is a major source of heat loss. The warm blankets may also be surrounded by plastic wrap or aluminum foil for additional heat retention. If stable, place the naked newborn against the mother, and cover both mother and child with blankets to prevent heat loss (Figure 5-3).

Since commercial warmers (Isolettes™) are usually not available in the prehospital setting, the provider must remember the potential heat loss from air conditioners used in the ambulance during the summer. These should be shut off for transport to the hospital. Depending on conditions, consider using the vehicle's heater.

 Tricks of the Trade

Turn off the air conditioner and consider using the heater in the ambulance when transporting a newborn to help maintain body heat.

Suctioning

As soon as the head is delivered, suction the mouth and then the nose. Although newborns are nose breathers, nasal suctioning may induce gasping or crying and lead to aspiration of secretions in the mouth. Suction the mouth and nose again following delivery.

Suctioning may be done using either a bulb syringe, suction catheter with a mucus trap, or mechanical suction using an 8 or 10 French suction catheter. Suction equipment available for neonatal resuscitation is shown in Figure 5-4. If using the bulb syringe, squeeze the bulb before inserting it into the mouth or nose. Suction catheters provide deeper suctioning of the oropharynx and may result in a vagal response leading to bradycardia and/or apnea. If mechanical suctioning is used, negative pressure should not exceed 100 mm Hg. Apply suction for no longer than three to five seconds per attempt, and monitor the newborn's heart rate. Allow time between suction attempts for the newborn to breathe spontaneously or for assisted ventilations if indicated.

Tactile Stimulation

Drying and suctioning are often enough to induce effective respirations. If these actions do not result in the newborn immediately beginning to breathe, there are two other safe and appropriate methods of providing

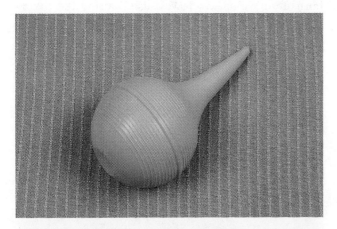
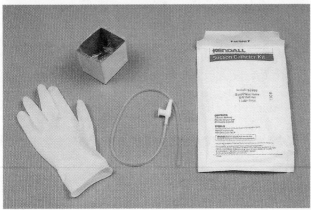

FIGURE 5-4 Equipment used for suctioning the infant.

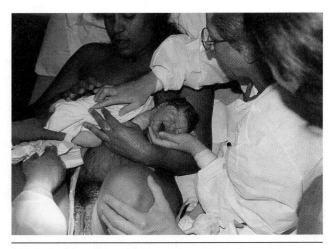

FIGURE 5-5 Firmly rubbing the newborn's back aids in lung expansion and initiation of spontaneous respirations.

tactile stimulation: (1) slapping the sole of the foot or flicking the heel or (2) firmly rubbing the newborn's back (Figure 5-5). One or two slaps on the sole or flicks of the heel OR rubbing the back once or twice will usually initiate spontaneous respirations. If spontaneous respirations do not occur, no further tactile stimulation should be done. Begin positive pressure ventilation immediately. Continued tactile stimulation after two attempts (5 to 10 seconds) may worsen the newborn's hypoxemia and will be a waste of precious time. The entire process of drying, warming, suctioning, and stimulation should take no more than 20 seconds.

Proper Positioning

In order to maintain a patent airway, position the newborn on the back or side with the neck in a neutral position. Due to the flexibility of the trachea, hyperextension or flexion of the neck may result in an airway obstruction. Elevate the body three-fourths to one inch by placing a rolled towel or blanket under the back and shoulders of the supine newborn. This action will help maintain the correct position. If there are a great deal of secretions, position the newborn on the side with the neck slightly extended to allow secretions to collect in the mouth instead of the back of the pharynx.

INITIAL ASSESSMENT

Initial assessment of the newborn should occur simultaneously with drying, warming, and suctioning. The initial assessment is based on three parameters: respiratory effort, heart rate, and color. The rate and depth of respirations should increase in the first few seconds after stimulation. The respiratory rate may be as high as 60 breaths per minute immediately following birth, then decrease to about 40 breaths per minute. If the newborn is apneic or has gasping respirations, begin positive pressure ventilation immediately.

Even though the newborn is breathing, do not assume that the heart rate is adequate. Normal heart rate for the newborn is 130 to 140 beats per minute, but may be as high as 150 to 180 beats per minute immediately following birth. Count the rate by feeling the brachial pulse or umbilical cord, or listening to the apical pulse (Figure 5-6). If the apical pulse is used, check for the presence of the brachial pulse to assure perfusion. If the heart rate is below 100 beats per minute, positive pressure ventilation should be initiated immediately. If the heart rate is above 100 beats per minute and respirations are spontaneous, assess color.

Two types of cyanosis may be present in the newborn. **Acrocyanosis** is a bluish discoloration of only the hands and feet. This peripheral cyanosis of the extremities is present in most newborns for the first few minutes following birth. It is caused by a combination of a cool delivery environment and initially decreased blood flow to the extremities. It is not due to a lack of oxygen and does not require treatment. **Central cyanosis** is cyanosis that involves the entire body, including the mucous membranes. It is due to a decreased level of oxygen in the blood. In some instances, it may be present even when respirations and heart rate are adequate. Central cyanosis occurs when there is adequate oxygen exchange to maintain the heart rate but not enough to fully oxygenate the newborn. In this situation administer free-flow or blow-by oxygen.

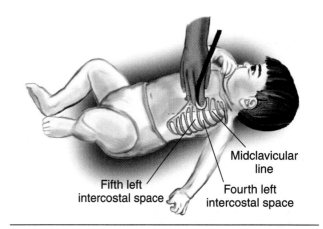

FIGURE 5-6 Apical pulse position for infant.

The **Apgar scoring** system is a standardized method for rating the condition of a newborn at one and five minutes following birth (Table 5-1). It involves five parameters:

- Appearance or skin color
- Pulse or heart rate
- Grimace or irritability
- Activity or muscle tone
- Respirations

The Apgar score is viewed only as an *indicator* for the need for resuscitation in the newborn. It should not be used to determine the *need* for resuscitation. ***Never withhold resuscitative measures in order to obtain the APGAR score.***

TABLE 5-1
Apgar Scoring

Heart Rate	Respiratory Rate	Tone	Reflex Irritability	Color
Absent = 0	Apnea = 0	Flaccid = 0	No response = 0	Cyanosis = 0
<100 = 1	Slow, irregular rate = 1	Some degree of flexion = 1	Grimace = 1	Body pink, extremities acrocyanotic = 1
>100 = 2	Crying vigorously = 2	Full flexion = 2	Crying = 2	Completely pink = 2

Exploring the Web

● What Web sites can you find related to medical care of the newborns? Are there any specific to prehospital care?

MANAGEMENT OF THE DISTRESSED NEONATE

Once the newborn has been delivered, it is critical to rapidly assess the baby and provide rapid intervention as necessary. The distressed neonate's outcome can be positively or negatively affected by actions taken or not taken immediately after birth.

Central Cyanosis with Respirations and Heart Rate above 100

The situation in which respirations provide enough oxygen to keep the heart rate up but do not fully oxygenate the newborn has been discussed. Congenital defects that interfere with pulmonary function or congenital heart disease may result in central cyanosis with respirations and a heart rate above 100 (see Chapter 7—Children with Special Health Care Needs). In this latter situation, administer blow-by or free-flow oxygen by blowing oxygen over the newborn's nose with either the oxygen tubing or oxygen mask. See Appendix C for a skills review.

Prehospital providers often express concerns about potential injury to a newborn from high concentrations of oxygen. Major complications of oxygen toxicity include **retrolental fibroplasia** (retinal detachment and blindness) and lung damage. It should be of some comfort to know that these complications occur as the result of high oxygen concentrations over a period of three to ten days. Therefore, *never withhold oxygen from a distressed newborn in the prehospital setting.*

Free-flow oxygen should be administered until the newborn's mucous membranes become pink. Once the mucous membranes are pink, gradually withdraw the oxygen by increasing the distance between the oxygen tubing and the nose until the newborn's color remains normal while breathing room air. If the newborn becomes cyanotic again as the oxygen is withdrawn, hold the tubing just close enough so the color remains normal.

Heart Rate below 100, Apnea, or Central Cyanosis Despite Maximal Oxygen

The most important intervention in resuscitating the depressed newborn is positive pressure ventilation. Positive pressure ventilation can be accomplished by using either a bag-valve mask (BVM) device or an endotracheal tube. For ventilation to be effective with the BVM, the newborn must be in the proper position, the appropriate size mask must be used, and a tight seal must be maintained (see Appendix C for a skills review).

If the newborn has not taken a breath since delivery, higher pressures will be required for the initial ventilation. These pressures range between 30 to 40 cm of water. Lower pressures (15 to 20 cm of water) are often adequate after the first breath, unless the newborn has an underlying pulmonary disease. Some bags may have pressure release (pop-off) valves which are set at 30 to 35 cm of water pressure. If the bag has a pop-off valve and the newborn requires higher pressures to ventilate, occlude the valve so pressure can carefully be increased.

The chest rise and fall should look like a shallow breath. If the chest is being expanded to its maximum diameter while bagging, the pressure is too high. Full expansion increases the risk for producing a pneumothorax. Do not mistake abdominal movement as an indication of effective ventilation. The abdomen may move as a result of air entering the stomach. It is also important to listen for air movement in the lungs. The newborn has little subcutaneous fat and structures to differentiate sound so breath sounds may echo from side to side.

The pulse rate should be reassessed after 15 to 30 seconds of ventilating. If the pulse rate is 100 beats per minute or greater, gradually discontinue ventilation. Gradual discontinuation of positive pressure ventilation increases the stimulation to resume spontaneous breathing. If spontaneous breathing is inadequate, continue positive pressure ventilation regardless of the heart rate.

If positive pressure ventilation with the BVM device is required for more than two minutes, gastric distention is likely to occur. Gastric distention may increase the pressure needed to adequately inflate the

Safety Tip

● When ventilating the newborn, increase tidal volume in small increments to help remove fluid from the lungs and prevent a pneumothorax.

chest. If it is within local system protocols, insert an oro-gastric tube.

Insertion of an endotracheal tube is indicated if unable to ventilate adequately with the BVM device or tracheal suctioning is required. Endotracheal intubation is also indicated when prolonged ventilation is required. This intervention prevents further gastric dissention and provides definitive control of the airway and ventilation. See Appendix C for a skills review of intubation.

Compressions

If the pulse rate is less than 60 beats per minute or 60 to 80 beats per minute and not rapidly increasing after 15 to 30 seconds of positive pressure ventilation, continue ventilations and begin chest compressions. Correct chest compressions apply pressure to the lower third of the sternum just below the nipple line. Compressions may be administered using either the thumb or the two-finger method.

Discontinue compressions when the heart rate reaches 80 beats per minute. Discontinue ventilations when the heart rate is above 100 beats per minute and spontaneous respirations resume. If the heart rate is below 80 beats per minute, continue compressions. If the newborn shows signs of improvement, check the heart rate frequently. These checks may be indicated as often as every 30 seconds. If the resuscitation is pro-longed, heart rate checks may be less frequent.

Venous Access

Venous access is desirable for medication and fluid administration. Although scalp veins can be used to do both, most prehospital providers are not trained in using this route and access to these veins is often difficult dur-ing resuscitation. Even the most familiar sites of extrem-ity veins may be difficult to access in a newborn. If a line cannot be established within 90 seconds or three attempts, the **intraosseous** (within the bone) route should be used. Even providers with minimal experi-ence can usually establish the intraosseous route in a brief period of time (30 to 60 seconds). See Appendix C for a skills review.

Medications

Medications may be administered to the distressed neonate depending on the condition at birth. Dosages must be properly calculated per the neonate's esti-mated weight.

Epinephrine

Epinephrine is a catecholamine with both alpha- and beta-adrenergic effects. These effects increase the rate and strength of myocardial contraction and cause vaso-constriction. Vasoconstriction results in an increase in coronary perfusion pressure and blood pressure. The rise in coronary perfusion pressure increases delivery of oxygen to the heart. Epinephrine is indicated in asystole and bradycardia (rate below 80 beats per minute) despite compressions and ventilation.

The dose of epinephrine for neonatal resuscita-tion is 0.01 to 0.03 mg/kg of a 1:10,000 solution. This dose can be repeated every three to five minutes. High-dose epinephrine may result in prolonged hypertension leading to intracranial bleeds in premature newborns. There is also inadequate data on the effects of high-dose epinephrine in neonates; therefore, the above dose should be used regardless of route of administration and for all subsequent doses.

Naloxone

Naloxone (Narcan®)is a narcotic antagonist that is indi-cated for the reversal of respiratory depression induced by narcotics. The dosage of naloxone is 0.1 mg/kg. It may be given intravenously, intraosseously, subcutaneously, intramuscularly, or via the endotracheal tube. The sub-cutaneous and intramuscular routes are not the pre-ferred methods of administration since the onset of action is much slower and there may be poor peripheral perfusion.

The administration of naloxone to a newborn born to an addicted mother may induce withdrawal and result in severe seizures. Consideration should be given to withholding naloxone and simply providing ventilatory support until the newborn can be assessed in the hospi-tal setting.

Other Medications

There is no evidence that atropine or sodium bicarbon-ate provide any beneficial effects during the initial stages of resuscitation of the newborn. Sodium bicarbonate is considered only when other therapies (e.g., ventilation, compressions, and epinephrine) are ineffective and the resuscitation period is prolonged.

 Exploring the Web

- Search the American Heart Association's Web site. What information is available related to resuscitation of the neonate? Create a flash card highlighting the proper protocols for resuscita-tion of the neonate.

MECONIUM STAINING/ ASPIRATION

Meconium is the newborn's first bowel movement. Normally, the first bowel movement does not occur until after birth. However, if the fetus suffers an asphyxial episode in utero, meconium may be expelled in the uterus prior to birth as a response to the distress. Asphyxial episodes may result from placental insufficiency or cord obstruction. Meconium is present in the amniotic fluid in approximately ten percent of all births. It may be present in the amniotic fluid in varying degrees causing the fluid to be thin and watery with a greenish color to thick with particulate matter, similar to the appearance of pea soup.

Etiology

The lung has the ability to move meconium to the periphery where it is reabsorbed; however, thick meconium can cause significant complications when aspirated. These complications include respiratory distress, aspiration pneumonia, air leak syndrome, and persistent pulmonary hypertension. Although meconium is considered sterile, it is a rich medium for the growth of bacteria which increases the risk of pneumonia.

As meconium is pulled into the lower airways, it may cause complete or partial obstruction of the bronchioles. If the obstruction is complete, the distal alveoli will collapse (i.e., atelectasis). If the obstruction is partial, a ball-valve effect occurs resulting in **air leak syndrome** from overinflation and rupture of alveoli (i.e., pneumothorax, pneumopericardium, or pneumomediastinum).

The underlying fetal hypoxic episode and the decreased ability to deliver oxygen to the alveoli cause pulmonary arterial vasoconstriction leading to **persistent pulmonary hypertension**. The hypertension causes blood to be shunted through the still open foramen ovale and ductus arteriosus resulting in severe hypoxemia.

Management

To prevent complications, it is critical to clear as much of the meconium as possible. Suction the mouth first, then the nose, with a bulb syringe as soon as the head delivers. Gasping, which results in aspiration, may occur due to stimulation of the nose with the bulb if the nose is suctioned first.

Following delivery, be prepared to provide tracheal suction to remove as much of the meconium as possible. If a newborn with thin meconium is active following oral and nasal suction, it is not necessary to intubate and suction. If the meconium is thick, use an

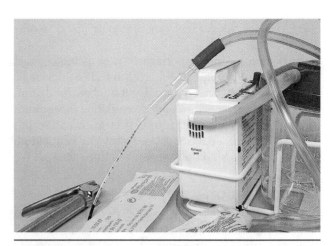

FIGURE 5-7 Meconium aspiration kit should contain a laryngoscope, blades, endotracheal tubes, and the meconium aspirator.

endotracheal tube with a meconium aspirator to suction (Figure 5-7). Attempting to use a suction catheter through the endotracheal tube is not effective. Meconium is too thick to be removed through the standard suction catheter.

Do NOT ventilate the newborn immediately. Ventilation will only force the meconium further into the lower airways, increasing the risk for the complications discussed above. Suctioning to remove the meconium MUST be done BEFORE the routine care of drying the newborn. Place a towel over the newborn to prevent heat loss, but do not waste time actively drying before dealing with the airway.

Suction the trachea using an endotracheal tube as the suction catheter. This procedure involves reintubating and suctioning with a new tube each time until clear. The newborn should then be re-intubated and ventilated with 100 percent oxygen. Complete this procedure even if the newborn has started to breathe. If the newborn is unstable or severely depressed, it may not be possible to clear all the meconium from the trachea. Do not withhold ventilation for a prolonged period to achieve complete clearing.

Prepare a kit containing all of the necessary equipment (e.g., pediatric laryngoscope, blades, six endotracheal tubes [two each of 2.5, 3.0, and 3.5], and the meconium aspirator) and keep it with the obstetric kit. When the procedure is required, there is not time to search through various kits to assemble the needed equipment.

If this procedure is not part of the local protocols, discuss its inclusion with the medical director. Proper airway management of the neonate with meconium staining can be a critical factor in the neonate's long-term morbidity and mortality.

Tricks of the Trade

Practice managing meconium aspiration as a team effort. One provider should intubate while the second provider attaches the meconium aspirator and suctions as the tube is removed. While suction is being applied, the first provider should prepare the next tube for immediate reintubation. Do not remove the laryngoscope between intubations.

Exploring the Web

● Search the Web using the key term *meconium aspiration*. What information is available? Is there any research on improving outcomes?

THE PREMATURE NEWBORN

The **premature newborn** is defined as one born before 37 weeks gestation and weighing 5.5 pounds or less. Premature newborns lose heat at a faster rate than full-term newborns under the same conditions. Be constantly aware of the need to provide and maintain a warm environment. Premature newborns are also at higher risk than are full-term newborns for developing respiratory problems. This risk increases significantly with younger gestational age. The more premature the newborn, the more likely the development of respiratory distress due to immature lung development and inadequate surfactant—the substance that regulates the amount of surface tension of the fluid lining the alveoli. Finally, the brain of the premature newborn is very vulnerable to

Exploring the Web

● Search for Web sites with information on premature infants. What information is available related to care in the prehospital setting? Is there any information available for the parents or families of premature infants?

bleeding when hypoxemia or rapid changes in blood pressure occur. Continually monitor the premature newborn for signs of respiratory distress and hypoxemia resulting in the need for immediate ventilation.

EMOTIONAL SUPPORT OF THE MOTHER

The challenge of a neonatal emergency causes the provider to focus on the newborn as the patient. Attention to the needs of the newborn is primary; however, the provider also has a responsibility to attend to the mother as well. She may be frightened, feel guilty, or be exhausted.

The unknown is frightening. Therefore, communication becomes a priority in dealing with the mother. Provide information, explanation, and instruction. Conversation with the mother should be conducted quietly, using clear diction and a slower pace of speaking. A calm, confident image, enhanced by a steady, relaxed tone of voice, will go a long way in providing comfort and conveying confidence in the ability to provide the best possible care to the newborn.

The anxieties of the unknown can overwhelm the mother's self control and lead to tears and sobbing. Support the mother and help her re-establish control by providing a gentle touch to her shoulder or arm. The parental instinct is one of the most powerful emotional reactions in the human being. Experiencing the thoughts or feelings of another is defined as empathy. Empathy is a worthy emotion. "Seeing" from the mother's perspective can help care for her emotional needs.

Exploring the Web

● Search the Web for professional journals that provide more information on the topics discussed in this chapter.

SUMMARY

Most neonates require only the routine care of suctioning, drying, warming, stimulation, and proper positioning for resuscitation. If assessment findings indicate a distressed newborn, the prehospital provider must be ready and capable of delivering immediate, appropriate intervention. Be familiar and comfortable with needed procedures and drug dosages required for additional interventions. Commercial charts can be purchased for reference.

Exposures to problems such as meconium aspiration are limited in the field setting. Practice the procedures required to deal effectively with these problems on a regular basis. Severe complications can be avoided if the prehospital provider is adept at procedures when they are required. In addition, work with the medical director to ensure that proper equipment, training, and protocols are in place before a potential neonatal resuscitation is encountered.

Management of Case Scenario

The initial immediate management of this newborn would include suctioning for secretions, position to allow for drainage of secretions, and drying and warming to decrease the risk of hypothermia. Based on the assessment findings, management would follow the interventions for central cyanosis with respirations and heart rate above 100.

This newborn's respiratory effort is enough to provide adequate oxygen to keep the heart rate up, but not fully oxygenate. You would administer blow-by oxygen over the newborn's nose with either the oxygen tubing or oxygen mask. In order to deliver approximately 80 percent oxygen, position the tubing 0.5 inch from the nose. You would hold the tubing steady to prevent decreasing the oxygen concentration delivered. If you use a mask, you would hold it firmly against the newborn's face using a minimum flow of five liters per minute. Keep the newborn wrapped (especially the head) and warm to prevent heat loss while administering oxygen and reassessing. Rapidly transport to the closest hospital.

REVIEW QUESTIONS

1. Compare and contrast acrocyanosis and central cyanosis.

2. Explain the function of the ductus arteriosus and foramen ovale.

3. List the four procedures involved in the routine care of a newborn.

4. List the parameters of the Apgar score.

5. The following actions should be performed for the depressed newborn.

   a. Immediately intubate the infant.

   b. Apply electrodes to monitor the infant's cardiac status.

   c. Begin compressions if the pulse is < 60 beats per minute.

   d. Suction the airway before ventilation.

6. List three complications of meconium aspiration.

7. Describe the pathophysiology of air leak syndrome as it relates to meconium aspiration.

8. You have just delivered a baby to a mother who admits she is a heroine addict. The newborn exhibits severe respiratory depression. How would you manage this newborn? Include your rationale.

REFERENCES

American Heart Association Guidelines 2000 for cardiopulmonary resuscitation and emerging cardiovascular care. *Journal of the American Heart Association, 102(8).* I-307-19.

BIBLIOGRAPHY

Emergency Nurses Association. (1997). *Emergency nursing pediatric course.* Chicago, IL: Kay Graphics.

Janing, J. (1993). Meconium staining and aspiration in the newborn. *Emergency Medical Services, 22(4),* 44–48.

Wertz, E. (1997a). Infants and children. In N. McSwain, R. White, J. Paturas, W. Metcalf, (Eds.), *The basic EMT—comprehensive prehospital patient care.* St. Louis, MO: Mosby-Year Book.

Wertz, E. (1993). Pediatric and newborn intubation. *Emergency, 25(12),* 53–56.

Wong, D. (1999). *Whaley & Wong's nursing care of infants and children* (6th ed.). St. Louis, MO: Mosby-Year Book.

Chapter 6

Medical Emergencies

OBJECTIVES

Upon completion of this chapter, the student should be able to:

- Identify causes, signs/symptoms, and initial field management of mild, moderate, and extreme dehydration in the pediatric patient.
- Identify causes of seizures in the pediatric patient.
- Identify the most common cause and field management of febrile seizures in the pediatric patient.
- Describe the management of status epilepticus.
- Compare and contrast the pathophysiology, signs/symptoms, and potential complications of viral and bacterial meningitis.
- Define and describe the assessment and field management of suspected sudden infant death syndrome (SIDS).
- Describe the pathophysiology, signs/symptoms, and field management of diabetic ketoacidosis (DKA) and hypoglycemia in the pediatric patient.
- Define and describe the signs/symptoms and field management of a child having a sickle cell crisis.
- Explain the assessment, possible complications, signs/symptoms, and management of childhood ingestions or poisonings.

KEY TERMS

absence seizure	dehydration	febrile seizure	Kussmaul respirations
activated charcoal	diabetes mellitus (DM)	generalized seizure	meningitis
antidote	diabetic ketoacidosis (DKA)	hypoglycemia	meningococcemia
aura	epilepsy	idiopathic	orthostatic hypotension
convulsive seizure	exudate	ketones	otitis media

partial seizure

petechiae

photophobia

polydipsia

polyphagia

polyuria

postictal

seizure

sickle cell anemia

sickle cell crisis

sickle cell disease

status epilepticus

sudden infant death

      syndrome (SIDS)

syrup of ipecac

Case Study

You are called to the home for an eight-year-old boy in pain. When you arrive at the house, the boy is lying on the couch writhing in pain and crying. His mother tells you, "We just moved into the neighborhood, and we don't have a doctor yet. He hasn't been this bad in a long time." You ask the child where he hurts, and he says "Everywhere!" What would you do?

INTRODUCTION

Many prehospital providers have little opportunity to gain experience treating the pediatric patient. Children under the age of 18 account for approximately ten percent of patients transported by ambulance. Although trauma represents approximately 60 percent of these transports, prehospital providers are still confronted with a wide range of pediatric medical problems.

DEHYDRATION

Dehydration is an acute loss of body fluids resulting from either increased fluid loss or decreased fluid intake. It occurs when the total output of fluids exceeds the total intake of fluids, regardless of the cause.

Incidence

Diarrhea is the leading cause of dehydration in children. Across the world, approximately 500 million children have diarrhea each year (Wong, 1999). Dehydration from acute diarrhea kills approximately 300 children per year in the United States (Wong, 1999). In addition, approximately 9.5 percent of all hospitalizations for children less than five years of age is due to diarrhea.

Etiology

Children are particularly susceptible to dehydration because a greater proportion of their body is water, and fluid maintenance requirements are much higher. Increased fluid loss can occur as a result of gastroenteritis, fever, diabetic ketoacidosis (DKA), or extensive burns. Reduced fluid intake can range from an error in formula preparation to the child being unable to eat or drink due to illness (American Heart Association, 1997).

Signs and Symptoms

The severity of dehydration is divided into mild (up to 5 percent loss of body weight), moderate (between 5 and 10 percent loss of body weight) and extreme (greater than 10 percent loss of body weight). Mild dehydration is characterized by pale skin due to vasoconstriction, pink lips due to hemoconcentration, normal to slightly decreased skin turgor, and a flat fontanelle in infants. Moderate dehydration is characterized by pallor, tachycardia, tachypnea, irritability, darkened or sunken eyes, decreased skin turgor and elasticity, a depressed fontanelle in infants, and decreased urine output. Extreme dehydration is characterized by cold extremities, absent peripheral pulses, tachycardia greater than 130 beats per minute, limpness and apathy, drowsiness to comatose, decreased urine output, and acidosis (Table 6-1).

Assessment

The history should focus on all intake and output. The amount, type, and content of intake should be ascertained as well as the child's ability to retain the ingested fluids. The amount, duration, and site of loss should also be documented. More specifically, ask about the number of wet diapers (in infants and toddlers) within a 24-hour period. Is the number less than usual for the child? Ask about the color and smell of the urine. Is it very dark and concentrated? Is there a foul smell to the urine? Questions regarding compounding factors such as vomiting, diarrhea, and fever should also be asked.

Management

Management of mild dehydration is aimed at providing supportive care. Most often, mild dehydration can be managed with oral fluids. The management of moderate and extreme dehydration in the prehospital setting is aimed at restoring tissue perfusion and increasing intravascular volume with an isotonic fluid bolus of either normal saline or Ringer's lactate. A 20 cc/kg fluid bolus is initially administered through intravenous access. If clinical reassessment shows no improvement

TABLE 6-1
Levels of Dehydration

Level	Signs and Symptoms	Management
Mild (5% loss of body weight)	• Normal vital signs • Alert • Flat fontanelles • Normal to slightly ↓ skin turgor • Mucous membranes dry • Warm and pale skin • Normal tears when crying • Increased thirst • Normal urine output	• Supportive • Child can usually take oral fluids • EMS not usually requested
Moderate (5–10% loss of body weight)	• ↑ HR and RR • Normal BP • ↓ peripheral pulses • Capillary refill of 2–3 seconds • Irritable • Depressed fontanelles • Decreased skin turgor • Mucous membranes very dry • Cool and pale skin • Some tears when crying • Sunken and darkened eyes • Intense thirst • Decreased urine output	• Restore tissue perfusion and ↑ intravascular volume • High-concentration O_2 • IV of NSS or LR • Bolus of fluid at 20 cc/kg • Transport • Repeat bolus if no improvement
Extreme (>10% loss of body weight)	• HR > 130 bpm • ↑ RR • Systolic BP < 80 • No peripheral pulses • Capillary refill > 3 seconds • Drowsy to comatose • Sunken fontanelles • Markedly ↓ skin turgor • Parched mucous membranes; no tears • Cold, clammy, and cyanotic skin • Sunken and soft eyes • Intense thirst (if responsive) • Decreased urine output	• True emergency requiring rapid transport • High-concentration O_2 • IV of NSS or LR en route ONLY • Bolus of fluid at 20 cc/kg • Repeat bolus if no improvement • Consider intraosseous route for fluid resuscitation

Abbreviations: BP, blood pressure; EMS, emergency medical services; HR, heart rate; LR, lactated Ringer's; NSS, normal saline solution; RR, respiratory rate; IV, intravenous; O_2, oxygen.

in pulse, skin color, capillary refill time, or mental status, the bolus should be repeated. Also, prehospital personnel should check a glucose level.

Transport

Extreme dehydration carries a significantly high mortality rate and is a true emergency. Time should not be wasted in the field in an attempt to establish intravenous (IV) or intraosseous (IO) access. The child should be transported immediately with an attempt at IV or IO access done en route.

Exploring the Web

- Search for information on dehydration in children. Can you find specific information related to care of the child with dehydration in the prehospital setting? Create flash cards on the care and management of dehydration based on the information you find.

SEIZURES

A **seizure** is a disturbance in the electrical activity of the brain (Epilepsy Foundation of America [EFA], 1999). Seizures are the result of an abnormal electrical discharge within the brain and are the most commonly observed neurological dysfunction in children (Wong, 1999). These discharges occur in various locations within the brain and spread in different directions and at different speeds. Seizures are not generally life threatening unless seizure activity is characterized as **status epilepticus**, which is a continuous seizure lasting for more than 30 minutes or a series of seizures from which the child does not regain consciousness (Wong, 1999). This condition is discussed later in this section.

Febrile Seizures

Febrile seizures (seizure resulting from a high fever) occur in approximately 3 to 4 percent of all children, and most children are between the ages of three months and five years when they occur (Wong, 1999). Boys are affected almost twice as much as girls. The cause of febrile seizures is not certain but it is believed that the height of the temperature elevation may be a factor. The seizure

actually occurs *during* the rise in temperature. The child's temperature is usually above 38.8° C (101.8° F).

Fever is the most common cause of seizures in children between six months and five years of age. The most common underlying cause is **otitis media** (inner ear infection). The most dangerous cause of a febrile seizure is meningitis.

Parents or caregivers are often upset by this event and may express serious concern about reoccurrence and long-term side effects. In approximately 95 to 98 percent of all children with a febrile seizure, epilepsy does not develop nor is there any neurologic damage (Wong, 1999).

Epilepsy

Epilepsy is a chronic seizure disorder and is usually defined as two or more seizures that are not provoked by any obvious cause (Epilepsy Foundation of America, 1999). Some children have uncontrolled epilepsy in that they continue to have frequent seizures despite aggressive medical, surgical, or diet therapy (see Chapter 7—Children with Special Health Care Needs). The child's ongoing growth and development may be affected by the seizures as well as the medications used in an attempt to control them. Prehospital providers may care for these children when injuries occur during the seizure activity (Figure 6-1).

Aura is the period of time right before the seizure begins. The length of time is different in each individual. The child may describe a certain sensation or feeling that serves as a warning that a seizure will occur. Children who have these warnings will actually have a short window of time to get to a safe position (e.g., get

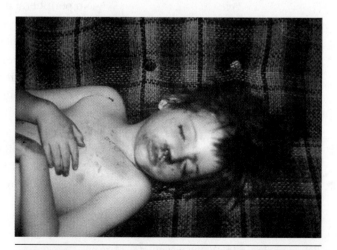

FIGURE 6-1   This child hit her face during the seizure activity resulting in a laceration and a bloody nose.

out of the swimming pool, sit down on the floor, or get off of a bike).

The **postictal** period is the time right after the seizure is over. The child may appear mildly confused to very tired and may actually sleep for some time. There may even be some short-term paralysis depending on the nature of the child's seizure disorder.

Seizures may be defined as either **partial** or **generalized** (Figure 6-2). With partial seizures, one particular area of the brain is affected, which usually causes specific symptoms. In generalized seizures, the electrical activity spreads throughout the entire brain resulting in various symptoms—those that involve some motor activity (known as **convulsive**) or those that involve some change in the child's level of consciousness (**absence** → pronounced "ab-saunce").

Incidence

More than two million people in the United States have some form of epilepsy (Epilepsy Foundation of America, 1999). Of that number, 30 percent are children under 18 years of age (EFA, 1999). About 180,000 new cases are diagnosed every year; and it is estimated that 1 in every 10 Americans, or 25 million people, have had, or will have, a seizure at some point in their lives (EFA, 1999).

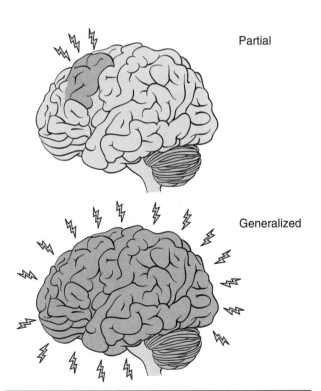

Partial

Generalized

FIGURE 6-2 Partial seizures only affect one area of the brain whereas generalized seizures result from electrical activity distributed throughout the brain.

Primarily, epilepsy affects children and young adults. However, any person can get epilepsy at any time. Approximately 20 percent of all cases develop in children under five years of age. Fifty percent of cases develop before 25 years of age (EFA, 1999).

Etiology

Seizures in children are either **idiopathic** or acquired. Idiopathic means that the cause of the seizures is unknown. Acquired seizures are the result of a brain injury during the prenatal, perinatal, or postnatal periods.

Pediatric seizures may result from head trauma, hypoxia, hypoglycemia, infections such as meningitis, toxic ingestions, tumors, drug overdoses, and electrolyte imbalances. Generally, anything that alters the brain's chemical and metabolic balance or somehow affects the structure of brain cells can cause a seizure.

Signs and Symptoms

Signs and symptoms will present depending on the location and spreading of the electrical storms in the brain (Table 6-2). Some examples include:

- Change in sensation (e.g., the child describes a particular smell or taste or has the feeling of "pins and needles" in an extremity)
- Change in the child's behavior (e.g., the child becomes very angry and begins to yell at a classmate for no apparent reason; the child begins repetitively smacking her lips or blinking her eyes)
- Muscle activity (e.g., shaking and stiffening of the arms, legs, or body as seen in a tonic-clonic or grand mal seizure)
- Change in the child's level of consciousness (e.g., the child seems to be "daydreaming" or collapses onto the floor)

Assessment

While obtaining the history, information related to the seizure should be gathered. Ask pertinent questions of anyone who was with the child or who witnessed the seizure activity.

- How long did the seizure last? (Remember, to a parent the time frame may seem like *forever*. Do not be insulted if the parents ask why it took so long to get to their house.)
- What part of the body was involved first? Did this activity stay the same, or were other body parts also involved? Was there any eye deviation?
- What was the child's level of consciousness during the seizure?

TABLE 6-2
Review of Seizure Types

Type	Presenting Signs and Symptoms	Treatment
Generalized tonic-clonic (used to be called grand mal)	• Change in level of consciousness • Sudden cry, fall, and rigidity followed by muscle jerks • Shallow breathing; lips or skin may be cyanotic • Possible loss of bowel and/or bladder control • Usually lasts 1–3 minutes • Confusion and/or fatigue usually occur after seizure finished	• DO NOT PUT ANYTHING IN THE MOUTH DURING THE SEIZURE ACTIVITY • Roll child to side to let saliva drain from mouth (unless trauma present). • Protect head and body from injury. • Time the seizure activity and document types and areas of movement. • Reassure child as consciousness returns. • Ventilate only if respirations absent after muscle jerks subside. • If first seizure, transport to hospital. • If ongoing seizure disorder, check with parent or caregiver regarding transport.
Absence (used to be called petit mal)	• Change in level of consciousness • Blank stare which begins and ends abruptly • Usually lasts only a few seconds • May see chewing movements of mouth or rapid eye blinking • Child is unaware of surroundings during seizure activity • Child quickly returns to full awareness once seizure is over	• Document level of consciousness during seizure activity. • Provide reassurance as child regains consciousness. • If first seizure, transport to hospital. • If ongoing seizure disorder, transport is usually not necessary. Check with parent or caregiver for instruction.
Simple-*partial*	• No change in level of consciousness • Limited to particular area of brain • Jerking may begin in one area of body, arm, leg, or face → child remains awake but cannot stop jerking • Jerking may spread to other body parts or may progress to tonic-clonic seizure • Other presentations may include nausea, sudden change in emotion, "funny" taste in mouth or feeling in stomach, or odd smell.	• None necessary unless seizure progresses to tonic-clonic seizure. • If first seizure, transport to hospital. Check with parent or caregiver for instruction. • If ongoing seizure disorder, transport is usually not necessary.
Complex-*partial*	• Change in level of consciousness • Usually starts with blank stare • Chewing and then random activity follow stare • Child may seem dazed or unaware of surroundings	• Protect child from injury or further injury. • Treat any injuries (i.e., laceration, head injury, etc.). • Time the seizure activity and document types of behavior.

(continues)

TABLE 6-2
(Continued)

Type	Presenting Signs and Symptoms	Treatment
Complex-*partial* (*cont.*)	• Child may appear afraid, try to run away, pick at clothes, or try to take clothes off • Confusion usually follows seizure • No memory of seizure	• Provide reassurance as child regains consciousness. • If first seizure, transport to hospital. • If ongoing seizure disorder, transport is usually not necessary. Check with parent or caregiver for instruction.
Atonic	• Change in level of consciousness • Child suddenly collapses and falls • After 10–60 seconds, child resumes previous activity (if not injured by fall).	• Protect child from injury or further injury. • Treat any injuries (i.e., laceration, head injury, etc.). • Time the seizure activity and document types and areas of movement. • Provide reassurance as child regains consciousness. • If first seizure, transport to hospital. • If ongoing seizure disorder, transport is usually not necessary. Check with parent or caregiver for instruction.
Myoclonic	• Change in level of consciousness • Sudden, brief, massive muscle jerks that involve one part of the body or whole body • Commonly occur as child is waking from sleep/nap or going to sleep • Usually occur in clusters (i.e., seizure activity occurs over and over with brief pause in between) • Movement may progress in strength as cluster of seizures continues; will decrease in strength as seizures end	• Protect child from further injury. • Treat any injuries (i.e., laceration, head injury, etc.). • Time the seizure activity and document types and areas of movement. • Provide reassurance as child regains consciousness. • If first seizure, transport to hospital. • If ongoing seizure disorder, transport is usually not necessary. Check with parent or caregiver for instruction.
Infantile spasms	• Change in level of consciousness • Clusters of quick, sudden movements • Usually start between three months and two years • If child is sitting, head will fall forward and arms will flex forward • If lying down, knees will draw inward toward body; arms and head will flex forward like baby or child is reaching for something • May resemble startle reflex in infants • Infant or child may be sleepy or confused once cluster of seizures is finished	• Protect child from injury. • Treat any injuries (i.e., laceration, head injury, etc.). • Provide reassurance as child regains consciousness. • If first seizure, transport to hospital. • If ongoing seizure disorder, transport may not be necessary. Check with parent or caregiver for instruction.

Epilepsy Foundation of America, 1999. *Epilepsy facts and figures [on-line]*. Available: http://www.efa.org/education/facts.html.

- Was there any urinary or fecal incontinence? If so, remember that the child may be embarrassed if he or she is already toilet trained.

- Was there any warning or aura before the seizure activity?

- Does the child remember the event?

- Is or was the child postictal?

- Does the child have an ongoing seizure disorder? If so, what medications are usually taken? When was the last dose taken? Was the dosage recently changed?

- Has the child used any drugs or substances that may have caused the seizure? This question should be asked when the child is of an older school age or an adolescent.

It is important to also gather information on events leading up to the seizure. Specific questions regarding the history of epilepsy, fever, head trauma, diabetes, recent headache or neck stiffness, irritability or lethargy, or infection should be asked. An infant's fontanelle should be checked for bulging, and any petechial or peripheral rashes should be noted.

Management

In general, prehospital management of pediatric seizures is aimed at preventing further injury and protecting the airway. DO NOT insert anything into the mouth, especially if the child is actively seizing. The child WILL NOT swallow his or her tongue.

- If the child is seizing, turn him or her onto the side as long as no spinal injury is suspected. Allow any saliva to drain out of the mouth. Suction is not necessary while the child is actively seizing. Support the head so that it is not injured during the seizure activity.

- Clear the area of hazardous objects such as desks if the child is in school. Move the child onto a soft surface if possible (and have ruled out the need for spinal immobilization) such as a carpeted floor instead of a cement or tile floor.

- A simple head tilt (as long as any cervical trauma has been ruled out) or nasal airway may be used if snoring respirations are heard.

- The child may be apneic for a brief period of time during a tonic-clonic seizure. Ventilations should only be assisted if the apnea lasts for more than two minutes.

- If the seizure is the result of a fever, remove the child's clothing. Check with medical control to see if sponging should be done in an effort to reduce the child's body temperature. This procedure is controversial in the prehospital setting as it usually works better AFTER a fever-reducing medication has been given. Without that medication, the child may begin to shiver, which will increase the metabolic rate and ultimately the fever.

- Management of febrile seizures is primarily supportive. The benign nature of these seizures and the low risk of recurrence outweigh the benefits of administering medications with their associated side effects. Remember to offer support to the parents or caregivers as they may be quite upset.

Status Epilepticus

Status epilepticus occurs when the seizure activity is continuous and lasts more than 30 minutes. Status epilepticus is also possible if the child has a series of seizures without regaining consciousness in between each seizure. Immediate intervention should consist of airway and breathing control. Monitor the child's cardiovascular status as well.

Consider nasal endotracheal intubation for definitive airway control especially if the child is vomiting. Assess a blood glucose level and consider the administration of diazepam (Valium®) for ongoing seizure activity. Diazepam can be administered intravenously or rectally. Intravenously, it is given in doses of 0.1 to 0.3 mg/kg every two to five minutes at a rate no greater than 1 mg/min. Rectally, diazepam (Diastat®) is given in doses of 0.5 mg/kg for children ages two to five, 0.3 mg/kg for children ages 6 to 11, and 0.2 mg/kg for children 12 and older. See Appendix D for a review of rectal administration. Consult your local protocols as well as medical control for specific administration guidelines.

Other drugs are being used to combat seizure activity. Lorazepam (Ativan®) is being used more often as the intravenous drug of choice. It causes less respiratory distress in children greater than two years of age and has a longer duration. In some cases, midazolam (Versed®) is given intranasally to treat acute seizures (Wong, 1999).

Transport

Any child with a first seizure should be transported to the hospital for further evaluation. If the child is stable, transport does not need to be urgent. If the child is postictal when transport begins, take time to orient her as she begins to wake up in the back of the ambulance. Reassess the child, and document her return to consciousness or any further seizure activity.

If the child is in status epilepticus, transport rapidly to the closest hospital. Monitor the respiratory status especially if any drugs have been given that may decrease respirations. Document all seizure activity.

Exploring the Web

● Search for information on febrile seizures, epilepsy, and status epilepticus. Can you find specific information related to care of the child having a seizure in the prehospital setting? Create flash cards on the care and management of each based on the information you find.

MENINGITIS

Meningitis is an infection of the central nervous system that affects the thin layers (meninges) surrounding the brain and spinal cord. Cerebrospinal fluid (CSF) lacks intrinsic immunity and, therefore, is particularly vulnerable to infection.

Incidence

The pediatric population between the ages of one month and five years account for approximately 90 percent of the cases of meningitis reported each year in the United States (Wong, 1999). The incidence of bacterial versus viral meningitis is discussed in detail later in this section.

Etiology

The causative organism of meningitis may be either bacterial or viral. Over 80 percent of the cases of viral meningitis result from seasonal enteroviruses (Wong, 1999). Mumps, herpes, and measles are some of the well-documented viral central nervous system organisms. Bacterial meningitis is caused primarily by three organisms and is discussed at length later in this section.

Signs and Symptoms

The definitive diagnosis of meningitis including the specific type can only be made by a lumbar puncture. Since that diagnostic procedure is not available in the prehospital setting, the child presenting with signs and symptoms of meningitis should be suspected to have the disease until proven otherwise.

The younger the child, the less obvious the signs and symptoms will be until late in the course of the disease. Neck stiffness is one of the most specific signs of meningitis. However, it is seen in less than 15 percent of children under 18 months of age. Specific signs and symptoms are discussed under each type.

Bacterial Meningitis

Bacterial meningitis is life threatening without antibiotic treatment. It carries a 5 to 10 percent mortality rate (Wong, 1999). The bacterial organisms causing meningitis are most commonly *Haemophilus influenzae* (type B), *Streptococcus pneumoniae*, and *Neisseria meningitidis* (meningococcus). These bacteria account for 95 percent of the bacterial meningitis seen in children older than two months (Wong, 1999). Most children now routinely receive the *H. influenzae* type B vaccine so that this type of meningitis is much less common. The most common bacterial meningitis in school-aged children and adolescents is meningococcal meningitis (caused by *Neisseria meningitidis*).

A thick **exudate** (pus or serum) forms and obstructs normal flow of cerebrospinal fluid (CSF) through the subarachnoid space. This exudate causes an inflammation and edema of the underlying brain tissue that may result in seizures, nerve palsies, coma, and/or death.

Signs and Symptoms

The onset of signs and symptoms of bacterial meningitis is usually rapid and can occur in as short as two hours. They may include:

- Upper respiratory infection (URI) symptoms
- Headaches
- Neck rigidity (may occur late with infant)
- Fever
- Seizures
- Nausea and vomiting
- Poor feeding in young infants
- **Photophobia** (abnormal sensitivity to light → especially in the eyes)
- An altered level of consciousness (may present as irritability with the infant or younger child not wanting to be held or comforted)
- Petechiae or dark blotching of the skin

The child may develop **meningococcemia**, which is a disease that occurs when the *N. meningitidis* bacteria spreads to the bloodstream. **Petechiae** (round, purple spots due to intradermal or submucosal hemorrhage) may appear on the child's extremities. The peripheral circulation eventually collapses, and shock occurs.

Assessment

In newborns and neonates, meningitis is extremely difficult to recognize. Symptoms may be vague and nonspecific such as poor feeding, poor sucking, vomiting, and diarrhea. Decreased muscle tone, lack of movement, and a poor cry may also be present. The fontanelle does not usually bulge until the later stages of the illness, and neck stiffness does not generally occur.

In infants and young children between three months and two years, the classic signs of meningitis may not always be present (Wong, 1999). Instead, the child may be extremely irritable with a fever, poor feeding, vomiting, and possible seizures. Some may have a high-pitched cry, and the most significant finding may be a bulging fontanelle. Stiffness of the neck usually occurs late in these age groups.

Management

If meningococcemia is present, treat for septic shock; and use body substance isolation including gloves, a gown, and a mask. Infants and children who survive this complication may become permanently disfigured when they lose skin and parts of their limbs that were damaged by the bacteria.

Transport

Rapidly transport the child to the hospital. Upon delivery of the patient, disinfect the ambulance before placing it back in service. Ask the emergency department staff to contact your service if the diagnosis of bacterial meningitis is confirmed. Prophylactic antibiotics may be necessary for all providers who were in contact with the child so that they do not get the disease.

The long-term outcome is dependent on age, causative organism, and rapidity of antibiotic therapy. Children with bacterial meningitis may have permanent complications including hearing loss (most common), motor impairment, seizure disorders, developmental and cognitive delays (mental retardation), hydrocephalus, or paralysis.

Viral Meningitis

Children with viral meningitis typically have a self-limiting illness without subsequent problems. Viral meningitis tends to run its course over several days with recovery in one week.

Signs and Symptoms

The signs and symptoms include headache, neck rigidity, fever, nausea and vomiting, and photophobia. Seizures are less common in children with viral meningitis. The level of consciousness is usually normal. For infants and toddlers, the onset is slower to develop.

Assessment

Again, the infant or younger child may have vague and nonspecific symptoms. In fact, the parents or caregivers may mention a change in their child's usual behavior that

was attributed to a minor illness. Once any meningeal signs appear, meningitis may be suspected.

Management and Transport

Prehospital management is primarily supportive. Since viral meningitis is not usually life threatening, transport does not need to be rapid.

Exploring the Web

● Search for information on bacterial and viral meningitis. Can you find specific information related to care of the child with meningitis in the prehospital setting? Create a flash card on the care and management of each based on the information you find.

SUDDEN INFANT DEATH SYNDROME (SIDS)

Sudden infant death syndrome (SIDS) or "crib death" is defined as the sudden death of an infant or young child that is unexpected by history and in which an autopsy fails to reveal an adequate cause of death. Ninety-five percent of SIDS cases occur in children before six months of age (Wong, 1999).

Incidence

SIDS is the third leading cause of death for all infants between 1 and 12 months of age (Anderson, Kochanek, & Murphy, 1997). The peak incidence is two to four months. Deaths from SIDS generally occur while the child is sleeping and mainly affect males.

In the United States the mortality from SIDS has decreased since 1988. From 1995 to 1996 alone, the incidence decreased 13 percent (Ventura, 1997). It was in 1996 that the American Academy of Pediatrics instituted the "Back to Sleep" campaign and began recommending that infants be placed on their backs instead of their sides or stomachs when sleeping. Evidence from England and New Zealand supported the increased risk of SIDS when infants were placed in the side-lying position because they could get to the prone position (Gershan & Moon, 1997).

The occurrence of SIDS is greatest in winter months and peaks in January (Wong, 1999). SIDS is not external suffocation, is not the result of aspiration, and is not child abuse. Table 6-3 outlines those infants at higher risk for developing SIDS.

Etiology

SIDS is not caused by sleep apnea (Wong, 1999). The exact cause of SIDS is not known, yet several theories exist. One theory is that there is an abnormality in the brainstem that regulates respiratory and cardiac control. Others theories include incidence of maternal smoking, young maternal age, poor prenatal care, suffocation from soft bedding, and co-sleeping or bed-sharing.

One other theory relates to the accumulation of carbon dioxide. When babies sleep on their stomachs or

TABLE 6-3
Infants at Higher Risk for SIDS

Males

Infants sleeping on stomach

Premature infants and low-birth-weight infants

Multiple births

Infants whose mothers smoked cigarettes or used cocaine, methadone, or heroin during pregnancy

Overheating during sleep (too many clothes or blankets)

Infants of mothers who did not receive adequate prenatal care

Infants exposed to second-hand smoke

Use of soft bedding in crib

Infants of young, unmarried mothers

Infants with CNS disturbances and respiratory disorders such as bronchopulmonary dysplasia (see Chapter 7—Children with Special Health Care Needs)

Neonates with low Apgar scores

Increased occurrence in lower socioeconomic class

Wong, D. (1999). *Whaley & Wong's nursing care of infants and children* (6th ed.). St. Louis, MO: Mosby-Year Book.

with soft bedding, they are unable to turn their heads to inhale oxygen and instead rebreathe their own carbon dioxide.

Signs and Symptoms

The infant may be limp or may be stiff if rigor mortis is present. If sufficient time has elapsed since death, the infant may feel cool or cold to the touch with signs of mottling or dependent lividity. It is common to see frothy, blood-tinged fluids in and around the nose and mouth. Autopsy findings show intrathoracic petechiae and pulmonary edema, which confirm the diagnosis of SIDS. Pulmonary congestion and microscopic inflammatory changes in the trachea are also common findings.

Assessment

Prehospital providers should focus their history on any health problems the baby may have had since birth. It is extremely important to elicit when the infant was put to bed, when the infant fell asleep, who discovered the infant, and what time the infant was discovered. The classic picture is that the parents find the infant in his or her crib after he or she has been put to sleep for the night. The infant usually appears to have normal hydration and nutrition.

Management

Assess and monitor the airway, breathing, and circulation. Begin cardiopulmonary resuscitation (CPR) usually with only basic life support (BLS) efforts. Consult with medical control regarding BLS, advanced life support (ALS) measures, and transport issues if the infant might have been dead for some time before initiating the resuscitation.

Support the parents and assist them during the grieving process. Refer to the infant by his or her name. Assure the parents that everything possible is being done for their baby. However, never offer false hope that the infant will recover. Parents should be given unconditional support.

If resuscitation is not started or is stopped at the residence, do not leave the parents alone. If the coroner is called, stay on the scene until his or her arrival or make arrangements to have someone else be in the house with the family.

Transport

If resuscitation is attempted, transport rapidly to the closest hospital. Continue to provide the parents with information on what is being done, and allow the parents to see and ride along with the infant to the hospital whenever possible.

Exploring the Web

● Search for information on sudden infant death syndrome. Can you find specific information related to care of the child and family in the pre-hospital setting? Create a flash card on the care and management of SIDS based on the information you find.

DIABETES MELLITUS

Diabetes mellitus (DM) is a chronic, systemic disease characterized by a disorder in the production of insulin. The result is an alteration in the metabolism of glucose and subsequently an alteration in the metabolism of carbohydrates, fat, and protein.

Two classifications of diabetes have been used in the past: Insulin-dependent diabetes mellitus (i.e., IDDM or type I) and non-insulin-dependent diabetes mellitus (i.e., NIDDM or type II). These terms were based on the treatment provided yet did not properly recognize the underlying problem. For instance, some people with type II diabetes actually used insulin.

In 1997, the American Diabetes Association stopped using those terms. Type 1 and type 2 are the new terms, using Arabic numbers to eliminate any confusion with the previous Roman numerals (Table 6-4). Type II was sometimes interpreted as "type eleven" (American Diabetes Association, 1998).

Incidence

Approximately 10 to 13 million people in the United States have diabetes mellitus with about 20 per 100,000 children and adolescents being affected (Wong, 1999). The peak incidence in children is between ages 10 and 15 years yet it can occur at any age. Approximately 75 percent of all children are diagnosed before they reach the age of 18. Boys are affected slightly more often than girls (Wong, 1999).

Etiology

When there is an insulin deficiency, glucose is blocked from entering the cells and the body breaks down fat and protein for energy. The by-product of fat metabolism is **ketones**.

Type 1 is considered to be an autoimmune disease and, in a genetically predisposed person, is usually a response to a precipitating event such as a viral infection. It is the predominant type of diabetes in children.

TABLE 6-4
Classifications of Diabetes Mellitus

Old Term	New Term	Characteristics
Type I or insulin-dependent diabetes mellitus (IDDM)	Type 1	• Pancreatic beta cells (that produce insulin) are destroyed • Usually results in complete insulin deficiency • Usually occurs in children and young adults who are slim but can occur in adults of any age
Type II or non-insulin-dependent diabetes mellitus (NIDDM)	Type 2	• Body does not use insulin properly • Some insulin deficiency present • Usually occurs in people over 45 years of age who: —Are overweight —Have a sedentary lifestyle —Have a family history of diabetes

Type 2 is rare in children but may occur in older children and those of Native American descent. Causes may include:

- Pancreatic secretion of insulin in a sluggish or insensitive manner resulting in an alteration in carbohydrate metabolism
- Problems with body tissues that may require an inordinate amount of insulin
- Insulin that, once secreted, is destroyed or inactivated in some way in those persons affected

Diabetic Ketoacidosis (DKA)

Diabetic ketoacidosis (DKA) is the buildup of ketones due to the metabolism of fat instead of glucose. It results in hyperglycemia, dehydration, electrolyte imbalance, metabolic acidosis, coma, and death. DKA occurs over several hours to several days.

DKA may be precipitated by several causes. In adolescents, noncompliance with insulin administration or diet is the primary cause. Infection and severe stress may also be precipitating factors.

Signs and Symptoms

Clinical signs and symptoms depend primarily on the severity of the hyperglycemia, metabolic acidosis, and dehydration. Signs and symptoms may include **polydipsia** (increased thirst), **polyphagia** (increased hunger), **polyuria** (increased urination), weight loss, weakness, nausea and vomiting, fruity breath odor, altered level of consciousness, flushed and dry skin with poor turgor, tachycardia, **Kussmaul respirations** (hyperventilation characteristic of acidosis), abdominal pain, and **orthostatic hypotension** (drop in blood pressure with a change in position).

Assessment

History should include whether the child has a history of diabetes, time of the child's last meal, the last insulin dose, and any recent illnesses. Try to determine if there has been a change in the eating or drinking patterns of the child or any stress-related events.

Management

Management of DKA consists of replacing fluid loss. Most children with DKA are 5 to 10 percent dehydrated. Therefore, treatment includes oxygen therapy, electrocardiogram (EKG) monitoring, blood glucose analysis, and fluid resuscitation with normal saline. In stable children, fluid should be administered at 20 cc/kg over one hour. If the child is in shock, fluid should be administered at 20 cc/kg as a bolus.

Transport

Rapidly transport the child in shock while continuing to monitor vital signs and the EKG. If the child's cardiovascular status did not improve from the initial bolus of fluid, a second bolus of 20 cc/kg should be administered en route.

Hypoglycemia

Hypoglycemia is defined as low blood sugar. Hypoglycemia is usually seen in newborns or a child with a known history of diabetes. The onset of hypoglycemia is fairly rapid, and it usually occurs before meals or when the effect of insulin is peaking. Increased amount of exercise without adequate food intake, an increase in administered insulin, or infections may precipitate hypoglycemia in the child with diabetes.

Signs and Symptoms

Clinical signs and symptoms of hypoglycemia include:

- Hunger
- Weakness
- Tachycardia
- Shallow tachypnea
- Diaphoresis
- Irritability
- Vertigo
- Vomiting
- Decreased level of consciousness
- Seizures

Assessment

Assess the child's level of consciousness. If the child is unresponsive, pay close attention to airway and breathing.

Try to determine when the child last had something to eat and when the last dose of insulin was given. Was the insulin dosage recently increased? Has the child been vomiting due to the flu? Are there any signs of infection present (e.g., ear infection or urinary tract infection)? Was the child participating in some rigorous physical activity without eating properly?

Evaluate any seizure activity if present. Document the specific body movements, level of consciousness, and postictal period if present.

Management

Management of hypoglycemia is aimed at returning the blood glucose level to within the normal range. After administration of oxygen, EKG monitoring, and blood glucose analysis, glucose should be administered. If the child is awake and oriented, glucose can be administered orally with a sugar solution or paste. If the level of consciousness is altered, an IV should be initiated and glucose administered intravenously. The dose of dextrose is 0.5 to 1 g/kg (2 to 4 cc/kg) of a 25 percent solution of dextrose in water ($D_{25}W$). A 50 percent solution of dextrose in water ($D_{50}W$) may be diluted 1:1 with sterile water to produce $D_{25}W$ and 1:4 to produce a 10 percent solution of dextrose in water ($D_{10}W$). In infants, the concentration of $D_{10}W$ is used, giving 5 to 10 cc/kg over 20 minutes.

Safety Tip:

• Remember that hypertonic glucose ($D_{25}W$ and $D_{50}W$) is very hyperosmolar. As a result, administration may cause sclerosis to the vein when administered peripherally. Observe the IV site and vein for any damage.

If an IV cannot be established, glucagon may be administered in a dose of 0.03 to 0.1 mg/kg intramuscularly. It takes approximately 15 to 20 minutes to produce any results and may be repeated after 20 minutes. Be aware that glucagon may cause vomiting. If the child is still unconscious, take precautions to prevent aspiration. Turn the child on his or her side and have suction equipment readily available. Document any changes in the child's level of consciousness and overall condition after any medication administration.

Transport

If there is any continuing alteration in the child's level of consciousness, transport immediately to the closest hospital. If the child responds to intervention and is now conscious, transport to the parent's hospital of choice. This child may be managed at a specific hospital because of chronic problems related to the diabetes.

Safety Tip:

• Glucagon may cause vomiting. If the child is still unconscious, take precautions to prevent aspiration. Turn the child on the side and have suction equipment readily available.

Exploring the Web

● Search for information on diabetes mellitus. Can you find specific information related to care of the child with diabetes in the prehospital setting? Create a flash card on the care and management of diabetes mellitus based on the information you find.

SICKLE CELL CRISIS

Sickle cell disease is a genetically determined disorder of the hemoglobin structure within red blood cells. **Sickle cell anemia** is the most common form of the disease.

Incidence

Sickle cell disease usually affects the African-American population with an incidence of about eight percent in American blacks (Wong, 1999). It has also been found occasionally in people of the Hispanic race and rarely affects whites (Wong, 1999).

Etiology

In sickle cell diseases, the normal hemoglobin cell (HgbA) is replaced completely or partially with sickle hemoglobin (HgbS). The irregular shape (i.e., sickled) of the red blood cells results in an increase in blood viscosity, thus obstructing blood flow and causing pain, tissue ischemia, and in some instances infarctions or cellular death (Figure 6-3). The sites most commonly affected include the bones, mesenteric vessels, liver, spleen, brain, lungs, and penis. Children with sickle cell disease are prone to sepsis and meningitis.

Children with sickle cell disease may also suffer a stroke when the sickled cells block major blood vessels in the brain. Cerebral infarction occurs and leads to a variable degree of neurologic impairment, depending on the area of infarction. In 47 to 93 percent of children who have suffered one stroke, repeated strokes occur and cause progressive brain damage (Wong, 1999).

Signs and Symptoms

Infection, physical exertion, and exposure to cold or stress may precipitate a **sickle cell crisis** (acute, episodic condition that occurs in children with sickle cell ane-

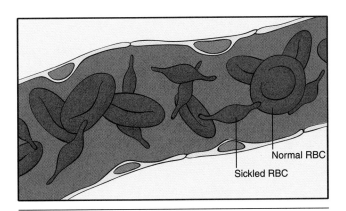

FIGURE 6-3 Regular red blood cell and "sickled" red blood cell.

mia). Clinical signs and symptoms of a sickle cell crisis include:

- Soft tissue swelling and tenderness over the affected site
- Pain in joints, abdomen, back, or chest
- Nausea and vomiting
- Headache
- Fever

Assessment

History should include inquiry regarding unexplained pain or swelling of the hands or feet, failure to thrive or frequent infections in infants, unexplained fever, family history, and known presence of the disease or trait.

Management

Management consists of hydrating the patient. Start an IV of normal saline, and administer a fluid bolus of 20 cc/kg. Give oxygen. Those children with chest pain can have acute chest syndrome and need oxygen. There is no contraindication for oxygen.

Follow local protocols for pain management. The child should be made as comfortable as possible.

Transport

If the child has been followed on a regular basis at a particular hospital, try to transport to that facility whenever possible. If the child's condition is critical, transport to the closest hospital for initial stabilization.

Continue to reassess the child throughout transport. Additional pain medication may be required to manage acute pain.

POISONING

Poisoning is the fourth leading cause of death in children. It is also a major cause of preventable death in children under the age of five years (Wong, 1999).

Incidence

More than 90 percent of poisoning occurs in the home. In addition, most cases occur in children less than six years of age (Wong, 1999).

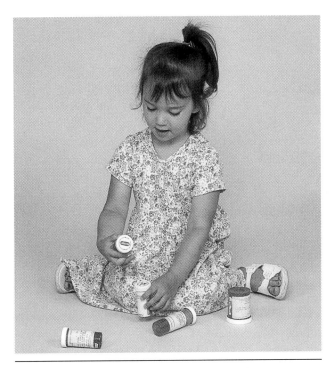

FIGURE 6-4 Accidental poisoning may occur if a child ingests prescription medicines.

Etiology

In young children, poisoning is caused by the ingestion of plants, household products, detergents, vitamins with iron, over-the-counter medications, prescription drugs, alcohol, insecticides, organophosphates, and corrosives. Also, poisonings can be caused by bites, stings, or envenomations. In older children, poisoning results from narcotics, depressants, stimulants, hallucinogens, and antidepressants. See Table 6-5 for the most commonly ingested poisons.

TABLE 6-5
Most Commonly Ingested Poisons

Type	Examples
Cosmetics and personal care products	• Perfume • Cologne • Aftershave lotion
Cleaning products	• "Household" bleach • Pine oil disinfectants
Plants	• Azalea • Buttercup • English ivy • Holly • Mistletoe • Philodendron
Foreign bodies/toys/miscellaneous	• Thermometers • Bubble-blowing liquid
Hydrocarbons	• Gasoline • Kerosene • Lighter fluid • Turpentine • Paint thinner

Litovitz, T., Smilkstein, M., & Felbert L. (1997). 1996 annual report of the American Association of Poison Control Centers Toxic Exposure Surveillance System. *American Journal of Emergency Medicine, 15*(5), 447–500; Wong, D. (1999). *Whaley & Wong's nursing care of infants and children* (6th ed.). St. Louis, MO: Mosby-Year Book.

Signs and Symptoms

Signs and symptoms are dependent on the specific poison ingested, inhaled, absorbed, or injected. Some of the more common signs are:

• Depressed or labored respirations
• Unexplained cyanosis
• Signs of shock
• Dizziness
• Sudden loss of consciousness
• Seizures
• Abdominal pain
• Vomiting
• Anorexia
• Diarrhea

Other signs and symptoms are outlined in Table 6-6.

Assessment

Questions in the history of suspected poisoning should focus on what was taken, how much was taken, and how long the substance was taken before the arrival of prehospital personnel. Ask about the route of exposure (ingested, inhaled, absorbed, or injected). Information regarding signs and symptoms that have appeared since the poisoning, treatment initiated prior to the prehospital provider's arrival, and whether vomiting was induced or occurred spontaneously should be determined. Assessment on the scene should include locating bottles, containers, or plastic bags that may contain traces of the substances. Any paraphernalia and environmental conditions should also be noted.

Management

Management of poisoning emergencies involves the principles of: (1) supportive care, (2) identification of the poison and the possible problems associated with the substance, (3) removal of the poison from the stomach (unless contraindicated) and (4) use of antidotes to counteract the effects of the poison. Supportive care begins with control of airway, breathing, and circulation, including oxygen therapy. Monitor the patient's level of consciousness and EKG. If shock is present, treat it with fluids. Diazepam (Valium®) should be considered for managing prolonged seizures.

Per local protocol, contact the poison control center or the medical control physician to confirm identification of the poison and possible problems associated with the substance. The poison may also be identified by recognition of signs and symptoms indicative of a partic-

TABLE 6-6
Signs and Symptoms of Poisons

Type of Poison	Signs/Symptoms
Salicylates	• Disorientation • Rapid respiratory rate • Dehydration • Diaphoresis • Fever • Ringing in the ears
Corrosives	• Severe burning in the mouth, throat, and stomach • Respiratory obstruction related to edema of lips, tongue, and pharynx • Violent vomiting and hemoptysis • Drooling and inability to clear secretions
Hydrocarbons	• Coughing, gagging, and choking • Altered level of consciousness • Tachypnea, grunting, retractions, and cyanosis due to pulmonary aspiration

Wong, D. (1999). *Whaley & Wong's nursing care of infants and children* (6th ed.). St. Louis, MO: Mosby-Year Book.

ular substance. If a poison control center is contacted, provide the center with the name of the poison, if known, as well as the dosage, time of ingestion, amount ingested, and signs and symptoms present.

For some poisons, **antidotes** (a drug or other substance that counteracts a specific poison) may be given. They may be:

• Mechanical (coat stomach or prevent absorption)
• Chemical (make toxin inert)
• Physiologic (oppose action of poison)

Removal or limiting the actions of the ingested poison is achieved by inducing vomiting or administering activated charcoal. DO NOT induce vomiting if

there is a decreased level of consciousness, vomiting has already occurred, seizures have occurred, signs of hypoperfusion or respiratory insufficiency are present, or the ingestion is one of corrosives, hydrocarbons, tricyclic antidepressants, or strychnine. The administration of activated charcoal is becoming the preferred treatment for ingested poisons.

Syrup of ipecac may be used to induce vomiting. Be aware that studies have shown that absorption of the poison is only reduced by about 30 percent. The standard dose is 10 cc for children 6 months to 1 year, 15 cc for children 1 to 12 years, and 30 cc for children over the age of 12 years. It is no longer necessary to force fluids after the dose as the volume of fluid does not alter ipecac's effectiveness (Wong, 1999). Vomiting will usually occur within 20 minutes. Any emesis should be transported to the hospital for analysis.

For children six months to one year, do not repeat administration of ipecac. For children over one year, repeat the dose once if there is no vomiting within 20 minutes after the first dose.

Do not induce vomiting if the child has ingested any corrosive substance or if the child is unresponsive, has no gag reflex, is seizing, or is in severe shock. Any condition that interferes with the child's ability to protect his airway is a contraindication to the induction of vomiting.

Activated charcoal is the indicated antidote for most ingested poisons. However, it should not be given if the child's level of consciousness is altered or the ingestion is one of alcohol, heavy metal, or caustics. The pediatric dose of activated charcoal is 1 g/kg (average 10 to 30 g). If the child needs activated charcoal, do not administer ipecac. Table 6-7 lists other drugs that can be used to counteract the effects of poisons. Consult local protocols for specific administration guidelines.

Exploring the Web

• Search for information on various types of poisoning. Can you find specific information related to care of the child with poisoning in the prehospital setting? What are your local protocols related to instances of poisoning? What is the phone number of your local poison control center? Create a flash card on the care and management of various types of poisonings you may encounter based on the information you find.

TABLE 6-7
Drugs Used to Counteract Poisoning

Name of Drug	Indications	Pediatric Dose
Atropine sulfate	Antidote for cholinergic poisoning (e.g., organophosphate and carbamate substances)	• 0.02 mg/kg • Minimum of 0.1 mg • Maximum single dose of 0.5 mg for a child and 1.0 mg for an adolescent • Repeat after five minutes for maximum TOTAL dose of 1.0 mg for child and 2.0 mg for an adolescent
Diphenhydramine (Benadryl®)	To reverse drug-induced dystonic reactions	1–2 mg/kg IV or IM
Flumazenil (Romazicon®)	Benzodiazepine antagonist (e.g., Valium® and Versed®)	0.01 mg/kg if > 20 kg
Naloxone (Narcan®)	Reverses the effects of narcotics (e.g., morphine sulfate, heroin, Dilaudid®, codeine, and Demerol®)	• If five years old or younger or up to 20 kg: give 0.1 mg/kg IV, IM, or subcutaneously • If >five years of age or > 20 kg: give 2 mg IV
Sodium bicarbonate	Tricyclic antidepressant overdose	1 mEq/kg of an 8.4% solution (1 mEq/ml) slow IV or IO push
Oxygen	Carbon monoxide	High-concentration via nonrebreather face mask or endotracheal tube

Transport

Urgency of transport depends on the clinical condition of the child. For a child that is unconscious, rapid transport to the closest facility is necessary. Monitor vital signs, and document any changes in the child's level of consciousness.

SUMMARY

Children under 18 years of age represent approximately 10 percent of patients transported by ambulance. Of the children transported by ambulance, about 40 percent of them present with medical emergencies. The limited exposure to medical emergencies in the pediatric patient may result in ambiguous and uncertain feelings when dealing with these situations. This chapter focused on providing an overview of those medical emergencies most commonly confronting the prehospital provider. Remember that the primary goal in any medical emergency is identification and management of life-threatening problems (airway, breathing, and circulation). If prehospital personnel are unsure of the specific problem, transport should never be delayed in an attempt to determine it.

Management of Case Study

Examination reveals a child in a great deal of pain. He is crying and is hyperventilating. You cannot hear breath sounds because of his crying. Pulse is strong and regular at 122 beats per minute with a blood pressure of 128/88. Mucous membranes are still pink at this point, and his skin is warm and diaphoretic. Skin turgor is good. He tells you his joints are aching and he cannot stand it any longer. The remainder of the exam is unremarkable.

Upon further questioning, the mother tells you that her son was quite upset about moving. He has sickle cell anemia, and she believes he is having a crisis because of the stress of moving, going to a new school, finding new friends, etc. He is not on any medications and does not have any allergies.

Provide as much emotional support as possible. Begin oxygen at 15 liters/minute via a nonrebreather face mask. Start an IV of normal saline solution or Ringer's lactate, and infuse a bolus of 20 cc per kg. Consider meperidine or morphine for pain relief per protocol or after consultation with the medical control physician.

Discuss with medical control the best destination for this child. Preferably, he should be taken to a center that can adequately treat children and provide comprehensive services.

Continue to reassess his condition and vital signs en route. Monitor his pain, and administer additional medication as ordered to make him comfortable. Watch for signs of decreased respirations if a narcotic is given.

REVIEW QUESTIONS

1. List the three levels of dehydration and three signs/symptoms of each.
2. When rehydrating a child, the dosage of fluid administration is:
   a. 20 cc/ml
   b. 20 cc/kg
   c. 20 cc/g
   d. 20 cc/lb
3. List three cause of seizures.
4. Define the following terms:
   a. Epilepsy
   b. Aura
   c. Postictal
5. An oral airway should be inserted into the mouth of a child who is seizing. True or False?
6. Define status epilepticus and list the treatment necessary.
7. A child with meningitis will present with a stiff neck. True or False?
8. Name the life-threatening complication of bacterial meningitis.
9. Name the campaign instituted in 1996 by the American Academy of Pediatrics to attempt to decrease the number of SIDS cases.
10. List four situations in which infants are at a higher risk for SIDS.
11. Describe the classifications and characteristics of diabetes mellitus.
12. Define diabetic ketoacidosis and hypoglycemia.
13. List three signs/symptoms of a sickle cell crisis.
14. _____ is the fourth leading cause of death in children and is a major cause of preventable death in children under the age of five years.
15. Syrup of ipecac is the indicated antidote for most ingested poisons. True or False?

REFERENCES

American Heart Association (2000). Guidelines 2000 for cardiopulmonary resuscitation and emergency cardiovascular care. *Journal of the American Heart Association. 120(8).* I-307-319.

American Diabetes Association: Clinical Practice Recommendations. (1998). Report of the expert committee on the diagnosis and classification of diabetes mellitus. *Diabetes Care, 21* (Suppl. 1), S5–S19.

Anderson, R., Kochanek, K., & Murphy, S. (1997). Report of final mortality statistics (1995). *Monthly Vital Stats Report, 45* (11, Suppl. l2).

Epilepsy Foundation of America. (1999). Epilepsy facts and figures. [on-line]. Available: http://www.efa.org/education/facts.html.

Gershan, N., & Moon, K. (1997). Infant sleep position in licensed child care centers. *Pediatrics, 100 (1),* 75–78.

Litovitz, T., Smilkstein, M., & Felbert, L. (1997). 1996 annual report of the American Association of Poison control centers toxic exposure surveillance system.

American Journal of Emergency Medicine, 15(5), 447–500.

Ventura, S. (1997). Births and deaths: U.S., 1996. *Monthly Vital Stats Report,* (1, Suppl. 2), 6, 29, 34.

Wong, D. (1999). *Whaley & Wong's nursing care of infants and children* (6th ed.). St. Louis, MO: Mosby-Year Book.

BIBLIOGRAPHY

Commission on Classification and Terminology of the International League Against Epilepsy (1989). *Epilepsia, 30,* 389–399.

Dieckmann, R. (1994). Rectal diazepam for prehospital pediatric status epilepticus. *Annals of Emergency Medicine, 23,* 216–224.

Wertz, E. (1997a). Infants and children. In McSwain, N., White, R., Paturas, J., & Metcalf, B., (Eds.), *The basic EMT—comprehensive prehospital patient care*. St. Louis, MO: Mosby-Year Book. 643–682.

Wertz, E. (1997b). Pediatric emergencies. In Shade, B., Rothenberg, M., Wertz, E., & Jones, S., (Eds.), *Mosby's EMT—intermediate textbook*. St. Louis, MO: Mosby-Year Book.

Wertz, E. (1997) The patient with special needs. In McSwain, N., White, R., Paturas, J., & Metcalf, B., (Eds.), *The basic EMT—comprehensive prehospital patient care*. St. Louis, MO: Mosby-Year Book. 770–785.

Jackson, P. & Vessey, J. (1996). *Primary care of the child with a chronic condition*. St. Louis, MO: Mosby-Year Book, 2nd ed. 400–419.

Santilli, N., Dodson, W., & Walton, A. (1991). *Students with seizures: A manual for school nurses*. Landover, MD: Epilepsy Foundation of America.

Chapter 7

Children with Special Health Care Needs

OBJECTIVES

Upon completion of this chapter, the student should be able to:

- Define the term *children with special health care needs*.
- Identify the most common physical disability of childhood.
- Recall the intent of the Emergency Information Form for children with special health care needs.
- Differentiate between congenital and acquired amputations.
- Define and describe management considerations for the following disabilities:

  Cerebral palsy
  Cleft lip
  Cleft palate
  Congenital heart disease
  Hearing impairment
  Muscular dystrophy
  Spina bifida
  Visual impairment

- Define and describe management considerations for the following chronic illnesses:

  Bronchopulmonary dysplasia
  Cancer
  Cystic fibrosis
  Hemophilia
  Human immunodeficiency virus infection (HIV)
  Acquired Immunodeficiency Syndrome (AIDS)
  Transplants

● Define and describe management considerations for the following disorders:
Mental retardation
Down syndrome
Fragile X syndrome
Attention Deficit Hyperactivity Disorder (ADHD)
Autism

KEY TERMS

acquired amputation
acquired immunodeficiency syndrome
    (AIDS)
amputation
anaplastic
ankle-foot orthoses (AFO)
antiretroviral drugs
Arnold-Chiari malformation
ataxic
atelectasis
athetosis
atlantoaxial instability
attention deficit disorder without
    hyperactivity (ADD-H)
attention deficit hyperactivity disorder
    (ADHD)
autism
bronchopulmonary dysplasia (BPD)
cancer
cerebral palsy (CP)
children with special health care needs
    (CSHCN)
clean intermittent catheterization (CIC)
cleft lip
cleft palate
cochlear implant
cognitive
cognitive impairment
congenital
congenital amputation
congenital heart disease (CHD)

congestive heart failure
contractures
cyanosis
cystic fibrosis (CF)
deaf
diplegia
Down syndrome (DS)
dyskinetic
early intervention (EI)
emphysema
encephalocele
epilepsy
fragile X syndrome
hard of hearing
hearing impairment
hemiplegia
hemophilia
human immunodeficiency virus (HIV)
hyaline membrane disease
hydrocephaly
hyperbilirubinemia
hypercyanotic
hyperleukocytosis
hypertonia
hypoxemia
hypoxia
idiopathic
immunosuppression
ketogenic diet
least restrictive environment (LRE)
meninges

meningocele
meningomyelocele
mental retardation
muscular dystrophy
myelomeningocele
neoplasm
neural tube
neurogenic
neuropathic
opisthotonic
osteogenic sarcoma
osteosarcoma
paraplegia
patent foramen ovale
phantom limb pain
polycythemia
prosthesis
quadriplegia
respiratory distress syndrome
retinopathy of prematurity
scissoring
spina bifida
strabismus
stump
superior vena cava syndrome
teratogens
transplant
trisomy 21
vesicostomy
visual impairment

Parent Perspective

Welcome To Holland

By Emily Perl Kingsley

I am often asked to describe the experience of raising a child with a disability—to try to help people who have not shared that unique experience to understand it, to imagine how it would feel. It's like this . . .

When you're going to have a baby, it's like planning a fabulous vacation trip—to Italy. You buy a bunch of guide books and make your wonderful plans. The Coliseum. The Michelangelo David. The gondolas in Venice. You may learn some handy phrases in Italian. It's all very exciting.

After months of eager anticipation, the day finally arrives. You pack your bags and off you go. Several hours later, the plane lands. The stewardess comes in and says, "Welcome to Holland."

"*Holland*?!?" you say. "What do you mean Holland?? I signed up for Italy! I'm supposed to be in Italy. All my life I've dreamed of going to Italy."

But there's been a change in the flight plan. They've landed in Holland, and there you must stay.

The important thing is that they haven't taken you to a horrible, disgusting, filthy place, full of pestilence, famine, and disease. It's just a different place.

So you must go out and buy new guidebooks. And you must learn a whole new language. And you will meet a whole new group of people you would never have met.

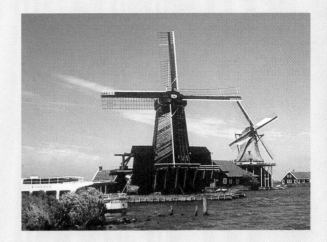

It's just a *different* place. It's slower-paced than Italy, less flashy than Italy. But after you've been there for a while and you catch your breath, you look around . . . and you begin to notice that Holland has windmills . . . and Holland has tulips. Holland even has Rembrandts.

But everyone you know is busy coming and going from Italy . . . and they're all bragging about what a wonderful time they had there. And for the rest of your life, you will say, "Yes, that's where I was supposed to go. That's what I had planned."

The pain of that will never, ever, ever, ever go away . . . because the loss of that dream is a very very significant loss.

But . . . if you spend your life mourning the fact that you didn't get to Italy, you may never be free to enjoy the very special, the very lovely things . . . about Holland.

Reprinted with permission

Case Scenario

You are dispatched around 4 p.m. to a local child care center for a child having a seizure. Upon arrival, one of the teachers directs you to a play area with a group of children crowded around a child on the floor. The teacher tells you the girl is ten-years-old and has an ongoing seizure disorder. Today's seizure started when she was taken off the bus after school, and it has continued for about 20 minutes, which is not her usual pattern. Another teacher has the girl positioned on her left side on a carpeted floor and is supporting her head. You notice blood on the girl's face around the nose and mouth. Another girl comes up to you and says, "I'm in first grade, and that is my sister." What would you do?

INTRODUCTION

I'm not the same
But then I'm not so different from the rest
I can proclaim
My needs are special
That's my challenge, my quest

I have a heart
I laugh and love and cry
Just like you
And I have a heart
Just want the chance to make my dreams
     come true

Just a matter of form and function
I will weather the storm with gumption
So just make one assumption . . .

I can do, I can
Shout it out across the land
I can do, I can

I've got a goal
I'll set my sights and push myself to achieve
With all my soul
Great things can happen, yes
For those who believe

So hear me out
There is a force within to fight off the fear
And I have no doubt
When all is said and done
The voices will cheer

Because I am determination
With drive and dedication
I'll be your inspiration
I will make my stand
I can do, I can

Dreams come true, they can
Yes they can

"I Can Do"
By Richard Obertots
© Obertunes, 1991. All rights reserved.

Due to vast improvements in medical procedures and technology, emergency medical services providers will encounter children in the community who have survived serious problems at birth as well as life-threatening illnesses and injuries. These children may have one or more ongoing conditions or disabilities that may influence their typical growth and development. However, they still may be at risk for the same hazards and emergent situations that harm children without additional challenges.

According to the Department of Health and

Developmental disability is a severe, chronic disability of an individual five years of age or older that:

- Is attributable to a mental or physical impairment or combination of mental and physical impairments
- Is manifested before the individual attains age 22
- Is likely to continue indefinitely
- Results in substantial functional limitations in three or more of the following areas of major life activity:
    a. Self-care
    b. Receptive and expressive language
    c. Learning
    d. Mobility
    e. Self direction
    f. Capacity for independent living
    g. Economic self-sufficiency
- Reflects the individual's need for a combination and sequence of special, interdisciplinary, or generic services, supports, or other assistance that is of lifelong or extended duration and is individually planned and coordinated, except that such term, when applied to infants and young children, means individuals from birth to age five, inclusive, who have substantial developmental delay or specific congenital or acquired conditions with a high probability of resulting in developmental disabilities if services are not provided.

The Developmental Disabilities Assistance and Bill of Rights Act as amended June 8, 1994; Department of Health and Human Services, Administration for Children and Families: Administration on Developmental Disabilities.

FIGURE 7-1 Definition of Developmental Disability.

Human Services Administration of Developmental Disabilities, more than 3 million individuals in the United States have developmental disabilities (Figure 7-1). Overall, 12.3 percent of children between the ages of 5 and 17 who live outside of an institution have difficulty performing one or more everyday activities such as eating, dressing, walking, communicating, and understanding school work (Centers for Disease Control and Prevention, 1999).

GENERAL CONSIDERATIONS

In 1994, the federal Maternal and Child Health Bureau's Division of Services for Children with Special Health

Care Needs (CSHCN) established a work group to discuss **children with special health care needs** and identify a definition. This diverse group included health care professionals, parents, and state CSHCN program directors. After several meetings and much deliberation, the following definition was developed:

> Children with special health care needs are those who have or are at increased risk for a chronic physical, developmental, or emotional condition and who also require health and related services of a type or amount beyond that required by children generally. (McPherson, 1998)

These needs may include physical disabilities, cognitive or mental disabilities, chronic illnesses, or forms of technology used to assist the child. It is estimated that anywhere between 2 and 32 percent of children in the United States have some type of disability or chronic illness. Even 12 years ago, in 1988, research studies showed 100,000 American children who were dependent on medical technology alone (Wallace, Biehl, MacQueen, & Blackman, 1997). That number has grown much higher since that time. See Chapter 8—Children with Special Health Care Needs Assisted by Technology for specific information on various devices used to assist children in the home or community.

Family Issues

Chronic illnesses may also require special adaptations in the daily activities of children, their families, and the people with whom they interact. Families may have less leisure time and face many interruptions to the usual routine of life. Siblings of children with special health care needs may feel neglected or jealous of the extra attention given to their brother or sister. They may simulate illness or injury just to get attention. Parents may not react to a serious situation with as much emotion because of the day-to-day crises they manage (Figure 7-2). In some instances parents or caregivers may be distant, unusually defensive, or just plain exhausted.

Earlier this week, a question was asked by some nit wit official as to why there weren't more parents (of kids with special needs) involved in the local PTA and other issues that have come up that directly involve our kids. His question, which was passed onto me was, "Where are the parents?"

They are on the phone to doctors and hospitals and fighting with insurance companies, wading through the red tape in order that their child's medical needs can be properly addressed. They are buried under a mountain of paperwork and medical bills, trying to make sense of a system that seems designed to confuse and intimidate all but the very savvy.

Where are the parents? They are at home, diapering their 15-year-old son, or trying to lift their 100 lb. daughter onto the toilet. They are spending an hour at each meal to feed a child who cannot chew or laboriously and carefully feeding their child through a g-tube. They are administering medications, changing catheters, and switching oxygen tanks.

Where are the parents? They are sitting, bleary eyed and exhausted, in hospital emergency rooms, waiting for test results to come back and wondering: "Is this the time when my child doesn't pull through?" They are sitting patiently, in hospital rooms as their child recovers from yet another surgery to lengthen hamstrings or straighten backs or repair a faulty internal organ. They are waiting in long lines in county clinics because no insurance company will touch their child.

Where are the parents? They are sleeping in shifts because their child won't sleep more than two or three hours a night and must constantly be watched, lest he do himself or another member of the family harm. They are sitting at home with their child because family and friends are either too intimidated or too unwilling to help with child care and the state agencies that are designed to help are suffering cutbacks of their own.

Where are the parents? They are trying to spend time with their non-disabled children, as they try to make up for the extra time and effort that is critical to keeping their disabled child alive. They are struggling to keep a marriage together, because adversity does not always bring you closer. They are working two and sometimes three jobs in order to keep up with the extra expenses. And sometimes they are a single parent struggling to do it all by themselves.

Where are the parents? They are trying to survive in a society that pays lip service to helping those in need, as long as it doesn't cost them anything. They are trying to patch their broken dreams together so that they might have some sort of normal life for their children and their families.

They are busy, trying to survive.

—Sue Stuyvesant, parent of a child with multiple disabilities
Written: 10/15/96
Reprinted with permission

FIGURE 7-2 Where are the parents?

Exploring the Web

- What sites can you find related to children with special health care needs?
- Explore the Emergency Medical Services for Children (EMSC) Web site. What information does this government site offer?
- Search for sites that pertain to specific disabilities and conditions.
- What professional organizations or journals could you search for information on children with special health care needs?

Legislation and Other Government Assistance

Many children with special health care needs are educated in local community schools. Several legislative efforts exist linking health care to these educational benefits. In 1975, Public Law 94-142, the Education for All Handicapped Children Act, gave children the constitutional right to receive an education that was publicly funded and that was conducted in the **least restrictive environment** (LRE). In other words, children with disabilities could receive an education alongside their peers without disabilities. They did not need to be segregated in separate institutions. Amendments were also developed.

In 1986, Public Law 99-457, Education of the Handicapped Act Amendments, established an **early intervention** (EI) system for infants and toddlers and their families. Early intervention is a federally funded program that provides early education for children with delays or disabilities or those at risk for disabilities. The policy was formed due to the following findings:

- Development of children will not be as delayed as it would be if services are delayed until age six or older
- The family's ability to meet the needs of their infants and toddlers with disabilities will be enhanced
- Over a period of time, these families and their children will use specialized education services that are less costly, the possibility of institutional-

ization will be minimized, and these children will have better opportunities to integrate and live socially within their own communities (Wallace et al., 1997).

In 1991, Public Law 101-476, the Individuals with Disabilities Education Act or IDEA, amended the two previous laws. Funds are provided through the Infants and Toddlers Program (Part H of IDEA) and through the Preschool Program (Section 619 of Part B of IDEA) for services to children ages three to five. This legislation also requires transportation and developmental, corrective, and other support services must be provided if determined necessary for the child to benefit from education.

As discussed in Chapter 1, the federal Emergency Medical Services for Children (EMSC) project sponsored by the Maternal and Child Health Bureau has been in existence since 1985. Within the last five years, they have funded many initiatives directly related to children with special health care needs.

Assessment and Treatment Factors

In some situations, walking through the front door of the home of a child with special needs may feel like walking into an intensive care unit. In addition to a crib or bed in the living room, there may be multiple devices, supplies, and other equipment needed to sustain the child's life (Figure 7-3). There may also be other health care providers present such as a visiting nurse, respiratory therapist, or physical therapist.

In other scenarios, the chronic illness or disability may not be the reason emergency care is required. For instance, a child with a serious seizure disorder and mental retardation may have fallen at school or at home and sustained a laceration requiring sutures. The chronic illness or disability will be secondary to the need for wound care. The presence of chronic illness or disability may, however, affect the assessment and treatment processes as the child may not understand the pain she is experiencing and why someone is pushing against her head with a bandage. She may not be able to verbalize her questions, fright, or level of pain.

Gathering an adequate history may also be difficult or time-consuming depending on the child's condition. The American College of Emergency Physicians (ACEP) in conjunction with the American Academy of Pediatrics (AAP) developed an Emergency Information Form (EIF) that standardizes information that would be helpful to emergency personnel inside and outside of

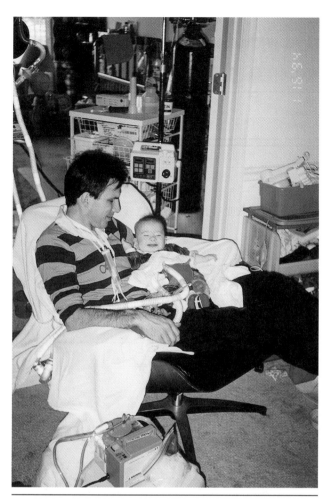

FIGURE 7-3 Children with complex medical needs are often cared for in the home by their parents. The EMT will often encounter equipment and medical supplies necessary to the care of these children.

 Exploring the Web

● Learn more about the development of the Emergency Information Form (EIF) for Children with Special Health Care Needs by searching the Web. Look for information at the American Academy of Pediatrics Web site and the American College of Emergency Physicians Web site. Are there any other sites you can find with additional information?

 Tricks of the Trade

Advocate for use of the Emergency Information Form for children with special health care needs in your service area. Copies may be downloaded from the Internet or purchased directly from the American Academy of Pediatrics. Work with school nurses to share this information with them.

the hospital setting (Figure 7-4). Both organizations have also developed formal policy statements regarding the use of this form (Figure 7-5).

During assessment, try not to be distracted by the child's disability or associated equipment. Assess the patient as you would any other child. Remember that *disability* still refers to the child's neurological status and not the chronic illness or condition. Consider asking the following questions of the patient or the family. Remember to direct your questions in a positive light. Focus on what the child CAN do instead of what the child CAN-NOT do (Table 7-1).

Utilize the parents, teachers, or other caregivers who may be with the child. They know the child well if they spend considerable time with him or her. There may, however, be circumstances when the parent or caregiver is not that familiar with the child or the child's medications, treatments, or the specifics of the disability such as in the case of a divorce or other marital strife. Do not be judgmental in that situation.

If a life-threatening injury or illness is discovered, begin intervention immediately. Focus on treating the acute problem since the chronic illness is usually an ongoing process.

For a child with any kind of cognitive disability, take a few extra minutes to explain what you are doing.

 Tricks of the Trade

Utilize the parents and caregivers to help with assessment and treatment of the child with special health care needs. In most instances, they have become experts at their child's care and know them better than any other medical provider.

Emergency Information Form for Children With Special Needs

American College of Emergency Physicians®

American Academy of Pediatrics

| Date form completed By Whom | Revised | Initials |
| Revised | Initials |

| **Name:** | Birth date: | Nickname: |

| Home Address: | Home/Work Phone: |

| Parent/Guardian: | Emergency Contact Names & Relationship: |

| Signature/Consent*: | |

| Primary Language: | Phone Number(s): |

Physicians:

| Primary care physician: | Emergency Phone: |
| | Fax: |

| Current Specialty physician: Specialty: | Emergency Phone: |
| | Fax: |

| Current Specialty physician: Specialty: | Emergency Phone: |
| | Fax: |

| Anticipated Primary ED: | Pharmacy: |

| Anticipated Tertiary Care Center: | |

Diagnoses/Past Procedures/Physical Exam:

1.

Baseline physical findings:

2.

3.

Baseline vital signs:

4.

Synopsis:

Baseline neurological status:

*Consent for release of this form to health care providers

FIGURE 7-4 Emergency Information Form for Children with Special Health Care Needs

Diagnoses/Past Procedures/Physical Exam continued:

Medications:

Significant baseline ancillary findings (lab, x-ray, ECG):

1.
2.
3.
4.
5.
6.

Prostheses/Appliances/Advanced Technology Devices:

Last name:

Management Data:

Allergies: Medications/Foods to be avoided   **and why:**

1.
2.
3.

Procedures to be avoided   **and why:**

1.
2.
3.

Immunizations

Dates						Dates					
DPT						Hep B					
OPV						Varicella					
MMR						TB status					
HIB						Other					

Antibiotic prophylaxis: Indication: Medication and dose:

Common Presenting Problems/Findings With Specific Suggested Managements

Problem	Suggested Diagnostic Studies	Treatment Considerations

Comments on child, family, or other specific medical issues:

Physician/Provider Signature: **Print Name:**

FIGURE 7-4 (Continued)

**American College of Emergency Physicians
Policy Statement**

Emergency Information Form for Children with Special Health Care Needs

Emergency physicians and pediatricians provide medical care to many children with special needs because of chronic, complex medical illnesses. Care of these children may be complicated by the lack of patient history information, and unusual and uncommon disease processes.

To optimize emergency care of children with special needs, the American College of Emergency Physicians supports these principles:

- A mechanism should be available to quickly identify the child with special health care needs when that child presents for emergency care.

- Records of each child's special needs should be maintained in an accessible and usable format.

- The exact form in which relevant information is stored may vary depending on individual physician and patient preference.

- A universally accepted form should be disseminated for use by prehospital providers, parents, physicians, and other child advocates.

Approved by the ACEP Board of Directors and the American Academy of Pediatrics, December, 1998

American College of Emergency Physicians (ACEP)
http://www.acep.org/policy/po400267.html

FIGURE 7-5   American College of Emergency Physicians Policy Statement

---

TABLE 7-1
Positive Questions for the CSHCN

Questions for the Child (modify based on age and level of understanding)	Questions for the Parents	Examples
• Are you taking any medicines? • Did you take them today like you usually do?	• Does your child take any medication for her seizure disorder? • Did she get her regular dose today? • Has the doctor recently changed her dosage? • Was she able to keep down the medication without vomiting?	A child with the flu may be vomiting or have a decreased appetite. When a child with a seizure disorder does not take her medication or that medication is not properly absorbed, breakthrough seizures can occur.
• Is it ok if I take off your braces so I can look at your legs? • Can you help me?	• Does your child wear these braces all the time? • Are they easily removable?	Consider a child with spina bifida. Hot water or grease may have splashed on the child's lap, and some of it may have dripped down onto the child's legs. • Children with spina bifida that wear braces on their lower legs may be injured and not be able to feel the damage due to a decreased sensation in their lower extremities. • If the brace itself is not damaged, it can be used as a splint.

(continues)

TABLE 7-1
(Continued)

Questions for the Child (modify based on age and level of understanding)	Questions for the Parents	Examples
• Can you "talk" to me with your special board?	• How does your child communicate?	Some children who are nonverbal may use a communication or picture board to let their needs be known. Other children may use sign language.
• Are you on a special diet?	• Is your child on any special diet?	For example, children on the ketogenic diet for severe seizures should only have IV fluid of normal saline. Any dextrose administration can throw these children out of the ketosis that is being meticulously maintained by the parents and caregivers. Any alteration to the ketosis could cause breakthrough seizures.
• I am going to tickle your legs. Tell me when you feel it. • Before today's accident, tell me what you were able to feel.	• What type of feeling did your child have in her legs before the accident?	The child with a spinal cord injury may have paralysis or decreased sensation in her legs before the injury. It is important to know the baseline function.
• When was your last operation to fix your shunt?	• How long ago was your child's shunt revised?	Children with hydrocephaly usually need shunt revisions as they grow. The signs and symptoms the child has during the emergency situation may be related to the need for another revision.
• What can we do for you today?	• What was different today that you needed to call for an ambulance?	Parents and caregivers become very knowledgeable in their child's care, especially in the child using various technological aids. The reason for the call to EMS may be because they are simply at the "end of their rope" or have encountered a new situation for which they feel unprepared.

*The situations mentioned in the examples will be discussed with more detail later in the chapter.

Avoid talking "over" the child to a parent or caregiver. Continue to address the child and explain procedures even if it seems that the child does not understand.

Some physical disabilities result in different body alignments such as **scoliosis** (curvature of the spine) or **contractures** (condition of a joint characterized by flexion and fixation—caused by atrophy or shortening of the muscles or by loss of usual elasticity of the skin). Do not try to force the child to conform to a certain piece of equipment. For instance, the child's back may not lie flat on the long backboard. Instead of trying to push her to lie flat, place additional padding under the back to compensate for the difference.

Limit exposure of the child when performing emergency treatments—especially those children with physical disabilities. Keep the child appropriately covered. Resist the temptation to "show" the child's unusual characteristic to other members of the team unless it is relevant to the child's treatment.

Some children with special health care needs will wear some type of identifying jewelry such as a Medic Alert™ bracelet or necklace. Older children may resist this identification as they do not want to point out their differences to their peers. While its absence does not rule out a disability or chronic condition, its presence can be quite helpful during assessment and treatment.

Latex Allergies

In 1989, latex allergy was found to be a serious problem in children with spina bifida (Wong, 1999). Due to repeated exposure to products containing latex (e.g., catheters and gloves), children become sensitive to the latex and develop life-threatening allergic reactions. Signs and symptoms include:

- Hives
- Watery eyes
- Itching
- Rashes
- Wheezes
- Respiratory difficulty
- Anaphylactic shock

Health care providers can also develop an allergy to latex because of their repeated contacts with products containing latex. Many hospitals and ambulatory facilities are switching to items that do not contain latex to minimize the risk to patients as well as staff.

It is important to know immediately if the child is sensitive to latex. If a sensitivity or allergy is present, the child must not come into contact with any latex products or even be near equipment with latex (Table 7-2). Assemble a latex-free kit that can be stored in the ambulance for use when needed.

TABLE 7-2
Items That May Contain Latex

Adhesive bandage strips
Airways
Blood pressure cuff and tubing
Bulb syringe
Catheters
Dressings
Elastic bandages
Electrode pads
Endotracheal tubes
Gloves
Intravenous tubing and bags
Medication vials
Nasogastric tubes
Oxygen masks and cannulas
Pulse oximeter
Spacer (from metered dose inhaler)
Stethoscope tubing
Suction tubing
Syringes (disposable)
Tape
Tourniquet

Exploring the Web

● Research the effects of latex allergies on patients and caregivers.

PHYSICAL DISABILITIES

Many children have physical disabilities that may limit their mobility or daily function in some way. Emergencies may occur that are not related to the physical disability yet the prehospital provider must have a brief understanding of the underlying condition.

Amputation

An **amputation** is the loss of a part of a limb or an entire limb. A **congenital amputation** occurs when a particular limb or part of a limb of a fetus does not develop completely while in utero. An **acquired amputation** is the loss of a limb or a part of a limb by accident or intentional surgery.

Incidence

It is estimated that congenital amputations occur in two to eight children in 10,000 births (Wallace et al., 1997). Variation occurs among communities. For instance, poor prenatal care and/or use of drugs that may cause birth anomalies may occur in underserved or low-income areas.

Etiology

In congenital amputation, children are born without part of a limb or an entire limb. Causes include infections to the mother during pregnancy (e.g., varicella or chicken pox) and drug use (e.g., Accutane® for acne treatment or thalidomide for nausea) as well as other genetic factors. Most commonly, the thumb is absent or the arm ends at the elbow (Wallace et al., 1997).

Exploring the Web

● Learn more about children who have amputations related to cancer. Are there specific complications or treatment guidelines of which the prehospital provider should be aware?

In some diseases, amputation is a form of treatment. For instance, in the child with **osteogenic sarcoma** or **osteosarcoma** (most common bone cancer in children), amputation is performed to stop the spread of cancer. The location of the cancer will determine how much of the extremity and joint is amputated.

Another form of acquired amputation is traumatic amputation as a result of an accident. Children who use heavy equipment at an early age or those who use power equipment in an unsupervised manner are prone to amputations. After an accident, surgery may be required to clean what is left of the extremity, remove fragments of tissue, and close the wound.

Signs and Symptoms

After a surgical amputation, the end of the limb or **stump** may become infected. The wound may be reddened, have purulent drainage, and have a foul odor. In addition, the child may have a fever and feel lethargic.

Phantom limb pain is very common after amputation due to disruption of the nerve endings. The child may complain of pain in the hand even though it is no longer present. To the child, the pain is very real. Tingling or itching may also be experienced.

Assessment

A temporary **prosthesis** (artificial replacement for some missing part of the body) may be used during the healing time to promote psychological adjustment to loss of the limb. Approximately four to six weeks after the surgery, the child is fitted for a permanent prosthesis. During assessment, examine the skin condition where the temporary or permanent prosthesis is attached. Look for signs of infection or tissue breakdown.

Management

Treat the child's illness or injury without undue attention to the amputation. Stabilize the emergency situation.

The child may also exhibit signs and symptoms of depression related to loss of the limb or the initial diagnosis (e.g., cancer of the bone). Allow the child an opportunity to express concerns about the current emergency as well as the long-term outcome related to the reason for the amputation.

Transport

If the child is receiving ongoing treatment at a specific facility, it may be most appropriate to transport to that facility, as long as it is able to handle the current emergency. For example, if a child is receiving chemotherapy at a local hospital yet suffers a traumatic event, that institution may not be qualified to handle pediatric trauma.

If the child is being transported with the prosthesis in place, note that fact in the written report. Do everything possible to make sure the prosthesis stays with the child if it has been removed for examination. These devices can be *very* expensive and are specifically fitted to the child. Loss of the prosthesis may be devastating to the child and family from both a financial and emotional aspect.

Cerebral Palsy

Cerebral palsy (CP) is a nonprogressive (does not worsen with age or growth) disorder of movement and posture caused by some injury to the brain during early development. The brain is unable to control muscle movement even though the muscles, peripheral nerves, and spinal cord are not damaged. Abnormal muscle tone and poor coordination are the primary symptoms. Intellectual involvement, language deficits, and perceptual problems may also be present.

Incidence

Cerebral palsy occurs in 1.9 to 2.3 per 1,000 live births. In areas with poor prenatal care and a greater number of premature births, the incidence is higher. Since technology has increased the infant survival rate, the actual number of cases in the community may be rising. It is the most common permanent physical disability of childhood (Wong, 1999).

Etiology

Most cases occur in utero or during delivery. Chromosomal abnormalities, maternal infections, or lack of oxygen to the brain because of placenta previa, toxemia, or a traumatic birth are causes of cerebral palsy. Birth asphyxia used to be considered the major cause yet now many researchers believe that prenatal brain abnormalities (e.g., intracranial hemorrhage, high bilirubin levels, or meningitis) play a greater role in causing the disorder (Wallace et al., 1997; Wong, 1999). Premature delivery occurs most often with very small infants and is the single, most important determinant of cerebral palsy. Approximately 24 percent of the cases are **idiopathic** in that no identifiable cause is found (Wong, 1999).

Signs and Symptoms

Some children may have cerebral palsy yet it may not be apparent for the first few months of life. Delayed development of certain motor milestones along with unusual movements and an unusual physical exam will develop during the first one to two years of life.

Cerebral palsy is classified based on the type of neuromuscular dysfunction. See Table 7-3 for a description of the classifications and the presenting symptoms.

Other disabilities are usually present including but not limited to: mental retardation (in 60 to 70 percent of children), learning disability, seizures (in 30 to 40 percent of children), feeding and growth problems, constipation (due to decreased mobility), dental disease (due in part to antiseizure medications), and behavior problems (Wallace et al., 1997). Visual, hearing, and speech-language impairment may also be present.

Assessment

Because cerebral palsy is not progressive, emergency treatment is usually not related to the CP. The child may be ill, injured, or going to the hospital for corrective surgery.

Increased salivation and tongue thrusting may make airway control more difficult. Coughing and choking while eating may also increase the risk of aspiration.

Children with cerebral palsy may have contractures caused by atrophy and shortening of muscle fibers. Examples include **"scissoring"** (legs in crossed position with stiff knees, hips, and ankles) or **opisthotonic** (exaggerated arching of the back) postures.

Many children with cerebral palsy wear **ankle-foot orthoses (AFOs)** or braces to help them walk. These devices are molded to fit the child's feet and fit down inside the shoes (see Figure 7-6). They help to reduce the existing deformity and prevent further deterioration. Leave the braces in place if they do not interfere with proper assessment or treatment of the lower extremities. If they are removed, make sure they are left at home or accompany the child to the hospital.

If the child has any speech difficulties, communication may be prolonged. Try to give the child enough time to finish a thought or a sentence. Whenever possible, ask "yes or no" questions so the child does not become frustrated trying to explain something or give a lengthy answer. Some children cannot speak at all and may use a computer with a voice synthesizer to "speak."

Management

Have adequate suction equipment available and use it as needed because of the potential for airway compromise. Continue to monitor the respiratory status throughout treatment and transport.

When immobilization is necessary, the child may not lie flat on the backboard because of postures such as scissoring or arching of the back. DO NOT force the child to conform to the equipment. Support the body as best as possible by padding those open areas that do not reach the board.

In another instance, a body part may be very stiff. Gently try to move the child into the position you need. Again, DO NOT try to force any movement! If the

TABLE 7-3
Types of Cerebral Palsy

Type	Involving	Major Manifestations
Spastic	Defined by: • **Diplegia**—trunk & all extremities; legs more involved • **Hemiplegia**—one side of body; most common • **Quadriplegia**—equal involvement of arms, legs, head & trunk • **Paraplegia**—only legs	• Reduced movement or stiffness due to **hypertonia** (increased muscle tone) • Poor control of posture, balance, and coordinated motion • Impairment of fine and gross motor skills • Active attempts at motion increase abnormal postures and overflow of movement to other parts of the body
Dyskinetic	Abnormal involuntary athetoid movements	• Athetosis → slow, writhing movements; usually involve extremities, trunk, neck, facial muscles, and tongue • Involvement of pharyngeal, laryngeal, and oral muscles cause drooling and difficulty articulating speech • Involuntary, irregular jerking movements • Disordered muscle tone • Movements increase with emotional stress and during adolescence
Ataxic	Wide-based gait	• Poorly performed rapid, repetitive movements • Difficulty balancing • When reaching for objects, movements of arms become disintegrated
Mixed type/ Dystonic	Varies	• Combination of spasticity and athetosis

Wallace et al., (1997). *Mosby's resource guide to children with disabilities and chronic illness*. St. Louis, MO: Mosby-Year Book; Wong, D. (1999). *Whaley & Wong's nursing care of infants and children*. (6th ed.). St. Louis, MO: Mosby-Year Book.

child's arm is bent, for example, it may be difficult to check a blood pressure if the arm cannot be straightened. Try the other arm, or use the popliteal artery with a cuff on the thigh. If unable to assess the blood pressure, notify medical control if necessary and document the reason in the written report.

In order to maximize mobility, children may have a special wheelchair that provides head, neck, and trunk support. Young children may even use small wheeled devices until they are large enough to use a wheelchair. Use caution when transferring the child from the wheelchair to the cot or long backboard.

Transport

Remember, this child may be seen routinely by physicians at a certain facility and the parents may prefer to have the child transported to that facility. Transport the child to the appropriate facility depending on the injuries or illness. The advantage to going to the "usual" place is that they may be very familiar with all of the child's ongoing needs. The disadvantage is that they may not be adequately prepared for the emergent condition (e.g., trauma).

Try to allow a parent to ride in the patient compartment whenever possible. These children may be

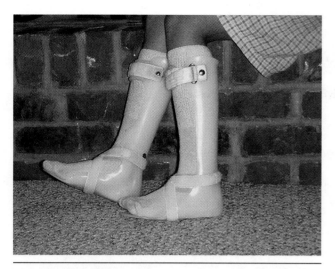

FIGURE 7-6 Children may wear ankle-foot orthoses to support the foot and ankle during walking.

more frightened because of the frequency of medical procedures in the past. In addition, the parent will feel much more comfortable being with the child as opposed to the front seat or in a separate car. Refer to Chapter 14—Interacting with Families and Caregivers for more information on parents riding in the back with their children.

Parent Perspective

"I was never allowed to ride in the back of the ambulance with my son when he was transported to the hospital. It was awful to have to hand your kid over to strangers like that. It was fine for me to take care of him through all of the other surgeries and problems."

—*Mother of a child with cerebral palsy*

Cleft Lip and/or Cleft Palate

Cleft lip is a congenital anomaly resulting in one or more clefts or openings in the upper lip. **Cleft palate** is also a congenital anomaly characterized by an opening in the midline of the palate.

Incidence

Cleft lip occurs in approximately 1 in 800 live births and is predominant in males. Cleft palate occurs in 1 in 2000 live births and is predominant in females (Wong, 1999). Cleft lip is also more common in people of Oriental or Native American descent and less common in people of African-American descent.

Etiology

Cleft lip occurs when the structures surrounding the oral cavity do not close or incompletely fuse in the embryo (see Figure 7-7a). The cleft or opening may be on one side or both sides of the upper lip and may range from an indentation in the lip to a deep and wide opening up to the nostril. Teeth may be missing, deformed, or abnormally placed where the cleft occurs. There is usually altered development of the nasal cartilages, nasal septum, and external nose.

Cleft palate occurs when the two sides of the palate do not fuse during development of the embryo (see Figure 7-7b). The cleft or opening may only affect the soft palate or may extend through the hard palate into the nostrils. Often a cleft lip is present with a cleft palate.

The combination of cleft lip and cleft palate is the most common craniofacial malformation and accounts for half of the total defects. Smoking by the mother during the first trimester of pregnancy is thought to be the cause of 11 to 12 percent of all cases of cleft lip and/or cleft palate (Wong, 1999).

Cleft lip is surgically repaired anywhere from 48 hours to 10 weeks after birth as long as the infant does not have any type of oral, respiratory, or systemic infection. There may be minimal scarring in some children or a larger deformity in children more severely affected.

Surgical repair of cleft palate usually takes place between 12 and 18 months of age so that the regular growth of the palate may be optimized. Some surgeons, however, believe strongly in early repair and may perform surgery as early as 28 days after birth. Others feel it is appropriate to wait until the child is between five and seven years of age. The timing for surgical repair remains controversial.

Signs and Symptoms

Feeding difficulty and maintenance of proper nutrition are primary complications, especially before the cleft is repaired. Before surgery, the infant is unable to suck adequately so that muscle development around the lips is delayed. Parents and caregivers are taught how to position the baby to minimize choking and may use adaptive nipples or a syringe to feed the child. Whatever mechanism is used, liquid going into the mouth can leak out through the cleft palate into the nose leading to choking and aspiration. The child also swallows a lot of air when feeding so that vomiting is common.

Frequent ear infections are also common due to improper draining of the middle ear. Psychologically, the

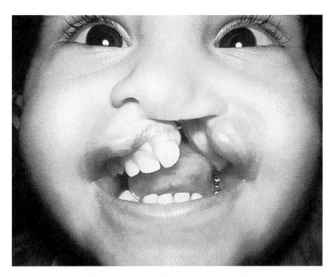

a.

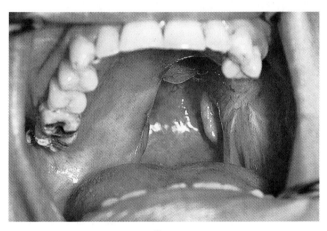

b.

FIGURE 7-7 a. Child with cleft lip
b. Child with cleft palate.

Assessment

For most parents, the birth of a child with a physical deformity is traumatic. Emphasize the positive aspects of the infant's or child's physical features. Do not show fear or disgust when treating the infant or older child who has not had the cleft lip or palate repaired.

Parent Perspective

"When my son was born, the initial site of him was so scary. A million things went through our minds during those first few days. The hardest part in the time before his first surgery was all of the staring—people would look at him and turn away. We wanted to try and enjoy our new baby just like other parents. One day, a woman came up to me and said, 'Your son has such beautiful eyes!' I was moved to tears! Finally someone could see past the large opening in his upper lip and nose and say something that would be said to a child WITHOUT a physical problem."

—*Father of a child with a cleft palate and cleft lip that were eventually repaired*

The boy grew to be a star Little League baseball player and does well in a regular school setting.

Assess the adequacy of the airway in addition to other complaints expressed by the child or parent. Gather information from the parents and/or caregivers as to what problems have arisen in the past before or since corrective surgery.

Management

Use caution when inserting anything into the oral cavity of a child with an unrepaired cleft lip or cleft palate. An oral airway or endotracheal tube may not position into the mouth properly because of the defect. Taping an endotracheal tube may require a different method so that the tube is stabilized adequately. Reassess airway and breathing frequently.

Be prepared to suction the airway since vomiting and aspiration are common in these children. Use caution not to injure the mouth during the procedure.

In a child with a recent surgical repair, most families are told to protect the surgical site at all costs. If the

child may have difficulty with social adjustment related to the remaining deformity and/or quality of speech. Parents may also have a difficult time adjusting to the presence of a physical deformity in their child.

Children with cleft palate usually develop some type of speech impairment due to insufficient palate function that interferes with the usual sounds of speech, improper tooth alignment affecting the development of clear speech, and hearing loss from frequent middle ear infections. Speech therapy is usually required.

Ongoing monitoring by a multidisciplinary team of physicians and specialists is common. The child will also undergo several stages of surgical repair and/or orthodontic procedures as he or she grows.

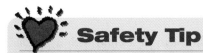

Safety Tip

• USE CAUTION when inserting anything into the oral cavity of a child with an unrepaired cleft lip or palate. An oral airway or endotracheal tube may not position into the mouth properly because of the defect.

child requires suctioning, ventilations, or intubation in an emergency, check with the family as to what they have been told to do. Remember, resuscitation of the child takes priority. If advanced airway control is necessary, intubate the child while trying as best as possible not to disturb the surgical site.

Assisting ventilations may be intimidating due to the presence of an uncorrected cleft lip or palate. Make sure the mask fits properly over the mouth and nose, and ventilate as usual.

Transport

Monitor the child's airway throughout the transport. Communicate with personnel at the receiving facility so that they can have specialists available when the child arrives.

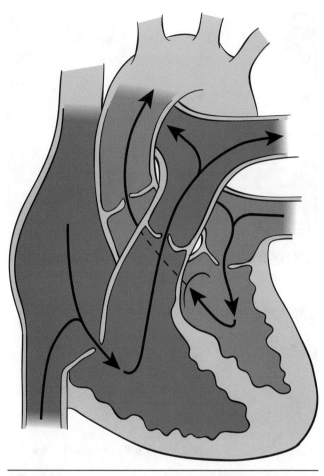

FIGURE 7-8 Circulation through the heart.

Exploring the Web

● Search for additional information about cleft palate and cleft lip on the Internet.

● Search for information related to parent support groups of children with cleft palate and cleft lip.

Congenital Heart Disease

Congenital heart disease (CHD) is the presence of any structural or functional defect (also called anomaly) of the heart or great vessels that is present at birth (Figure 7-8 shows circulation through the heart). Many of these problems are not discovered until well after birth. Types of CHD are outlined in Table 7-4.

Incidence

Generally, 4 to 10 in 1,000 live births result in congenital heart disease. Except for prematurity, congenital heart disease is the major cause of death during the first year of life. Approximately 32 percent of all defects are ventricular septal defects (Wong, 1999).

After one child is born with CHD, there is a 2 to 6 percent chance of having another child with CHD. In addition, children with CHD have up to a ten percent chance of having a future child with CHD (Wallace et al., 1997).

Etiology

In more than 90 percent of all cases, the cause of CHD is unknown (Wong, 1999). Of the remaining 10 percent, the following factors are contributory during pregnancy:

• Rubella (measles) in the mother during pregnancy

• Active alcoholism

• Maternal age over 40 years

• Diabetes type 1 in the mother

TABLE 7-4
Types of Congenital Heart Disease

Heart Anomaly	Description	Other Associated Problems
Ventricular septal defect (VSD)	• Opening in the septum or wall between the left and right ventricles • Most common defect	• Down syndrome • Fetal alcohol syndrome
Pulmonic stenosis	• Narrowing of the pulmonary artery	• Rubella syndrome • Noonan syndrome
Patent ductus arteriosus	• Opening between the pulmonary artery and aorta • Usual finding only during prenatal life • Fetal ductus arteriosus fails to close	• Rubella syndrome • Down syndrome
Patent foramen ovale	• Opening in the atrial septum • Usual finding during prenatal life • Fetal foramen ovale fails to close	• None
Atrial-septal defect (ASD)	• Opening in the septum or wall between the right and left atria	• Noonan syndrome • Down syndrome • Fetal alcohol syndrome
Coarctation of the aorta	• Localized narrowing of aorta • Increased pressure before the defect • Decreased pressure past the defect	• Turner syndrome • Apert syndrome
Tetralogy of Fallot	Four defects include: • Pulmonic stenosis (narrowing of the pulmonary artery) • Ventricular septal defect • Malposition of the aorta (arises from septal defect or the right ventricle) • Right ventricular hypertrophy (enlarged right ventricle)	• Down syndrome • Fetal alcohol syndrome
Atrioventricular valve defect	• Defect in valve in which blood flows from the atria to the ventricles • Left atrium to left ventricle → mitral valve • Right atrium to right ventricle → tricuspid valve	Down syndrome
Tricuspid atresia	• Failure of the tricuspid valve to develop • No communication from right atrium to right ventricle	N/A
Hypoplastic left heart syndrome	• Incomplete or underdeveloped left side of the heart	N/A

(continues)

TABLE 7-4
(Continued)

Heart Anomaly	Description	Other Associated Problems
Transposition of great vessels (also known as *blue baby*)	• Pulmonary artery arises from the left ventricle • Aorta arises from the right ventricle • No communication between systemic and pulmonary circulations	• Diabetes • Prediabetes in mother

Anderson, K., Anderson, L., & Glanze, W. (1998). *Mosby's medical, nursing, & allied health dictionary.* 5th ed. St. Louis: Mosby-Year Book. Wong, D. (1999). *Whaley and Wong's nursing care of infants and children* (6th ed.). St. Louis: Mosby-Year Book.

Teratogens (substance, agent, or process that interferes with normal prenatal development) also contributes to the development of congenital heart disease. The fetus is most vulnerable during the 3rd through 12th weeks of gestation. It is during this time that the major organs and systems are differentiated. Any infections such as rubella, any drugs such as alcohol, or exposure to radiation during that period can negatively affect the developing cardiovascular system.

Many children with CHD also have a chromosomal abnormality such as Down syndrome (trisomy 21). Many children with Down syndrome require heart surgery to correct a congenital heart defect.

Assessment

Congenital heart disease can be classified by whether or not the child is cyanotic. Since the presence of cyanosis has been used as the distinguishing symptom, the defects are considered either cyanotic or acyanotic. Examples are given in Table 7-5.

Congestive Heart Failure

One of the primary complications that can occur in children with cardiac defects is **congestive heart failure (CHF)**. CHF occurs when the cardiac defect causes an increase in volume or workload of the ventricles. An

TABLE 7-5
Classification of Congenital Heart Disease

Type	Characteristics	Defects
Acyanotic (no cyanosis present)	Increase in blood flow through pulmonary artery	Atrial-septal defect Ventricular-septal defect Patent ductus arteriosus
	Blood flow from ventricles is obstructed	Coarctation of aorta Aortic stenosis Pulmonic stenosis
Cyanotic (cyanosis present)	Decrease in blood flow through pulmonary artery	Tetralogy of Fallot Tricuspid atresia
	Mixed blood flow (deoxygenated blood goes back out to the body without receiving oxygen from the lungs)	Transposition of great arteries Hypoplastic left heart syndrome

Wong, D. (1999). *Whaley & Wong's nursing care of infants and children* (6th ed.). St. Louis, MO: Mosby-Year Book.

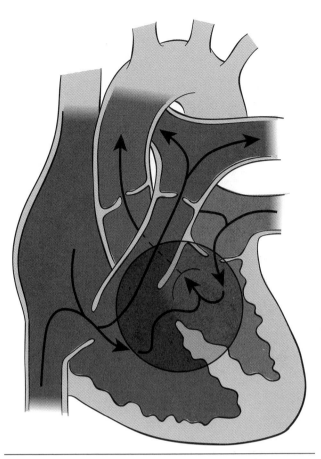

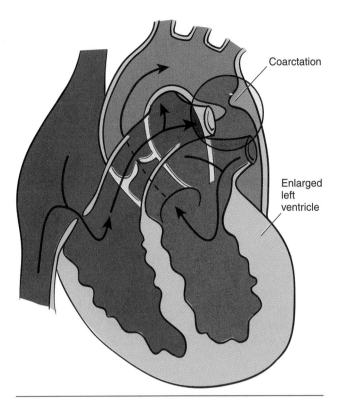

FIGURE 7-10 Coarctation of the aorta with an enlarged left ventricle.

FIGURE 7-9 In a child with a ventricular-septal defect, oxygenated blood (red) is pumped back into the right ventricle and mixes with unoxygenated blood (blue).

opening in the septum (e.g., ASD or VSD as previously described in Table 7-4) causes an increase in volume in the right ventricle because of the left-to-right shunt of blood (see Figure 7-9). Right-sided heart failure results. Coarctation of the aorta causes a higher pressure in the left ventricle because it has to push harder against a narrowed aorta (Figure 7-10). The left ventricle is then not able to pump an adequate amount of blood out to the systemic circulation (i.e., left-sided heart failure).

These children may already be on several medications to counteract congestive heart failure until the defects are surgically repaired. Digoxin (Lanoxin®) and furosemide (Lasix®) are routinely used. ACE inhibitors such as captopril (Capoten®) and enalapril (Vasotec®) are also used in pediatric patients.

Signs and Symptoms

Signs and symptoms of the child in congestive heart failure may include the following:

- Tachycardia (>160 beats/minute in sleeping infant)
- Tachypnea (>60 breaths/minute in infants)
- Dyspnea
- Costal retractions
- Diaphoresis (especially with exertion)
- Edema
- Distended neck veins (difficult to see in infants) and peripheral veins
- Cold extremities, weak pulses, slow capillary refill, hypotension, and mottled skin due to poor perfusion

Management

Treatment should be aimed at reducing respiratory distress and decreasing the cardiac demand. Provide oxygen and position the infant or child in a sitting position of at least 45° to maximize chest expansion. Make sure clothing and/or diapers do not restrict the chest. In younger children, ensure the abdomen is not restricted by clothing or straps from the stretcher. Use the cardiac monitor to document the heart rate and rhythm.

Tricks of the Trade

Limit stress on the infant or child to decrease cardiac demand. Allow a parent or family member to be present whenever possible. Allow the infant to use a pacifier, and explain procedures to older children to decrease their anxiety.

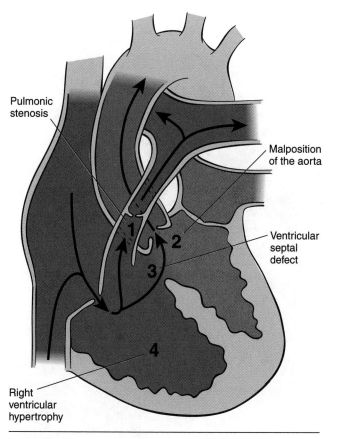

FIGURE 7-11 Tetralogy of Fallot.

One method of decreasing cardiac demand is to limit stress on the infant or child. Allow the parent or another familiar caregiver to be with the infant or child whenever possible. Allow the infant to suck on a pacifier to provide comfort. For an older child, explain what is being done to decrease the level of anxiety. Provide reassurance whenever possible.

Transport

Another strategy to decrease cardiac demand is to monitor the infant or child's temperature. Fever increases oxygen demands and increases the cardiac workload. If the child has a fever, remove extra clothing whenever possible and keep the ambulance cool in hot weather. A cold environment causes shivering and again increases the demand on the heart. Make sure the child is kept warm with blankets or increase the heat in the compartment of the ambulance during transport in cold weather.

Hypoxemia

Hypoxemia is a deficiency of oxygen in the arterial blood. **Hypoxia** is inadequate oxygen at the cellular level. **Cyanosis** is a blue discoloration of the skin, nail beds, and mucous membranes that occurs in the child with a reduction in oxygen saturation.

In children with congenital heart disease, cyanosis may occur from pulmonary stenosis that severely restricts blood flow through the pulmonary artery to the lungs. Blood shunting from the right side of the heart to the left side also causes cyanosis. Unoxygenated blood does not get to the lungs and is pumped back out into the body. **Tetralogy of Fallot** most commonly produces these problems (Figure 7-11).

In the child with transposition of the great vessels or arteries, blood that has been oxygenated goes to the lungs, and unoxygenated blood is pumped out to the body. Most newborns have another defect such as a **patent foramen ovale** (opening in the atrial septum that does not close after birth), a septal defect, or a patent ductus arteriosus that allows some oxygenation of the blood (Figure 7-12)

Children with chronic hypoxemia also develop **polycythemia** or increase in the number of red blood cells. The body tries to make more red blood cells to increase the oxygen-carrying capacity of the blood. These additional cells also make the blood thicker than usual and put the infant or child at risk for stroke.

Signs and Symptoms

Upon assessment, look carefully at the hands and feet. Many children will have clubbing from the ongoing hypoxemia and polycythemia. The tips of the fingers and toes become thickened and flattened (Figure 7-13).

Children with unrepaired tetralogy of Fallot will often squat in an attempt to relieve chronic hypoxia, especially during exercise or times of stress. This position reduces the return of deoxygenated blood from the legs and increases systemic vascular resistance, forcing more blood flow into the pulmonary artery. Placing an infant in a knee-chest position accomplishes the same hemodynamic benefits.

Infants with unrepaired tetralogy of Fallot may have **hypercyanotic** or "tet" spells because the heart is

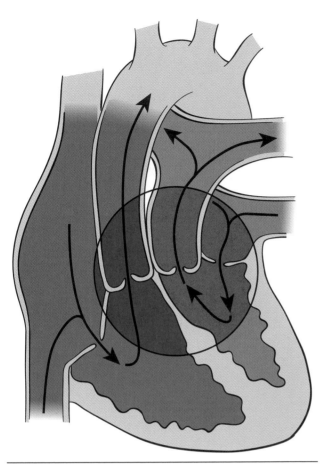

FIGURE 7-12 Patent Ductus Arteriosus (PDA).

unable to meet an increased need for oxygen. Acute cyanosis and rapid, shallow respirations occur which quickly lead to cerebral hypoxia if not treated quickly. This phenomenon is rarely present before two months of age, is most common during the first year of life, and

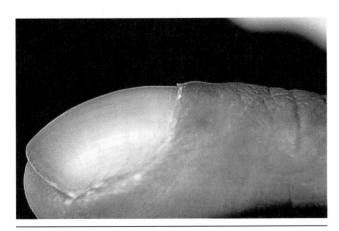

FIGURE 7-13 Clubbing of toes and fingers in child with congenital heart disease.

Parent Perspective

"All of the other children would be playing, and our son would be in the corner squatting. We kept asking him if he had to go potty! Here he was having trouble breathing and keeping up with everyone else."

—*Parents of a boy with tetratology of Fallot (had multiple surgeries to correct the defects; now grown with four children of his own!)*

occurs more often in the morning. Feeding, crying, or having a bowel movement may trigger a spell.

Children with ongoing hypoxemia may have significant adverse effects. Poor growth as well as delayed motor and cognitive development occur due to the lack of appropriate oxygenation of the brain and other related organs and tissues. Consider these factors during assessment and treatment.

Management

Treatment focuses on increasing oxygenation. Calm the infant as much as possible, utilizing family members whenever possible. Hold the infant with knees up against the chest, and provide supplemental oxygen via a nonrebreather face mask or blow-by method. Use of a pulse oximeter is beneficial to monitor the oxygen saturation. However, do not expect normal values in children with cyanotic heart disease. If these measures do not improve the respiratory status, assist ventilations and consider intubation. Also use a cardiac monitor to watch the baby's heart rate.

In an older child, allow him or her to squat during assessment and treatment if that position produces some relief. Provide oxygen with a nonrebreather face mask if the child will tolerate it. If not, use the blow-by method. Consider letting a parent or other familiar caregiver hold the oxygen to attempt to calm the child. Use electrocardiogram (EKG) monitoring to document the heart rate.

 Tricks of the Trade

In children with cyanotic heart disease, do not expect normal pulse oximetry values.

If the child's immediate past history includes sudden paralysis, altered speech (if old enough to talk), extreme irritability, extreme fatigue, or seizure activity, suspect a cerebrovascular accident or stroke. Provide airway and breathing support and transport for immediate evaluation. Carefully document all neurological changes as described by the family or bystanders.

Transport

Once on the stretcher, secure one strap around the child's waist without constricting the chest or abdomen. Allow the child to continue to have his or her knees up against the chest to promote comfort during transport.

If a stroke is suspected, document any neurological changes that occur during transport. Reassess the child frequently and notify the receiving facility. Diversion to a tertiary pediatric center may be necessary.

Exploring the Web

- Search the Internet for more information about children and congenital heart disease.

- Find ways that your organization can work with other community leaders to promote healthy lifestyles for children with congenital heart disease. Look for Web sites related to Kiwanis clubs, rotaries, not-for-profit organizations, parent support groups, etc. in your service area.

Hearing Impairment

Hearing impairment is the reduction in the ear's responsiveness to loudness and pitch. It can be mild to profound. **Deaf** indicates that the child could not hear before he or she learned to talk. **Hard of hearing** indicates the child has some hearing ability, generally with the use of a hearing aid. Several classifications exist depending on the location of the problem (Table 7-6).

Incidence

One of the most common disabilities in the United States, hearing impairment affects about 1 million children from birth to age 21. Approximately one-third of those children have additional disabilities such as cognitive or visual problems. An estimated 1 in 1,000 infants is born deaf, and the number of infants who are deaf rises to about 1 to 3 per 100 neonates admitted to a neonatal intensive care unit (Wong, 1999)

TABLE 7-6
Classifications of Hearing Loss

Conductive	• Related to problems of the outer or middle ear • Most common • Interference with loudness of sound
Sensorineural	• Result of problems with inner ear or auditory nerve • Also called *perceptive* or *nerve deafness* • Distortion of sound and problems with discrimination of sound (identifying one sound from another)
Mixed	• Combination of conductive and sensorineural • Interference with transmission of sound in the middle ear and along the neural pathways

Etiology

Hearing impairment can be present at birth or acquired as a result of infections, complications of prematurity, head trauma, **hyperbilirubinemia** (high bilirubin concentration in the bloodstream), or drugs that are toxic to the eighth cranial or auditory nerve or the organs of hearing and balance (e.g., aspirin, some antibiotics, furosemide, and quinine). Older children may suffer irreversible hearing loss from sounds loud enough to damage sensitive cells in the inner ear (Wong, 1999).

Signs and Symptoms

The child's level of hearing may range from total loss to a small decrease in the usual transmission of sound. Many children have difficulty with regular speech and language as a result of the hearing loss.

Some children with conductive hearing loss may wear a hearing aid that amplifies the sound, enabling them to hear. These devices may be worn in or behind the ear or be attached to a child's eyeglass frame. A whistling sound may occur if the aid is not properly fitted into the ear.

Children with sensorineural loss may have a surgically placed device or **cochlear implant** which converts sounds to electrical impulses and sends them directly to the auditory nerve. This process allows the brain to process the information and interpret the impulses as intelligible sounds.

Other children compensate for the loss by learning to read lips or use sign language. With lipreading, the child may only understand about 40 percent of the words spoken (Wong, 1999). Sign language using hand signals that relate to specific words and concepts requires much less concentration and is used quite effectively by many children, their families, and their significant others (i.e., friends, teachers, therapists, etc.).

Assessment

The child with a hearing impairment may be more frightened during an emergency due to the inability to communicate adequately. Try to determine the child's usual method of communication from the child's family, teachers, school nurse, etc.

If the child reads lips, face the child when speaking. Move down to the child's level so that your face and mouth can be clearly seen. Try to talk at a slow and even pace, and do not use large words or complicated language.

For a child who signs, use support people as translators. Remember that an injury to the upper extremities or hands may inhibit the child's ability to use signs to communicate.

Do not be tempted to shout at the child. Speak in a louder voice than usual if the child can hear louder sounds.

Regardless of the communication method, use gentle touch and a calm, reassuring manner to help the child adjust to the emergent situation. Establish eye contact and show you are interested in what the child is trying to say.

Management

Treat the emergent condition while maintaining communication as best as possible. Use parents and care-

Tricks of the Trade

Face the child who reads lips, and move down to eye level so that your face and mouth can be seen. Try to talk at a slow and even pace, and do not use large words or complicated language.

Exploring the Web

● Look for programs on the Internet that promote safety and integration into the community for children with hearing impairments.

givers to help prepare the child for potentially painful procedures (i.e., intravenous lines).

Transport

During transport, provide reassurance. Remember, the child with a hearing impairment may not be able to hear the siren or any of the commotion in the back of the ambulance. However, the reaction of the providers to certain situations is easily observed. A gentle touch and a simple "It's ok" (of course, only if the situation really *is* ok) in front of the face may help to keep the child calm during transport.

Muscular Dystrophy

Muscular dystrophy is a genetic muscle disorder that is usually progressive and disabling. Muscle fibers gradually degenerate causing muscle weakness and wasting, loss of strength, deformity, and increasing disability. Muscular dystrophies are the largest and most important group of muscular dysfunctions in childhood (Wallace et al., 1997; Wong, 1999).

Incidence

Duchenne muscular dystrophy (DMD) is the most common and occurs in approximately 1 in 3,500 live male births (Wong, 1999). Other types occur in 3 to 5 of 100,000 male births (Wallace et al., 1997). A gene defect in the X chromosome makes the disorder affect males almost exclusively.

Etiology

Duchenne muscular dystrophy begins in early childhood, usually between the ages of one and three. Its progression is rapid, and it ultimately involves all voluntary muscles. Most children die between the ages of 15 and 25.

Other types exist that usually develop after the age of eight years. They are slower in progression and do not usually cause death. They do, however, cause considerable disability as the child grows due to the progressive muscle weakening and wasting. Some children become completely incapacitated within 20 years of onset.

Signs and Symptoms

Most children require the use of a wheelchair by the ages of 12 to 14 and even earlier in Duchenne muscular dystrophy. Due to the decreased mobility, pulmonary compromise occurs leading to frequent infections and pneumonia. As the respiratory muscles weaken, children may require ventilatory assistance and then progress to full-time ventilator dependency. **Contractures** (flexion and fixation of a joint caused by atrophy and shortening of the muscle fibers) also occur from muscle disuse and weakness.

Airway compromise may be evident in older children because of the inability to clear the airway due to muscle weakness. The child requiring ongoing ventilatory support will have a tracheostomy (see Chapter 8—Children with Special Health Care Needs Assisted by Technology).

Assessment

Many of these children know that the disease is eventually going to make them completely dependent on others for all care and then kill them. They may be angry and resent ongoing medical treatments. They may be isolated socially due to the progression of the disease. Use care and compassion when responding to their questions and the concerns of their families.

Management

Contractures may make treatment and immobilization more difficult. Again, use care in moving the extremities; and do not force the child to conform to the equipment. Pad all open areas if the injuries require the use of a backboard.

Transport

Children with muscular dystrophy may already have a relationship with a certain hospital. Transport to that institution whenever possible.

Tricks of the Trade

Many children with muscular dystrophy know they are going to be completely dependent and then die. They may be angry and resent ongoing medical treatments. Use care and compassion when responding to their questions and the concerns of their families.

Exploring the Web

● Visit the Muscular Dystrophy Association of America, Inc. Web site to learn about the muscular dystrophy telethon and where it might be supported in your community.

Spina Bifida (Myelomeningocele)

Spina bifida is a neural tube defect that develops during the first 28 days of pregnancy. The spinal cord is usually encased in a protective sheath of bone and **meninges** (three membranes enclosing the brain and spinal cord—dura mater, pia mater, and the arachnoid). The **neural tube** (the tube that becomes the brain, spinal cord, and other neural tissue of the central nervous system) in the embryo fails to close and fuse thus leaving an open area for spinal tissue to protrude as the embryo grows.

A **myelomeningocele** (also called **meningomyelocele**) is synonymous with spina bifida and forms when the sac contains meninges, spinal fluid, and a portion of the spinal cord with nerves (Figures 7-14a and 7-15a). Other types of neural tube defects include a meningocele or encephalocele. A **meningocele** forms when the sac-like cyst contains meninges and cerebrospinal fluid (Figures 7-14b and 7-15b). This form is not usually associated with neurological deficits. An **encephalocele** forms when the brain and meninges herniate through a defect in the skull as a fluid-filled sac on the back of the neck (Figures 7-14c and 7-15c).

Incidence

Spina bifida occurs in approximately 1 in 1,000 live births, although the rate has been declining due to women of childbearing age taking folic acid before conception and during pregnancy. Female children and those of English and Irish descent are more susceptible to spina bifida. If other family members are affected, the chances are higher that an infant in the same family will be born with spina bifida (Wallace et al., 1997).

Myelomeningocele accounts for 90 percent of all spinal cord lesions. Approximately 90 to 95 percent of all children with myelomeningocele also have **hydrocephaly** or an accumulation of cerebrospinal fluid in the ventricles of the brain (Figure 7-16). Most children also have an Arnold-Chiari malformation as explained below (Wallace et al., 1997).

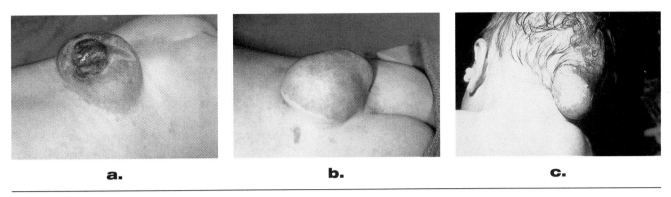

FIGURE 7-14   **a.** Myelomeningocele.   **b.** Meningocele.   **c.** Encephalocele.

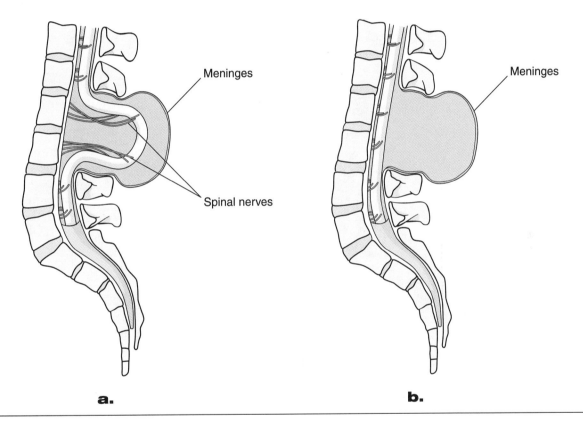

FIGURE 7-15   **a.** Illustration of mylelomeningocele.   **b.** Illustration of meningocele.

Etiology

Spina bifida is detected in utero or at birth and can occur anywhere along the spinal column. It is most common at the lumbar or lumbosacral area. The protruding area or sac may be covered by a thin membrane and leak cerebrospinal fluid or be covered by dura, meninges, and skin.

    With **Arnold-Chiari malformation (ACM)**, the child's small cerebellum, medulla, pons, and fourth ventricle herniate down through an enlarged foramen magnum (Figure 7-17). The flow of cerebrospinal fluid is obstructed resulting in hydrocephalus.

    The newborn undergoes neurosurgery within the first 24 to 72 hours after birth to repair the defect. This surgery helps to prevent infection and preserve as much neurological function as possible. A scar will be noticeable on the infant's back after the repair.

Signs and Symptoms

The nature and extent of any neurological impairment are determined by the location and magnitude of the defect. Below the level of the lesion, the child may lose voluntary muscle movement, sphincter control (causing

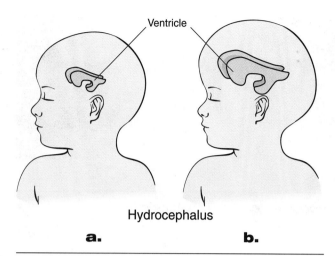

FIGURE 7-16 a. Brain with regular ventricles. **b.** Brain with hydrocephalus.

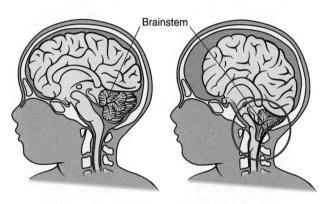

FIGURE 7-17 a. Brain in child without spina bifida. **b.** Brain with Arnold-Chiari malformation.

loss of bladder or bowel control), and skin sensation. In these situations, the child is not able to feel pressure or other sources of tissue injury (e.g., cold, heat, direct trauma, or irritation from braces). Pressure sores may develop, especially over bony prominences.

Most children have a surgical procedure in which a shunt is inserted into the ventricle of the brain to drain the fluid into another part of the body, most often the abdominal cavity or peritoneum. This shunt may be palpable behind one of the child's ears and feel like intravenous tubing underneath the skin. See Chapter 8—Children with Special Health Care Needs Assisted by Technology for information on shunts and potential problems.

Children with malfunctioning shunts will act as if they have sustained a head injury and may exhibit signs and symptoms of increased intracranial pressure. In tod-

dlers, for instance, headache and lack of appetite are the earliest signs of shunt failure.

Myelomeningocele is one of the most common causes of **neuropathic** (inflammation or degeneration of the peripheral nerves) or **neurogenic** (originating in the nervous system) bladder dysfunction in children. Urinary incontinence, stress incontinence, incomplete bladder emptying, and recurrent urinary tract infections are common. Many children as young as six years of age practice **clean intermittent catheterization (CIC)** in which they catheterize themselves at routine intervals to empty the bladder. Other children empty urine directly through a **vesicostomy** in which a stoma is created by bringing the anterior wall of the bladder to the abdominal wall. See more information on an ostomy in Chapter 8—Children with Special Health Care Needs Assisted by Technology.

Assessment

Pay close attention to any areas of decreased sensation. The child may have also injured the legs and not know that there has been an injury due to lack of feeling in the area. In any traumatic situation, assess the extremities to look for potential swelling and/or deformity even though the child does not complain of any pain in the area.

Ask the child how he or she moves from place to place. Some children are ambulatory with the assistance of braces or crutches. Other children are mobile through the use of a wheelchair.

Management

Once you know the child has spina bifida, assume that he or she also has an Arnold-Chiari malformation. Hyperextending the head may cause episodes of apnea due to pressure on the brain stem and cerebellum. Other complications include stridor and a hoarse cry from vocal cord paralysis during the hyperextension. *Avoid hyperextending the child's head for ANY airway maneuvers.* Use in-line stabilization, even though the child has not suffered any cervical trauma, to decrease the likelihood of apneic episodes.

 Safety Tip

- When treating the child with spina bifida, DO NOT hyperextend the child's head for ANY airway maneuvers. Hyperextension may cause episodes of apnea due to pressure on the brain stem and the cerebellum as a result of the Arnold-Chiari malformation.

Exploring the Web

● Search the Internet for more information about spina bifida. Search for the Web site of a local organization in your community that provides assistance to children with spina bifida. Make arrangements to visit the organization to interact with children who have spina bifida during a non-stressful time. Provide education about emergency medical services (EMS) and the types of equipment used to decrease the children's stress when an actual emergency does occur.

Transport

Children with spina bifida have usually undergone extensive medical and surgical management since birth. Whenever possible, transport the child to the facility that is currently managing his or her care. If that destination is not possible, contact the receiving facility during transport; and give them the name of the facility where the child receives the majority of care. Provide the name of the child's pediatrician, neurosurgeon, or other physicians so that personnel at the receiving hospital may make telephone contacts for additional information.

Visual Impairment

Visual impairment is a general term that refers to varying degrees of sight ranging from complete loss of sight (i.e., blindness) to blurred vision. Many children are able to use books with large print to continue in school.

Incidence

Approximately 1 in 4,000 children are blind and 1 in 20 have significant but less severe loss of sight. About 30 percent of children with multiple disabilities have visual defects (Wallace et al., 1997).

Etiology

There are many genetic, prenatal, and postnatal conditions that can cause visual impairment. See Table 7-7 for

TABLE 7-7
Causes of Visual Impairment

Genetic or inherited conditions	• Congenital cataracts • Chromosomal anomalies such as Down syndrome • Congenital infections such as rubella
Perinatal events (immediately after birth)	• Infections such as herpes, chlamydia, gonorrhea, rubella, syphilis, or toxoplasmosis • Retinal damage in premature infants (known as **retinopathy of prematurity**)
Postnatal events	• Trauma such as penetrating wounds or closed head injuries • Infection such as meningitis • Connective tissue diseases (e.g., Marfan syndrome) • **Strabismus** or misalignment of the eyes → may cause progressive loss of vision in one eye • Sickle cell disease • Juvenile rheumatoid arthritis • Tay-Sachs disease • Albinism • Retinoblastoma

Wallace et al., (1997). *Mosby's resource guide to children with disabilities and chronic illness*. St. Louis, MO: Mosby-Year Book; Wong, D. (1999). *Whaley & Wong's nursing care of infants and children* (6th ed.). St. Louis, MO: Mosby-Year Book.

examples. Some children may exhibit self-stimulating activity such as rocking, eye pressing, and light gazing. Others may have additional disabilities such as cerebral palsy, mental retardation, or hearing impairment.

Assessment

Children who cannot see for any reason may be very frightened during an emergency. Try to orient the child to what is happening and explain all procedures. As you touch the arm, tell the child that you are putting a cuff on the arm to measure blood pressure. The child may also be particularly sensitive to sounds and smells.

Management

It is again important to explain anything being done to the child since he or she cannot anticipate the treatment. For example, touch the child and explain how the intravenous line will be started in the left arm. Tell the child as you open the alcohol wipe since the child may be acutely aware of new smells.

Transport

The sound of the siren may be extremely loud because of the increased sensitivity to sounds. Reassure the child throughout transport as much as possible.

Exploring the Web

● Search the Internet for more information about visual impairments. Are there guidelines for communicating with a child who is blind?

CHRONIC ILLNESSES

Many children have chronic illnesses for which they receive ongoing treatment. Several of the more common illnesses are discussed below.

Asthma (Reactive Airways Disease)

Asthma is a chronic inflammatory disorder of the airways. It is discussed in detail in Chapter 4—Respiratory Emergencies.

Bronchopulmonary Dysplasia (BPD)

Bronchopulmonary dysplasia (BPD) is a chronic lung disease that occurs in the lungs of premature infants treated with positive-pressure ventilation and oxygen for respiratory distress syndrome. It is a pathologic process related to the therapies provided after birth.

Incidence

In the United States, BPD is the leading cause of chronic lung disease in infants (Jackson and Vessey, 1996). As more infants are born before 28 weeks of gestation and weigh less than 1,500 g survive, the incidence of BPD increases. Of those infants that survive respiratory distress syndrome, approximately 20 to 30 percent develop BPD (Wong, 1999).

Etiology

Respiratory distress syndrome is respiratory dysfunction that occurs in preterm infants because their lungs are not fully matured when they are born. It is also called **hyaline membrane disease**. At birth, the lungs are not ready to serve as efficient organs for gas exchange and need assistance in the form of high oxygen concentration, positive-pressure ventilation, and endotracheal intubation.

Other causes of BPD include:

- Meconium aspiration syndrome
- Persistent pulmonary hypertension
- Pneumonia
- Cyanotic heart disease

Damage and death occur at the local cellular level of the lungs from the oxygen and mechanical ventilation. The severity ranges from the child who needs bronchodilators and diuretics to treat pulmonary symptoms to the child who has a tracheostomy and is ventilator dependent at home.

Signs and Symptoms

Signs and symptoms of respiratory distress are common (see Chapter 4—Respiratory Emergencies). Pulmonary edema may occur because of increased lung permeability when the child is adequately hydrated. If fluids are then restricted, signs of dehydration may be present due to a restriction as well as the loss of large amounts of fluid through increased respiratory effort. These infants use a lot of energy just to breathe and they also tire very easily.

Infants with BPD may develop other problems as outlined in Table 7-8. These problems may precipitate an emergency situation for which EMS is requested. For instance, the child may have had an upper respiratory

---

TABLE 7-8
Ongoing Problems Associated with Bronchopulmonary Dysplasia

Airway complications	• Structural damage from endotracheal intubation and positive pressure ventilation • Loss of cilia → decreased cleansing ability of the lungs (may require daily chest physiotherapy and postural drainage)
Infections	• Increased during first year of life • Major cause of rehospitalization, late morbidity, and mortality
Poor growth and nutrition	• Fluid restrictions • Frequent respiratory infections • Elevated metabolic rate • Feeding disorders (as a result of negative oral stimuli such as suctioning and endotracheal intubation)
Gastroesophageal reflux	• Lower esophageal sphincter allows acidic gastric contents to move back into the esophagus • Symptoms include: emesis, apnea, bradycardia, recurrent pneumonia, delayed growth, and esophagitis
Cardiac conditions	• Occur because of chronic low PaO_2 and numerous hypoxic insults • Pulmonary hypertension leads to right ventricular hypertrophy and congestive heart failure
Neurodevelopmental conditions	• High risk for developmental delays • Hypotonia (low muscle tone), hypertonia (high muscle tone), and delayed motor development are most common in the first year of life. • Physical, cognitive, language, and sensorimotor skills can be affected
Seizures	• Occur due to hypoxic insults and intraventricular hemorrhages in the newborn period
Visual problems	• Retinopathy of prematurity • Blindness from severe hypoxia and severe intraventricular hemorrhage
Renal conditions	• Renal calcification due to chronic furosemide (Lasix®) therapy

---

Jackson, P., & Vessey, J. (1996). *Primary care of the child with a chronic condition.* St. Louis, MO: Mosby-Year Book.

infection that progressed to pneumonia. The child now needs treatment and transport because of increased respiratory distress.

Older children who have had BPD as an infant may exhibit the following:

• Growth failure
• Overall decreased pulmonary function
• Airway hyperreactivity
• Hyperexpansion of the lungs
• Increased incidence of respiratory infections
• Airway obstruction
• Lower bone mineral density (prone to fractures)
• Lower intelligence scores

Assessment

During assessment of the infant or child, the parent or caregiver may explain that the child was born prematurely. Ask if the child received any oxygen or ventilatory support after birth or if he or she was ever diagnosed with bronchopulmonary dysplasia. If the child usually has some form of stridor or retractions, ask if the current condition is more severe than usual.

If BPD was present and the child now requires aggressive airway management, pay particular attention to the structures of the airway when attempting resuscitation. Difficulty may be encountered during intubation because of structural damage during the early neonate period.

Most infants with BPD are discharged home once they begin to gain weight and their oxygen need is low. Since they have a low respiratory reserve, even a minor illness can be life threatening. Many parents are taught cardiopulmonary resuscitation and how to manage simple emergencies due to the high mortality rate during the first year of life.

If the child has a tracheostomy and is at home on a ventilator, get the settings and other pertinent information from the parents or other caregivers available in the home. They have become experts in this child's 24-hour care and must be considered as valuable members of the treatment team!

 Tricks of the Trade

Use the parents as additional resources for patient care. Remember, most of them have become experts at ventilating and suctioning their child's tracheostomy.

> ## Parent Perspective
>
> "The first few times my daughter had to be transported to the hospital by ambulance, we resented the EMTs almost pushing us out of the way to 'do their jobs.' They didn't realize that our 'jobs' were the everyday activities we performed to keep her alive WITHOUT their help!"
>
> —*Father of a child with a tracheostomy and multiple disabilities*

Infants with BPD often have delayed growth and development due to the problems associated with feeding and nutrition. Being in the hospital for long periods of time also deprives the infant of the usual sensory and physical stimulation necessary to develop properly. Parent-child bonding may also be negatively affected.

Management

Airway management and oxygenation are critical for infants with BPD. The use of a pulse oximeter and cardiac monitor may be helpful in managing the child's overall status. In addition, involve the parents or caregivers in the treatment whenever possible.

Transport

If the transport time will be longer than 10 to 15 minutes and the infant or child requires positive pressure ventilation, consider the use of a portable ventilator. A parent can also ride in the patient compartment to assist with ventilations if personnel resources are limited and a portable machine is not available. Remember, most parents become experts at ventilating and suctioning their child's tracheostomy.

Cancer

Cancer is clinically defined as a "neoplasm characterized by the uncontrolled growth of anaplastic cells that tend to invade surrounding tissue and metastasize to distant body sites" (Anderson, 1998). A **neoplasm** or tumor is an abnormal growth of new tissue that can be either benign (noncancerous) or malignant (cancerous). **Anaplastic** refers to a change in the structure or orientation of cells.

Incidence

In children ages 1 to 14 years, childhood cancer is the second leading cause of death and occurs in approximately 129 per million children. In all pediatric age groups, leukemia is the most common followed by brain tumors and lymphomas (Wong, 1999).

In blacks, tumors of the kidney and soft tissue are more common. In whites, tumors of the bone are more common. Young males have an increased risk for acute lymphoid leukemia, lymphoma, and medulloblastoma and are affected more often by cancer than females at a rate of 1.2:1 (Wong, 1999).

Most encouraging is that the prognosis for childhood cancer has improved over the last 30 years. A survival rate of more than five years is seen in approximately 70 percent of all children with malignant neoplasms who were treated at a major cancer center (Wong, 1999).

Etiology

Cancer occurs when the body is not able to regulate the production of cells. Abnormal cells develop, multiply, and spread. The cause is not known. If untreated, the host (infant or child, in this case) will die. Children with immune deficiencies from either a disease (e.g., acquired immunodeficiency syndrome [AIDS], discussed later in this chapter) or suppression of the immune system (e.g., after an organ transplant, discussed later in this chapter) are more prone to developing cancer.

Signs and Symptoms

Signs and symptoms vary based on the type of cancer and the location of the tumors. For instance, bone cancer may cause aching in the back if it is located in the spine or pain in the leg if the tumor is in the femur.

Children actively undergoing cancer treatment may also have specific signs and symptoms related to the drugs used for chemotherapy or the radiation used to shrink the tumor (Table 7-9). Nausea, vomiting, de-

creased appetite, hair loss, and burns to the skin from the radiation are common (Figure 7-18).

Assessment

Children being treated for cancer may be managed at home in between therapies. Complications can occur, however, that may require emergency care and immediate return to the hospital. Obtain baseline information as well as what changed or occurred that necessitated EMS intervention.

Children with cancer as well as their families need extra emotional support. Be supportive when asking questions and do not ask for more details than are necessary to manage the current emergency.

Many families use the hospice team so that the child can die at home. There are times, however, when family members may disagree about what is best for the child or simply cannot face the actual death as it approaches. EMS may be summoned to the house, yet the services may be refused. When assessing the situation,

---

TABLE 7-9
Types of Therapy for Childhood Cancer

Type	When Used	Side Effects
Surgery	• To obtain biopsy • To remove all traces of tumor and restore regular body function • Most successful when tumor is encapsulated and confined to the site of origin	• Depends on type of surgery performed • Example: removal of bone tumor may result in amputation of extremity
Chemotherapy	• May be primary form of treatment or used in combination with surgery and/or radiation therapy • Several drugs may be used in combination for minimum toxic effects and optimum cell cycle destruction • Many children have a central venous access device (see Chapter 8 Children with Special Health Care Needs Assisted by Technology) • Examples include: —Oncovin® (vincristine) —Adriamycin® (doxorubicin) —Cytoxan® (cyclophosphamide) —Corticosteroids	• Nausea and vomiting • Decreased appetite • Hair loss • Diarrhea • Local phlebitis • Bone marrow depression • Neurotoxicity (mostly from vincristine) • Fever; chills • General malaise • Constipation • Oral ulcers • Ulcers anywhere along the alimentary tract • Hemorrhagic cystitis (inflammation of the bladder) • Heart failure (Adriamycin® only) • Moon face and fluid retention from steroids • Allergic reactions

(continues)

TABLE 7-9
(Continued)

Type	When Used	Side Effects
Radiation therapy	• Usually used in conjunction with chemotherapy and/or surgery • Often used to relieve symptoms by shrinking the size of the tumor • High-dose radiation produces most serious side effects • Total body irradiation used to prepare the immune system for bone marrow transplantation	• Most effects are specific to the area undergoing radiation • Nausea and vomiting • Anorexia • Burns to skin • Hair loss • Ulcers along the gastrointestinal tract (e.g., esophagitis)
Bone marrow transplantation (BMT)	• Malignancies that are unlikely to be cured by other forms of treatment • Lethal doses of chemotherapy often combined with radiation are given to rid the body of all cancer cells • Previously stored cells from the patient or marrow or stem cells from a donor are infused intravenously back into the patient	• Suppression of immune system • Infections due to immune system suppression

Wong, D. (1999). *Whaley and Wong's nursing care of infants and children* (6th ed.). St. Louis, MO: Mosby-Year Book.

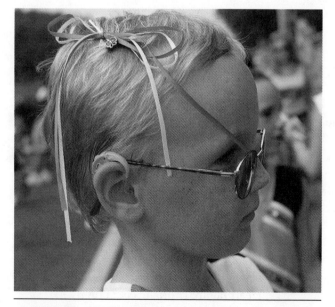

FIGURE 7-18 This child's hair is growing back after another round of chemotherapy.

Safety Tip

• If there is any confusion at the house regarding resuscitation of the child, make every effort to identify a parent or legal guardian who is responsible for making the decision. Whenever possible, ask for a written document if conflict continues. If in doubt, begin resuscitation.

identify the parents or legal guardians to receive information about possible resuscitation or Do Not Resuscitate orders. Try to get a written document if the disagreement is out of hand. If there is any doubt, begin resuscitation realizing that some of the family may be devastated with any attempts to prolong the child's death.

In other instances, the family may not feel comfortable at home and want the added support of the team of professionals at the hospital. EMS may be called to transport the child to the hospital to die.

Management

Support the child's airway, breathing, and circulation. Offer pain control without hesitation. Provide emotional support to the child and the family, but *do not* offer false hope.

Transport

Whenever possible, transport the child to the hospital that is providing the cancer treatment. The child and family will be most familiar with this facility and the personnel at the hospital will have all pertinent records on the child.

Complications

Several complications may occur from the cancer itself or the treatment used to try to fight it. Several examples are outlined below.

Superior Vena Cava Syndrome

Some lesions that occupy a specific space in the chest, such as those from Hodgkin's disease and non-Hodgkin's lymphoma, may cause **superior vena cava syndrome** as they enlarge. The mediastinal structures are compressed which causes airway compromise and possible respiratory failure.

Signs and Symptoms

The child will look like someone with traumatic asphyxia and have cyanosis of the face, neck, and upper chest. Dyspnea (from airway obstruction), upper extremity edema, and distended neck veins will also be present.

Management

Maintain a patent airway, provide high-concentration oxygen, and ventilate as necessary. Keep the child in an upright position to try to maximize respiratory effort.

Transport

Rapidly transport the child to the hospital. The child should be taken to a tertiary center with pediatric cardiovascular capabilities whenever possible.

Increased Intracranial Pressure

As brain tumors grow within the child's closed skull, intracranial pressure increases. This increase may be subtle and occur over a prolonged period of time. In some children, the tumor growth may cause bleeding and quickly produce increased pressure within the cranium related to the blood loss.

Signs and Symptoms

Signs and symptoms of increased intracranial pressure will be present (see Chapter 9—Head and Spinal Trauma). As the child's neurological status deteriorates, respiratory compromise may occur.

Management

Support the child's airway, provide high-concentration oxygen, and ventilate as necessary. If herniation of the brainstem occurs, the child may also become bradycardic and require cardiac resuscitation.

Transport

This child also requires rapid transport. The destination should be a tertiary facility with pediatric neurosurgical capabilities whenever possible.

Hyperleukocytosis

Hyperleukocytosis is a peripheral white blood cell count that becomes greater than 100,000 cells/mm. This massive production of white cells leads to capillary obstruction, small infarctions of the tissue, and organ dysfunction.

Signs and Symptoms

Children will be cyanotic with respiratory distress. Neurological changes include an altered level of consciousness, agitation, confusion, ataxia, delirium, and visual disturbances.

Management

Support the child's airway, breathing, and circulation. Provide high-concentration oxygen and ventilate as necessary. Intubation may be necessary especially if the child is unconscious.

Transport

This child will need rapid transport to the hospital. Treat ongoing respiratory distress while en route and continue to monitor the child's neurological status.

Acute Tumor Lysis Syndrome

During the initial treatment of some malignancies such as acute leukemia, intracellular metabolites are rapidly released causing a rise in serum potassium, a decrease in serum calcium, and possible renal failure. These changes are known as **acute tumor lysis syndrome**.

Signs and Symptoms

Children may complain of flank pain, nausea and vomiting, and itching. They may show an altered level of consciousness. The parent may state that the child has not wet any diapers that day.

Management

Provide high-concentration oxygen and assist ventilations as necessary. Start intravenous therapy of D₅W at a keep vein open (KVO) rate.

Transport

Make the child as comfortable as possible during the transport. Contact personnel at the receiving facility to inform them of the child's ongoing treatment for cancer. Whenever possible, transport the child to the hospital at which he or she has been treated for the malignancy.

Infections

Infections present an ongoing threat to children receiving treatment for cancer. Many of these children are immunosuppressed from the treatment and are at risk from even the smallest cold.

Signs and Symptoms

General signs and symptoms of infection include fever, chills, diaphoresis, tachycardia, decreased appetite, difficulty breathing if the lungs are involved, and possibly pain. Septic shock may be present if the infection has progressed without treatment (see Chapter 3—The Critically Ill Child for more information on septic shock).

Exploring the Web

● Search the Internet for additional information on children with cancer.

● Visit Web sites that support children with cancer and their families.

● The national Make-a-Wish Foundation grants wishes to children with life-threatening illnesses and has local chapters in many cities. Learn about their activities and see what you can do in your own community to support their efforts.

Management

Provide oxygen as necessary and start an intravenous line of normal saline or lactated Ringer's as needed for hydration and/or support of the child's circulation. If the child has a fever, remove clothing as appropriate (e.g., snowsuits on babies in the winter). Keep the child as comfortable as possible and provide reassurance.

Transport

If the child is in shock, immediate transport is necessary. Again, notify personnel at the receiving facility so appropriate specialists might be available.

Cystic Fibrosis

Cystic fibrosis (CF) is a condition in which the exocrine or mucus-producing gland does not function properly. The disease usually involves multiple systems throughout the body, is progressive, and is incurable. Examples of exocrine glands are the sebaceous glands and sweat glands.

Incidence

In white children, adolescents, and young adults, cystic fibrosis is the most common lethal genetic illness. It occurs in 1 in 3,500 white births, 1 in 11,500 Hispanic births, 1 in 14,000 black births, and 1 in 25,000 Asian births. Approximately 3.3 percent of whites in the United States are asymptomatic carriers. Individuals born with CF in the 1990s are expected to survive into their forties as compared to the median life expectancy of 7.5 years in 1966 (Wong, 1999).

Etiology

Cystic fibrosis is an inherited disease with the child receiving the defective gene from both parents. The mutated gene was discovered in 1989. Ongoing research continues to study the multisystem effects of CF on the body.

The disease has several unrelated features:

- Increased viscosity of mucous gland secretions
  —Progressive chronic obstructive lung disease associated with infection as mucus thickens and accumulates
  —Pancreatic enzyme deficiency occurs from duct blockage as mucus thickens and accumulates
- Sweat gland dysfunction → causes high sodium and chloride concentrations in the sweat
  —Present from birth throughout life → unrelated to severity of disease or extent of other organ involvement

- Increase in several constituents of saliva (sodium and chloride elevated)
- Abnormalities in autonomic nervous system function

Almost all children with CF have pulmonary complications, depending on the onset and extent of involvement. Mucus lies in the airways, bacteria colonize, and lung tissue is eventually destroyed. The thick mucus is difficult to remove and eventually obstructs the bronchi and bronchioles, causing areas of **atelectasis** (collapse of lung tissue preventing the exchange of carbon dioxide and oxygen) and **emphysema** (overinflation and destructive changes in alveolar walls causing a loss of lung elasticity and decreased gases). Drug-resistant infections develop from the stagnant mucus and are fatal in 20 percent of patients with mild to moderate CF (Wong, 1999).

The gastrointestinal tract involvement is variable, depending on the blockage of the pancreatic ducts. Pancreatic enzymes do not get to the duodenum so that digestion and absorption of nutrients are markedly impaired. Fats, proteins, and some carbohydrates are mainly affected. The child is usually given pancreatic enzymes with all meals and snacks to combat this problem.

Signs and Symptoms

Pulmonary symptoms include a dry, nonproductive cough and wheezing respirations. Dyspnea increases with bronchial and bronchiolar obstruction and the cough may become paroxysmal (severe attack of coughing). The child may have a barrel chest from the emphysema. Cyanosis and clubbing of the fingers and toes may also be seen due to significantly impaired gas exchange. Repeated episodes of bronchitis, bronchopneumonia, sinusitis, and nasal polyps are common. Pneumothorax may be seen in those children with more advanced disease.

Sometimes a bacterial infection of the airway will cause streaks of blood in the sputum of children with CF over 10 years of age. If the child has hemoptysis of more than 300 ml within a 24-hour period, the child needs to be treated at the hospital.

Affected children may not be able to maintain weight despite a healthy appetite and diet. Because of the pancreatic enzyme deficiency, nondigested food is excreted (mainly unabsorbed fats and protein). The infant may have large, loose stools or chronic diarrhea while older children have excessively large stools that leave both groups prone to dehydration.

Many of these children will have distended abdomens, thin extremities, and sallow skin with marked wasting of tissues. Fat-soluble vitamins such as A, D, E, and K are not absorbed which causes easy bruising. Anemia is also common.

Exploring the Web

- Search the Internet for more information on cystic fibrosis.

Assessment

Assessment of the child with CF will focus on the child's respiratory status. Regardless of the type of emergency, this infant or child may have respiratory compromise because of the underlying disease.

Once airway and breathing have been adequately assessed (and treated if life-threatening problems are discovered), move to the reason for the request for EMS (if another reason exists). Complete the assessment pertinent to the chief complaint.

Management

To treat chronic respiratory infections, intravenous antibiotics may be given at home through a central venous access device (see Chapter 8—Children with Special Health Care Needs Assisted by Technology for information on venous access devices). In addition, parents and caregivers maintain a twice daily regimen of chest physiotherapy and postural drainage to help loosen the secretions in the lungs and facilitate expectoration of the mucus. This therapy is increased when a pulmonary infection is present.

Provide oxygen as necessary during acute respiratory distress. In CF, the body is accustomed to chronic carbon dioxide retention so frequent monitoring is necessary. Start an intravenous line for fluid resuscitation according to local protocol.

Transport

Transport the child to the hospital for additional management. Reassess airway, breathing, and circulation en route; and provide adequate notice of arrival to the receiving hospital.

Epilepsy/Seizure Disorder

One of the most common complications in children with disabilities and chronic illnesses, especially those with a neurological focus, is the occurrence of seizures (see Chapter 6—Medical Emergencies for a full discussion of Epilepsy and Seizure Disorders). Ongoing seizures

Tricks of the Trade

Some children with uncontrolled seizures are on a special diet called the *ketogenic diet*. Only use normal saline solution (NSS) or lactated Ringer's (LR) as the IV fluid of choice since any dextrose products will throw the child out of ketosis and possibly cause breakthrough seizures.

become a chronic illness when they cannot be controlled despite aggressive medical and surgical interventions. The seizures interfere with the daily lives of the children and their families, affecting them at school as well as during leisure times. In addition, the child's growth and development may be adversely affected by the number of seizures as well as the side effects of multiple medications and/or surgical procedures.

Some children with uncontrolled seizures may be on the **ketogenic diet** if they have not responded to other conventional therapies. This diet is high in fat, low in carbohydrates, and low in protein. It is meticulously maintained by the parents, caregivers, school nurse, child care provider, and any other individual responsible for the child's care and feeding. The diet is thought to offer some seizure control through the ketosis that results from the breakdown of fat instead of glucose. *Children on this diet should not be given any glucose solutions either intravenously or orally.*

Exploring the Web

- Search the Web for more information on seizure disorders.

Hemophilia

Hemophilia is used to describe a group of hereditary bleeding disorders. One of the factors necessary for coagulation of the blood is deficient.

Incidence

In most cases, female carriers pass the disease on to their sons. One form, hemophilia A, involves a defi-

ciency of factor VIII and is known as classic hemophilia. This form is most common and accounts for approximately 75 percent of all cases. Hemophilia B or "Christmas disease" involves a deficiency of factor IX. Approximately 60 to 70 percent of children with hemophilia have the severe form (Wong, 1999).

Etiology

Prolonged bleeding can occur anywhere *from* the body or anywhere *inside* the body. In the severe form of the disorder, spontaneous bleeding occurs without any trauma. In the moderate form, bleeding occurs from direct trauma. In the mild form, bleeding only occurs with severe trauma or surgery. In children with hemophilia, the loss of a tooth or a slight fall or bruise may cause uncontrolled bleeding.

The primary long-term treatment is to replace the missing clotting factor. In fact, many children over ages two to three years receive home infusion therapy. Once the child reaches 8 to 12 years of age, he or she is taught to give the infusions.

Signs and Symptoms

Several areas of bleeding can be life threatening to the child. See Table 7-10 for signs and symptoms related to the site of bleeding.

Bleeding into joint cavities like the knees, ankles, and elbows is the most frequent type of internal bleeding. Over the long term, range of motion is decreased or lost in those joints most often affected. The child may know when bleeding is occurring into the joint as it will feel stiff, tingle, ache, and become increasing more difficult to move. Warmth, swelling, redness of the joint, and severe pain may also indicate bleeding.

Assessment

Children who were treated with blood and blood products before 1985 may have been exposed to HIV. Approximately 50 percent of those exposed are now human immunodeficiency virus (HIV) positive, and approximately 30 percent actually have acquired immunodeficiency syndrome (AIDS) (Wong, 1999). Use universal precautions if HIV or AIDS are suspected.

Treatment

During treatment, avoid giving any medication through the intramuscular route to minimize the potential for bleeding into the muscle. Substitute the subcutaneous route whenever possible. For blood samples, use a venipuncture instead of finger or heel punctures to again minimize ongoing bleeding. Treat other sites of bleeding as outlined in Table 7-11.

TABLE 7-10
Signs and Symptoms Related to Area of Bleeding

Site	Signs and Symptoms
Neck, mouth, or thorax	• Airway obstruction • Respiratory distress to respiratory arrest
Intracranial hemorrhage	• Signs and symptoms of increased intracranial pressure • Seizures • Decreased level of consciousness
Gastrointestinal tract	• Vomiting of blood • Anemia • Bloody diarrhea or stool
Retroperitoneal cavity	• Back pain or hypotension due to accumulation of large amount of blood in the retroperitoneal space
Around spinal cord	• Numbness • Tingling • Decreased sensation • Paralysis

Wong, D. (1999). *Whaley & Wong's nursing care of infants and children* (6th ed.). St. Louis, MO: Mosby-Year Book.

Transport

In most instances, rapid transport is necessary because of current or impending shock. Start the intravenous line during transport to minimize time wasted at the scene.

Safety Tip

• Avoid any intramuscular (IM) injections because of the risk of bleeding into the muscle. If blood needs to be collected, use a venipuncture instead of finger or heel punctures to minimize ongoing bleeding.

Exploring the Web

• Research hemophilia and learn more by viewing the National Hemophilia Foundation Web site.

Human Immunodeficiency Virus and Acquired Immunodeficiency Syndrome

Human immunodeficiency virus (HIV) is the virus that is the primary cause of **acquired immunodeficiency syndrome (AIDS)**. AIDS is a disease that involves a defect in cell-mediated immunity and is manifested by various opportunistic infections. It has a long and debilitating course as well as a poor prognosis.

Incidence

The first cases of AIDS were identified in adult homosexual males and intravenous drug users in the early 1980s. Currently, about 3.5 million women and more than 1 million children are infected with HIV throughout the world. Of those numbers, about 500,000 children have already developed AIDS. It is estimated that 7,000 infants are born in the United States each year to women infected with HIV. In 1995 in children ages one to four years of age, HIV infection was the sixth leading cause of death. During that same year in children ages 5

TABLE 7-11
Common Treatments for Bleeding in Children with Hemophilia

Site	Assessment Findings	Treatment
Neck, mouth, or thorax	• Airway obstruction • Respiratory distress to respiratory arrest	• Aggressive suctioning of oral cavity • High-concentration oxygen • Ventilations as necessary • Rapid transport • IV of LR or NSS en route
Intracranial hemorrhage	• Signs and symptoms of increased intracranial pressure • Seizures • Decreased level of consciousness • Major cause of death	• Provide patent airway and assist ventilations as necessary with high-concentration oxygen • Intubation as needed • Rapid transport • Frequent monitoring of neuro status
Gastrointestinal tract	• Vomiting of blood • Anemia • Bloody diarrhea or stool	• High-concentration oxygen • Intubation as needed • IV of LR or NSS at scene or en route depending on severity of bleeding or presence of hypovolemic shock • Rapid transport for shock
Retroperitoneal cavity	• Back pain or hypotension due to accumulation of large amount of blood in the retroperitoneal space	• High-concentration oxygen • Intubation as needed • IV of LR or NSS at scene or en route depending on severity of bleeding or presence of hypovolemic shock • Rapid transport for shock
Around spinal cord	• Numbness • Tingling • Decreased sensation • Paralysis	• High-concentration oxygen • Intubation as needed • Immobilize body as done for trauma patient • Treat for shock • Rapid transport

Wong, D. (1999). *Whaley & Wong's nursing care of infants and children* (6th ed.). St. Louis, MO: Mosby-Year Book.

to 14 years, HIV infection was the seventh leading cause of death (Wong., 1999).

Etiology

HIV is a retrovirus (any one of a family of ribonucleic acid [RNA] viruses containing the enzyme reverse transcriptase) and is transmitted through contact with an infected person's blood, semen, cervical secretions, cerebrospinal fluid, breast milk, or synovial fluid. It infects the T-helper cells of the immune system and results in an infection after an incubation period averaging ten years.

Children less than seven years of age represent the majority of children infected with HIV. These children were either born to mothers who were HIV positive, received infected blood products before HIV screening became mandatory in 1985, or were infected as adolescents after participating in high-risk behaviors. Through 1996, perinatal transmission was responsible for 90 percent of the cases of HIV infection in children (Centers for Disease Control and Prevention[CDC], 1999).

In children infected perinatally, about 20 percent develop AIDS during the first year of life and die by 4 years of age. The other 80 percent may not develop AIDS until they begin school or reach adolescence and survive to 5 years of age and greater (Wong, 1999).

Children are treated with **antiretroviral drugs** that prevent reproduction of new virus particles and slow the growth of HIV. Antibiotics are used prophylactically as well as to treat active infections with *Pneumocystis carinii* pneumonia, seen most frequently in infants between three and six months of age.

Signs and Symptoms

Most children with AIDS will have central nervous system problems and many of them are developmentally delayed. Motor skills, communication, and behavior are most commonly adversely affected. Children have more trouble expressing themselves through language than understanding what is spoken to them.

Assessment

The complications associated with HIV in children are potentially painful (Table 7-12). Assess the child for pain and follow local protocols regarding pain relief (e.g., nitrous oxide in older children to morphine sulfate intravenously). Remember that children who cannot speak or whose development is delayed may not be able to adequately express their true level of pain.

Management

Utilize universal precautions when in contact with any of the child's body fluids to prevent any spread of the virus. If accidentally exposed to blood or other body fluids, follow local protocols for testing and routine follow-up.

Use the same compassion for the child or family as appropriate for any ill or injured child. Be as supportive to the family as possible yet realistic about outcomes.

Sibling Sensitivies

"Thank you for treating my little brother so nicely when you came to school with the ambulance. I know that you were afraid of getting his HIV. Don't worry. I see him every day and I don't have it."

—*10-year-old sister of child with HIV*

TABLE 7-12
Causes of Pain in Children with HIV

Cause	Examples
Infections	• Middle ear infection leading to ear pain • Dental abscess leading to mouth and jaw pain • Pneumonia leading to chest pain
Encephalopathy	• Spasticity
Side effects of medications	• Peripheral neuropathy
Treatments	• Venipunctures • Lumbar punctures • Biopsies
Unknown sources	• Deep musculoskeletal pain
Other signs of pain	• Emotional detachment • Lack of interactive play • Irritability • Depression

Wong, D. (1999). *Whaley & Wong's nursing care of infants and children* (6th ed.). St. Louis, MO: Mosby-Year Book.

Limit the source of exposure to infections. Wear a mask if necessary to avoid spreading potentially infectious droplet nuclei to the child.

Transport

Provide rapid transport if the child's airway, breathing, or circulation are compromised. Most importantly, notify personnel at the receiving hospital without violating the patient's right to confidentiality.

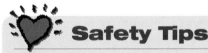 **Safety Tips**

• Use universal precautions when treating a child with HIV or AIDS. However, do not scare the child or treat him or her as an outcast.

Exploring the Web

● Search the Web for more information about pediatric HIV and AIDS. One source is the national Pediatric HIV Resource Center. What other sources can you find?

Transplants

The word **transplant** means to transfer an organ from one person to another or from one body part to another. Transplants are done to replace a diseased organ or structure, restore function, or change appearance.

Incidence

In 1998, 11 percent of all heart transplants in the United States were performed on children. Pediatric patients received 7 percent of all lung transplants, 19 percent of all heart-lung transplants, and 13 percent of all liver transplants (UNOS, 1999). The United Network for Organ Sharing (UNOS) estimates the following number of children were on waiting lists for transplants in 1998:

- 648 for kidney
- 854 for liver
- 267 for heart

Etiology

Organ transplants are performed in children that have life-threatening problems as the result of structural defects (e.g., birth anomalies) or organ failure. Renal, liver, and heart transplants are most commonly done in pediatric patients. The surgical procedure is complex and brings a lifelong list of additional complications.

In some children, two organs may be transplanted at one time. Examples are heart-liver, heart-lung, or liver-kidney. Congenital heart disease associated with end-stage pulmonary vascular disease and primary pulmonary hypertension is the most common reason for heart-lung transplants in children (Jackson & Vessey, 1996).

The most common complication after transplant is **immunosuppression**. Drugs are given to suppress or lessen the body's response to a foreign body (i.e., rejection of the transplanted organ). Cyclosporine is the most common anti-rejection drug given and has been used since 1981. Corticosteroids are also used.

Infection is a major cause of graft failure and death due to destruction of the organ tissue by bacteria, fungi, viruses, and protozoa (cause of *Pneumocystis*

carnii). In addition to preventing rejection of the transplanted organ, the suppressed immune system is unable to respond adequately to ordinary infections. Symptoms of the infection may not be obvious until the child is critically ill and the transplanted organ is at risk.

Rejection of the transplanted organ is also a serious complication. If acute, the rejection usually occurs within six months of the transplant and is reversible. A chronic rejection is much slower and can take from months to years to surface. The chronic form of rejection is the most common cause of late failure of the transplanted organ.

Signs and Symptoms

Signs and symptoms will depend on the etiology of the child's problem and subsequent transplant. For instance, corticosteriods are used to suppress the child's immune system so that it does not fight off the transplanted organ. Children on these drugs will have the characteristic "moon face" (Figure 7-19).

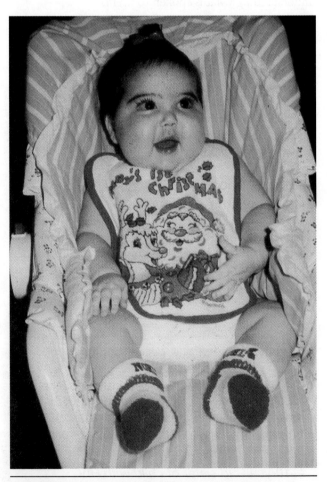

FIGURE 7-19 This infant is being given steroids. Notice the "moon face."

Other children will be seen because their bodies are actively rejecting the transplanted organ. Table 7-13 shows various signs and symptoms of organ rejections.

Assessment

Gather information from the child and the family regarding the transplant, when it occurred, what medications the child is currently taking, and what types of complications have been present in the past, if any. If rejection is present, the family may tell you the child is on the waiting list for another organ.

Providers should wear a mask if they have any illness because of the child's susceptibility to infection resulting from the immunosuppressant drugs. Even routine colds and flu can make these children extremely ill.

TABLE 7-13
Rejection of Transplanted Organs

Organ	Signs and Symptoms
Heart	• Symptoms of heart failure (dyspnea, jugular venous distention, swollen extremities) • Tachycardia • Cardiac dysrhythmias • Fever • Irritability • Poor feeding in infants
Liver	• Fever • Abdominal pain • Irritability • Lethargy and fatigue • Fluid retention
Kidney	• Fever • Swelling and tenderness over transplant area • Hypertension • Irritability • Lethargy and fatigue • Dark, concentrated urine or no urine output

Jackson, P., & Vessey, J. (1996). *Primary care of the child with a chronic condition*. St. Louis, MO: Mosby-Year Book.

Wong, D. (1999). *Whaley & Wong's nursing care of infants and children* (6th ed.). St. Louis, MO: Mosby-Year Book.

Exploring the Web

● Research the issue of transplants and organ availability.

● Research Web sites related to hospitals and organizations in your area to learn their policies about organ donation. Advocate for organ donation whenever possible.

Management

Provide oxygen, ventilations, and circulatory support as necessary. If rejection is occurring, provide treatment as outlined in Table 7-14.

Transport

In all instances of organ rejection, the child should be transported to a tertiary facility whenever possible. Ideally, the child should go to the center where the transplant was performed.

COGNITIVE IMPAIRMENTS

Cognitive refers to the mental processes of comprehension, judgment, memory, and reasoning. As a child develops cognitively, he or she becomes an intelligent person through the acquisition of knowledge and the ability to think, learn, reason, and abstract. **Cognitive impairment** is a general term that refers to any type of alteration in these previously mentioned processes. Several types are evident in children.

Mental Retardation

Mental retardation is defined by the American Association on Mental Retardation (AAMR) as a mental difficulty or deficiency that "has three components: subaverage intellectual functioning, deficits in adaptive behavior, and onset before 18 years of age." The child's intelligence quotient (IQ) is usually below 70, and the level of impairment can be mild to profound. Limitations must occur in two or more of the following areas:

• Communication
• Self-care
• Home living
• Social skills

TABLE 7-14
Treatment of Rejection of Transplanted Organs

Organ	Signs and Symptoms	Treatment
Heart	• Symptoms of heart failure (dyspnea, jugular venous distention, swollen extremities) • Tachycardia • Cardiac dysrhythmias • Fever • Irritability • Poor feeding in infants	• High-concentration oxygen • Cardiac monitoring • IV KVO • Transport to tertiary facility when possible
Liver	• Fever • Abdominal pain • Irritability • Lethargy and fatigue • Fluid retention	• High-concentration oxygen • Cardiac monitoring • IV KVO • Transport to tertiary facility when possible
Kidney	• Fever • Swelling and tenderness over transplant area • Hypertension • Irritability • Lethargy and fatigue • Dark, concentrated urine or no urine output	• High-concentration oxygen • Cardiac monitoring • IV KVO • Transport to tertiary facility when possible

• Leisure
• Health and safety
• Self-direction
• Functional academics
• Community use

The AAMR strongly emphasizes the positive things about individuals with mental retardation—abilities, environments, support, and empowerment. Children may need intermittent, limited, extensive, or complete support to participate in the usual activities of daily life. The overall goal is to help the child so that his or her ability to function will improve over time (AAMR, 1999).

Incidence

It is difficult to detect mental retardation at birth so that the incidence may actually be higher than the current estimate of 150,000 births per year. Approximately one

Parent Perspective

"Hearing the words 'mental retardation' used to make me cry for about the first five or six years of my daughter's life. 'Retardation' is such an ugly word. We heard it when she was first diagnosed as an infant and then saw it every year on all of her IEPs [individualized education plans] at school. A friend of mine used to call his dogs retarded, and the word would cut right through me. I prefer to think of her as 'developmentally delayed' even though I know her mental 'delay' is almost profound. It is still painful . . . even now . . . even after all of this time."

—*Mother of a 13-year-old child with multiple disabilities including severe "developmental delay"*

to three percent of all children are affected with the mild level found more in lower socioeconomic areas. Moderate to severe cases are evenly seen in all classes (Wallace et al., 1997).

Etiology

The cause of many cases of mental retardation is unknown. Severe mental retardation is more likely to have an identifiable etiology. In children in which the cause is known, it may have occurred before the baby was born, during the birth itself, or after the child was older. See Table 7-15 for specific causes.

Signs and Symptoms

There are no "classic" signs and symptoms of mental retardation as with many other conditions. The child can be classified, however, through his or her level of function as outlined in Table 7-16.

Assessment

Assess the child's abilities and level of understanding. Explain treatments and procedures in simple words that the child can follow.

Verbal skills are often delayed more than motor skills and can lead to problems with communication.

TABLE 7-15
Causes of Mental Retardation

Cause	Result	Examples
Infection and exposure to toxins	• Anything encountered that could cause abnormalities or malformations	• Rubella • Syphilis • Toxoplasmosis (by handling cat feces while pregnant) • Alcohol use by the mother during pregnancy leading to fetal alcohol syndrome • Drug intake by the mother during pregnancy • Exposure to industrial chemicals • Increased levels of lead in the blood (i.e., children eating lead-based paint) • Rh incompatability • Eclampsia during pregnancy
Trauma	• Any injury to the brain during pregnancy, during delivery, or after birth	• Physical injury (e.g., direct trauma to the abdomen during pregnancy resulting in fetal head injury) • Lack of oxygen • Exposure to radiation
Metabolism or nutrition	• Metabolic or endocrine disorders • Inadequate nutrition	• Congenital hypothyroidism • Phenylketonuria
Postnatal brain disease	• Skin eruptions • Lesions • Tumors	• Tuberous sclerosis • Neurofibromatosis • Infantile spasms • Severe cerebral palsy
Unknown prenatal influence	• Malformations	• Microcephaly • Hydrocephaly • Myelomeningocele

(continues)

TABLE 7-15
(Continued)

Cause	Result	Examples
Chromosome abnormality	• Radiation • Viruses • Chemicals • Parental age • Genetic mutations	• Down syndrome • Fragile X syndromes
Psychiatric disorders	• Onset during development	• Autism
Environmental	• Deprived environment • History of MR among parents and siblings	• Low socioeconomic areas may have limited educational opportunities, parenting skills, nutrition, etc.

Wong, D. (1999). *Whaley & Wong's nursing care of infants and children* (6th ed.). St. Louis, MO: Mosby-Year Book.

Abbreviations: MR, mental retardation.

TABLE 7-16
Classification of Mental Retardation

Level	Birth–5 Years (Preschool)	6–21 Years (School-Aged)
Mild (IQ of 50–75) • Also known as educable mentally retarded (EMR) • 85% of all people with mental retardation	• Slow to walk and feed self • Slower to talk • Not always noticeable to observers	• Can acquire practical skills • Can learn reading and math to a third- to sixth-grade level with special education • Can be guided toward social appropriateness • Achieves mental age of 8–12 years
Moderate (IQ of 35–50) • Also known as trainable mentally retarded (TMR) • 10% of all people with mental retardation	• Obvious delays in motor development and speech • Can learn self-help activities	• Can learn simple methods to communicate and simple manual skills • Can learn elementary health and safety habits • Does not progress in reading or math • Achieves mental age of three to seven years
Severe (IQ of 20–35)	• Large delay in motor development • Minimal to no communication skills • May respond to basic self-care training (e.g., feeding self)	• Usually walks if no other disability present to prohibit walking • Some understanding of speech; may have some response • Achieves mental age of toddler
Profound IQ below 20	• Gross delay • Requires total care	• Obvious delays in all developmental areas • Basic emotional response present • Needs close supervision • Achieves mental age of young infant

American Psychiatric Association. (1994). *Diagnostic and statistical manual of mental disorders (DSM-IV).* 4th ed.

Sibling Sensitivity

"Even though she is 13, someone always has to be with her to help her walk, feed her, give her medicine, change her diaper, and make sure she doesn't get hurt during her seizures. It is not the first thing that I talk about when I meet new people. I don't know how to even bring it up. I still love her and all, but sometimes it is embarrassing when she slobbers and makes noises."

—*16-year-old brother of child with multiple disabilities including severe mental retardation*

Some children do not speak at all. Alternate methods of communication may be used, depending on the child's cognitive level and physical abilities. Signing or a picture board where the child points to what is wanted can help the child to express needs. Some communication devices are computerized and produce a voice so that the child can "talk" in short phrases or sentences.

Management

The most important concept when treating a child with mental retardation is to have respect for what the child can do. Take a few extra minutes (if there is no life-threatening condition) to explain everything that is being done. Involve the family and caregivers whenever possible as they know the child best.

Transport

Explain the reason for transport in terms the child can understand. Also explain why the siren has to be on if it is used since it may frighten the child. Inform personnel at the receiving hospital that a social worker might be helpful for the family to provide assistance and ongoing support.

 Exploring the Web

- Research how far individuals with mental retardation have progressed over the years. What additional information can you find that may help you communicate and treat children with mental retardation?

Down Syndrome

Down syndrome (DS) is a congenital condition with varying degrees of mental retardation and other physical characteristics. It is also called **trisomy 21**.

Incidence

Down syndrome occurs in 1 in 800 to 1,000 live children born each year and is the most common chromosomal abnormality of a generalized syndrome. It is primarily linked with maternal age over 35 years. In women over 40 years, the incidence is as high as 1 in 100 live births. In women 30 years of age, the incidence drops to 1 in 1,500 live births. Despite these commonly known facts, the majority of infants with Down syndrome are born to women under the age of 35 (Wong, 1999).

Etiology

Although the exact cause of Down syndrome is not known, about 92 to 95 percent of all cases show an extra chromosome 21 in the child's DNA. The other name of trisomy 21 is based on the additional chromosome 21 (Wallace et al., 1997).

The most common congenital anomaly associated with Down syndrome is congenital heart disease. Approximately 30 to 40 percent of these children have various heart defects with septal defects being the most common. Respiratory infections are also common and, when combined with cardiac anomalies, are the chief cause of death during the first year of life (Wong, 1999).

Signs and Symptoms

Physical appearance of the child includes a flattened occiput, eyes that slant, depressed nasal bridge, low-set ears, and a large, protruding tongue (Figure 7-20). The infant is usually small with low muscle tone. The hands are short and broad with stubby fingers.

The older child will be short with weight gain more rapid than increases in height. By the age of three years, most children with Down syndrome are overweight. Growth of those children that also have mild to moderate congenital heart disease is more adversely affected.

Other problems include an altered immune system, chronic respiratory infections, visual problems, and abnormalities in tooth development. Acute leukemia is much more frequent than what is seen in children without Down syndrome.

Children with Down syndrome have large, protruding tongues that may interfere with airway maneuvers. Intubation may be particularly difficult due to problems visualizing the vocal cords because of the large tongue.

Sibling Sensitivity

A feather is magic!
It can help you make a wish.

I wish _my sister was not_

disabled

Then I would _be happy_

Ashley

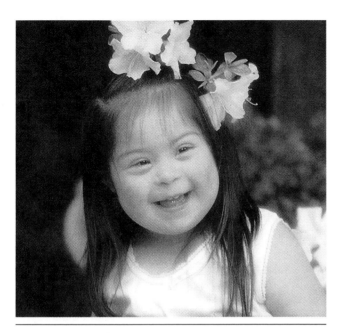

FIGURE 7-20 © Marijane Scott, Marijane's Designer Portraits, Down Right Beautiful 1996 Calendar. **Young girl with Down Syndrome.**

Assessment

The most significant feature of Down syndrome is mental retardation, which can be quite variable. The average IQ is 50 to 60 and might be related to parental intelligence. Many children do quite well, attend school in the local neighborhood, and can function somewhat independently in the community by early adulthood.

Management

About 15 to 20 percent of children with Down syndrome have **atlantoaxial instability**. The first two cervical vertebrae are unstable causing neck pain and weakness. These children are at risk for spinal cord compression during hyperextension of the head. Airway maneuvers should be done with the head and neck immobilized if the child is unconscious or awake enough to complain of neck pain or weakness even WITHOUT any evidence of cervical trauma.

 Tricks of the Trade

Just like the child with spina bifida, do not hyperextend the head of a child with Down syndrome. Spinal cord compression can result because of the atlantoaxial instability.

Transport

Whenever possible, transport the child to a tertiary center with pediatric cardiovascular capabilities if any cardiac concerns are present. If the child is being seen for a minor procedure (e.g., stitches or splinting of a broken finger), the local hospital should be adequate. Use good judgment when selecting the destination.

Fragile X Syndrome

Fragile X syndrome is a condition that causes cognitive impairment that can range from mild learning disabilities to severe mental retardation. It is the most common inherited cause of mental retardation and, after Down syndrome, is the second most common genetic cause of mental retardation (Jackson & Vessey, 1996).

Incidence

Fragile X syndrome affects 1 in 1,250 males and 1 in 2,000 females. In addition, 1 in 700 females are carriers. Its classification as a disorder is relatively new (Jackson & Vessey, 1996).

Etiology

The syndrome is caused by an abnormal gene on the X chromosome. Direct DNA analysis has been used since 1991 to identify both affected individuals as well as carriers.

Signs and Symptoms

Various physical and behavioral features are present. They include:

- Long, wide, and/or protruding ears
- Long, narrow face with prominent jaw
- High, arched palate → food may become wedged in palate, predisposing child to choking and possible airway obstruction
- Mitral valve prolapse
- Low muscle tone
- Mild to moderate mental retardation
- Speech delay; speech may be rapid with stuttering and repetition of words → allow child ample time to finish sentence; ask questions that only require one- and two-word answers
- Short attention span; hyperactivity
- Intolerance to change in routine; autistic-like behaviors
- May exhibit aggressive behaviors

TABLE 7-17
Treatment Considerations for Children with Fragile X Syndrome

Feature	Treatment Considerations
Long, narrow face with prominent jaw	Oral intubation may be more difficult.
Mitral valve prolapse	Monitor cardiac status.
Mild to moderate mental retardation	As described in text above
Short attention span; hyperactivity	• Be concise with treatment. • Allow child to participate in care as much as possible.
Intolerance to change in routine; autistic-like behaviors	See section on Autism
May exhibit aggressive behaviors	Ensure safety of child, emergency personnel, family, and bystanders

Wong, D. (1999). *Whaley & Wong's nursing care of infants and children* (6th ed.). St. Louis, MO: Mosby-Year Book.

Assessment

Approach the child with developmental delay or mental retardation as previously described. In children with aggressive behaviors, assess for potential escalation of frustration. End the questioning if possible before the child becomes highly agitated.

Management

Treat the airway, breathing, and circulation problems as usual. Monitor the child's respiratory and cardiac status. Several features may cause challenges in treatment as described in Table 7-17.

Transport

Be prepared to use restraints during transport if the child displays any aggressive behavior. Explain the reason for transport in terms the child can understand.

BEHAVIORAL DISABILITIES

Behavioral disabilities will affect the manner in which the child interacts with people and things in his or her surroundings. The most common disabilities are outlined as follows.

Attention Deficit Hyperactivity Disorder (ADHD)

Attention deficit hyperactivity disorder (ADHD) is defined by the American Psychiatric Association as a "persistent pattern of inattention and/or hyperactivity-impulsivity that is more frequent and severe than is typically observed in individuals at a comparable level of development" (APA, 1994). Some of the hyperactive and impulsive behaviors must have been present before the age of seven years and have occurred for at least six months. **Attention deficit disorder without hyperactivity** (ADD-H) refers to children who have deficits in their attention spans but no hyperactivity.

Incidence

Approximately three to five percent of school-age children have ADHD, and boys are diagnosed three times more often than girls (Wong, 1999). Some girls may be less aggressive or hyperactive and therefore not be diagnosed as often.

Etiology

Most cases of ADHD do not have an identifiable cause. Contrary to the popular notion of sugar or food additives causing ADHD, no research has demonstrated any relationship. Diet as a factor remains controversial since some children do show improvement when certain foods are eliminated from their diets.

Signs and Symptoms

Children with ADHD have great difficulty with sustained attention, impulse control, and motor activity. Their behavior is not appropriate for their particular age; and their performance at school, home, or a child care facility is adversely affected.

In an emergency, these children may not be able to concentrate on the situation at hand. They may not be able to answer questions during the assessment phase and may be easily distracted by extraneous stimuli (e.g., flashing lights of ambulance, medical equipment, badge on shirt, etc.).

Assessment

Approach the child from the front in a slow, methodical manner. Do not abruptly change positions or make sudden movements that may frighten the child any more than he or she is already frightened. Ask simple questions that can be answered without elaborate explanations.

Treatment

Redirect the child's attention as much as possible. Explain procedures and treatments repeatedly if the child asks. Utilize the parents or caregivers to help reassure the child.

Transport

Explain the transport to decrease anxiety. Make sure the child is adequately restrained on the stretcher so that the child is not able to harm himself or herself or the other prehospital providers.

Autism

Autism is a complex disorder that is usually detected within the first 30 months of life. It is a pervasive developmental disorder in which the child has deficient social interaction, impaired communication, and a limited range of play interests and activities (Wallace et al., 1997).

Incidence

Autism occurs in 1 in 2,500 children and is approximately 4 times more common in males than in females. Females, however, are more severely affected. Race, socioeconomic level, and parenting style do not affect the incidence (Wallace et al., 1997).

Etiology

In many cases, the actual cause of autism is unknown. It does occur sometimes with other syndromes or diseases such as fragile X syndrome, tuberous sclerosis, or congenital rubella. It is more common in brothers and sisters of children already affected. Some children also have a history of difficulty during the prenatal or perinatal period.

Most children with autism require lifelong adult supervision, and it is usually a severely disabling condition. Those children with an IQ of at least 50 who were able to communicate through speech by age 6 before diagnosis seem to respond most favorably to intervention and education.

Signs and Symptoms

The most common characteristic of autism is the inability of the child to maintain eye contact with another person. Infants may not want to be cuddled and may show minimal social imitation. Toddlers and older children may seem completely unaware of other children and not pay any attention to them. Approximately half of all children with autism are nonverbal. These children also do not adapt well to any change in their routines.

Examples of repetitive behaviors include rocking, spinning in circles, flipping a light switch, and lining up toys over and over again. Some children may speak but only use words to repeat what another person said or what may have been heard in the recent past (e.g., something on the radio or television).

Assessment

Ask the parents or caregivers how the child best responds to emergency situations or strangers. Unless the child is unconscious, he or she will probably be uncooperative and quite frightened. Speak in a soft tone, and use people with whom the child may be familiar whenever possible.

Management

Explain all treatments to the child and the family. Be prepared for the child to resist touch.

Transport

Consider sedation for safety during transport as necessary per local protocol. Discuss transport and possible sedation with the family whenever possible.

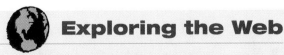

Exploring the Web

● Learn more about autism and what can be done to support individuals with autism.

SUMMARY

Due to increased survival rates from life-threatening illness and injury, more children with special health care needs are being integrated into the communities and schools where they live. Prehospital providers will encounter these children as they become ill and injured or need additional medical care at the hospital for their existing conditions.

Education about the unique characteristics of children with special health care needs before an emergency will greatly benefit the prehospital provider. In addition, interaction with these children whenever possible will contribute to the provider's skills and confidence when called to render assistance.

Management of Case Scenario

Your partner gets information from the director of the center while you start the assessment. The child is having very small, intermittent, jerking movements of her arms only; and she looks like she is sleeping. Her airway is patent with some saliva down the side of her face. She is breathing deeply at 12 times per minute, and breath sounds are clear in all fields.

There is blood coming from a laceration on the bottom of her chin. Bleeding was controlled by the teacher with a clean towel. The laceration is about 3 cm long and will probably need some stitches. No other sites of bleeding are noted. You put 4 × 4's on the child's chin, and ask the teacher to continue to hold some light pressure against the wound.

The child's skin is pink and warm to the touch. Her hands are diaphoretic and slightly purple. Pupils are 6 mm, sluggishly reactive to light, and equal in size. Heart rate is rapid and regular at 140. Blood pressure is 122/78. No other injuries are found. The remainder of the exam in unremarkable.

You speak to the patient's sibling who tells you that her sister cannot talk or walk by herself. She also tells you that her sister has seizures every day. You ask the little girl to sit beside you and hold her big sister's hand so she might feel better when she wakes up.

Your partner shows you an emergency form completed by the child's parents with all of the necessary information. The mother has requested that her daughter be transported to the Emergency Department a few miles away. She will meet you at the hospital.

You secure the pressure dressing with some tape, and move the child to the stretcher. As you apply oxygen via a face mask, the child begins to wake up. She pulls off the mask and begins to cry. You ask the little sister to help you comfort her big sister while your partner continues preparing the child for transport.

As you go out the door, you allow the little sister to give her big sister a kiss on the cheek. "Tell her you will see her when she gets home," you say.

During transport, you switch to a nasal cannula as the child continues to awaken. She is content and begins to look around the back of the ambulance. Per her parents' information sheet, you notice that the child's baseline neurological status includes the inability to squeeze your hands (even before the long seizure). Repeat vitals are within normal limits, her pupil size has reduced to 2 mm, and they are reactive to light. You notify the receiving hospital and provide an updated report on arrival.

► REVIEW QUESTIONS

1. Define *children with special health care needs.*

2. Name the document that standardizes information that would be helpful to emergency personnel inside and outside of the hospital setting.

3. Who developed the document described above?

4. Define the following terms:
   a. Amputation
   b. Congenital amputation
   c. Acquired amputation

5. Phantom limb pain is not very common after amputation. True or False?

6. Define cerebral palsy.

7. Name two factors that may make airway control difficult in the child with cerebral palsy.

8. What is the best procedure to use when immobilizing a child with cerebral palsy who has contractures?

   a. No special accommodations are necessary.

   b. Straighten one arm as much as possible to strap it to the long backboard.

   c. Pad the open areas to support the body as much as possible.

   d. Pull apart the legs so that each one fits tightly against the long backboard.

9. Define cleft lip and cleft palate.

10. A child with a surgically repaired cleft palate should not be intubated. True or False?

11. Define congenital heart disease.

12. Congenital heart disease can be classified as _____ and _____. List characteristics of each type and give two examples of each.

13. Explain why congestive heart failure occurs in infants and children with congenital heart disease.

14. List two strategies to decrease cardiac demand for an infant.

15. Differentiate between hypoxemia, hypoxia, and cyanosis.

16. What is the classic position used by children with an unrepaired tetralogy of Fallot in an attempt to relieve chronic hypoxia, especially during exercise or times of stress? Explain the physiology. What position can be used in an infant?

17. Define the following terms: hearing impairment, deaf, and hard of hearing.

18. A cochlear implant converts electrical impulses into sound so the child can hear. True or False?

19. Define muscular dystrophy.

20. Why does airway compromise occur in older children with muscular dystrophy?

21. Define the following terms: spina bifida, neural tube, hydrocephalus, Arnold-Chiari malformation, myelomeningocele, meningocele, and encephalocele.

22. To obtain the best position for intubation in a child with spina bifida, hyperextend the neck before inserting the laryngoscope. True or False?

23. List five items that contain latex.

24. Define visual impairment.

25. Define bronchopulmonary dysplasia and explain how it occurs.

26. Airway complications may occur in the infant with BPD because of structural damage related to early endotracheal intubation and positive pressure intubation. True or False?

27. Define cancer, neoplasm, and anaplastic.

28. Name the syndrome that occurs in children with cancerous lesions in the chest as they enlarge. List the signs and symptoms.

29. When treating a child undergoing chemotherapy, the prehospital provider should wear a mask if she or he has any cold symptoms. True or False?

30. Define cystic fibrosis and list two pulmonary complications from CF.

31. Define hemophilia.

32. Name the most frequent type of internal bleeding for a child with hemophilia.

33. To minimize bleeding, finger or heel sticks should be used to collect blood from children with hemophilia. True or False?

REFERENCES

American College of Emergency Physicians. (2000). *Emergency Information Form for Children with Special Needs*. ACEP OnLine.

Anderson, K., Anderson, L., & Glanze, W. (1998). *Mosby's medical, nursing, & allied health dictionary*. St. Louis, MO: Mosby-Year Book.

Centers for Disease Control and Prevention (1999).

Developmental Disabilities Assistance and Bill of Rights Act as amended June 8, 1994; Department of Health and Human Services, Administration for Children and Families: Administration on Developmental Disabilities.

McPherson, M. (1998) A new definition of children with special health care needs. *Pediatrics, 102 (1),* 137–139.

U. S. Department of Health and Human Services, Health Resources and Services Administration, Office of Special Programs, Division of Transplantation. (1999). *1999 Annual Report of the U. S. Scientific Registry for Transplant Recipients and the Organ Procurement and Transplantation Network: Transplant data: 1989–1998.* Rockville, MD.

Wallace, H., Biehl, R., MacQueen, J., & Blackman, J. (1997). *Mosby's resource guide to children with disabilities and chronic illness*. St. Louis, MO: Mosby-Year Book.

Wong, D. (1999). *Whaley and Wong's nursing care of infants and children* (6th ed.). St. Louis, MO: Mosby-Year Book.

▶ BIBLIOGRAPHY

American Academy of Pediatrics, Committee on Pediatric Emergency Medicine (1999). Emergency preparedness for children with special health care needs. *Pediatrics, 104 (4),* 53.

Estes, M. E. Z. (1998). *Health assessment and physical examination.* Albany, NY: Delmar Thomson Learning.

Jackson, P. L., & Vessey, J. A. (1996). *Primary care of the child with a chronic condition.* St. Louis, MO: Mosby-Year Book.

Krajicek, Marilyn J. (1998). *Instructor guide for the care of infants, toddlers, and young children with disabilities and chronic conditions.* Austin, TX: PRO-ED.

Maternal and Child Health Bureau, Health Resources and Services Administration, U. S. Department of Health and Human Services (2000). Press Release—National center established to improve care for children with special needs.

Mitchell, N. A. (1997). Innovative informations: Latex allergy—accessing information on the Internet. *Journal of Emergency Nursing, 32 (1),* 51–52.

National Association of EMTs. (1998). *Prehospital trauma life support.* St. Louis, MO: Mosby-Year Book, Inc.

Porter, S., Haynie, M., Bierke, T., Caldwell, T.H. & Palfrey, J.S., (1997). *Children and youth assisted by medical technology in educational settings.* Baltimore, MD: Paul H. Brookes Publishing Company.

Wertz, E. (2000). Children with special health care needs. In L. Bernardo and D. Thomas, (Eds.), *Core curriculum for pediatric emergency nursing.* Des Plaines, IL: Roadrunner Press.

Wertz, E. (1997). The patient with special needs. *The basic EMT—comprehensive prehospital patient care.* St. Louis, MO: Mosby-Year Book.

Wertz, E. (1997b). Pediatric Emergencies. In *Mosby's EMT—intermediate textbook.* St. Louis, MO: Mosby-Year Book. 484–517.

Chapter 8

Children with Special Health Care Needs Assisted by Technology

OBJECTIVES

Upon completion of this chapter, the student should be able to:

- Identify two indications for a tracheostomy in an infant or child.
- List three causes of tracheostomy obstruction.
- List three types of tracheostomy tubes.
- Describe the treatment of a child with a tracheostomy.
- Describe the assessment of a child using a mechanical ventilator.
- List three reasons for a central venous access device.
- Identify at least two types of central venous access devices used in children with special health care needs.
- List two types of artificial pacemakers.
- Describe the vagus nerve stimulator and assessment findings related to the device.
- List two types of feeding tubes used in children.
- State the procedure for treating a dislodged feeding tube that was originally surgically placed.
- Identify signs and symptoms related to a child with a malfunctioning shunt.
- Define the following terms: stoma, colostomy, and urostomy.

KEY TERMS

air embolism	dermatitis	granulation	jejunostomy tube
cellulitis	dislodgement	ileostomy	lead
cerebrospinal fluid (CSF)	epicardial	intracranial pressure	lumen
colostomy	fenestrations	(ICP)	multilumen
continuous positive airway	fungal infection	intractable	nasogastric tube
pressure (CPAP)	gastrostomy	jejunum	nasojejunal tube

negative-pressure ventilation

obturator

orogastric tube

orojejunal tube

percutaneous endoscopic gastrostomy (PEG) or button

positive-pressure ventilation

pulse generator

shunt

stoma

tracheostomy

transvenous

urostomy

vagus nerve stimulator (VNS)

ventricular-septal defect (VSD)

ventriculoatrial shunt (VA shunt)

ventriculoperitoneal shunt (VP shunt)

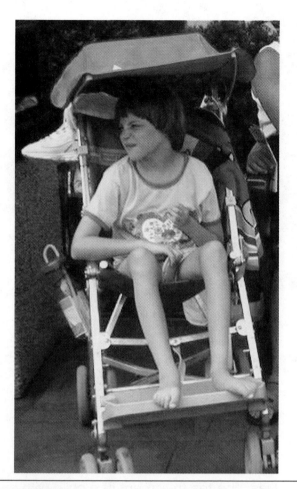

FIGURE 8-1 This child has special health care needs and uses assistive technology to live at home and in the community.

Case Scenario

You are dispatched at 10 a.m. to an elementary school for a child with difficulty breathing. When you arrive, you find a seven-year-old boy with a tracheostomy sitting in a wheelchair. You hear gurgling from his tracheostomy site and notice his tube is connected to a portable ventilator on the back of his chair. The school nurse tells you she is substituting for the regular school nurse and does not have much experience with children who are ventilator dependent. Jimmy seemed to be having trouble breathing, and she was not sure what to do so she called for the ambulance. How would you approach the assessment of this child?

tion, central intravenous catheters, pacemakers, vagus nerve stimulators, feeding tubes, shunts, and ostomies.

It is important for EMS providers to become familiar with the special medical needs of these children. Familiarity with the details of their specialized types of equipment and the unique types of intervention required can be lifesaving.

GENERAL APPROACH

When one encounters a child with special health care needs assisted by technology, it is natural to feel overwhelmed by the complexity of the situation and the associated equipment. However, the same management goals and approaches are maintained. It is helpful to remember that the parents or other caregivers have a wealth of information about these children and most likely have performed some intervention prior to arrival of prehospital personnel.

INTRODUCTION

Children assisted by technology represent a growing segment of the pediatric population (Figure 8-1). Up to one quarter of pediatric Emergency Department (ED) visits are related to complaints associated with chronic illness (see Chapter 7—Children with Special Health Care Needs—Chronic Conditions). This increase is due to the larger number of children being discharged from intensive care nurseries and pediatric intensive care units. Numerous children are now managed in the home, utilizing private duty nursing and significant parental involvement. Forms of technology discussed in this chapter include tracheostomies, mechanical ventila-

Tricks of the Trade

Ask the parents or other caregivers about a concise form with emergency information. If one is not currently used, provide a copy of the Emergency Information Form and encourage them to work with the child's pediatrician to finalize the information for future requests for assistance.

History taking in this population may be challenging due to things like developmental delay, communication difficulties, and the long list of previous treatments, surgeries, and/or medications. Growing numbers of children with special health care needs have computerized or paper-based histories in their local Emergency Departments, or parents and nurses in the home may provide a concise summary of the child's complex history (see Emergency Information Form in Chapter 7—Children with Special Health Care Needs).

Physical assessment can also be difficult due to the complexity of the equipment and the multifaceted nature of the disease entities. Vital signs and mental status may differ significantly from other children of the same chronological age.

Exploring the Web

● What sites can you find related to children with special health care needs who use specialized technology?

● Explore the Emergency Medical Services for Children (EMSC) Web site.

● Review sites that pertain to specific equipment.

● What professional organizations or journals could you search for information on children with special health care needs assisted by technology?

TRACHEOSTOMIES

Some children may breathe through a **tracheostomy** or **stoma** as it may also be called (Figure 8-2). A stoma is a surgically created opening. A tracheostomy is a surgical

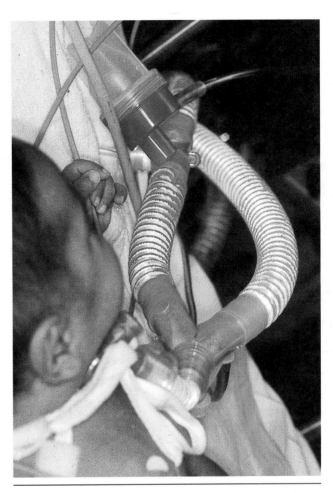

FIGURE 8-2 This child breathes with the assistance of a tracheostomy.

opening into the trachea on the front of the neck. A tracheostomy tube is then inserted into the opening to provide an artificial airway. Breathing then occurs either partially or completely through this airway.

Etiology

Children may require a tracheostomy for reasons outlined below:

● Need for long-term mechanical ventilator support (e.g., a child with a head injury who is unconscious for a prolonged period or unable to breathe independently)

● Muscular or neurological disease or injury (e.g., paralysis)

● Need for assistance with removal of secretions from the trachea (e.g., children with cerebral palsy may not be physically able to cough up secretions due to muscle weakness)

Equipment Overview

Tubes that fit into the tracheostomy are available in many different types and sizes depending on the manufacturer. In most situations, the family or primary caregiver will have extra tubes available in case of emergency. Whenever possible, the same size and type of tube should be used for replacement (Table 8-1).

The opening of the tube is usually compatible with a bag-valve device. This device, therefore, can be connected directly to the tracheostomy tube to ventilate the child. If the bag-valve device does not fit, ask if an adapter is available.

All tubes include an **obturator** or a rigid guide inside the tube to help with insertion. Think of it as a device similar to a stylet used for endotracheal intubation. The obturator keeps the tracheostomy tube rigid and is removed after the tube is inserted into the stoma. It may also be helpful during an emergency to help clear secretions that are obstructing the tube.

Tracheostomy tubes are available with or without cuffs except for the neonatal size. No cuffs are used for neonates because the pliable trachea seals around the tube. Cuffed tubes are primarily used in adults although they may be used in children to reduce an air leak or help reduce aspiration for a child who cannot adequately protect his or her airway. In cuffed tubes, the cuff is inflated with air or sometimes foam to create a seal in the trachea so air flow through the mouth and nose is reduced or eliminated.

The tracheostomy tube is usually secured around the child's neck with cloth ties made of material that is durable and will not fray. Ties with self-adhering clo-sures are also available and are more popular since they cause less skin breakdown. These ties are changed daily or when soiled. When in place, they should be snug around the neck yet allow at least one finger to be inserted between the neck and the ties (Figure 8-3).

Single Lumen or Cannula

One hollow tube is used for breathing and suction of secretions. They are available with and without cuffs and look similar to a short endotracheal tube. The most common tubes used for infants and children are uncuffed, single lumen tubes (Figure 8-4).

Double Lumen or Cannula

The hollow, outer tube is like the single lumen tube. The second tube is a removable inner cannula that can be taken out for cleaning (Figure 8-5). The outer tube stays

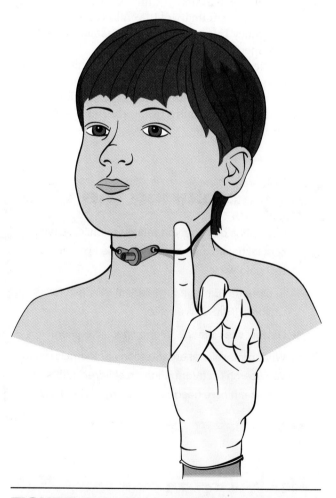

FIGURE 8-3 The tracheostomy ties should be snug around the child's neck yet allow one finger to be inserted between the ties and the neck to minimize neck irritation.

TABLE 8-1
Tracheostomy Tube Sizes

Age	Tube Size
Neonatal (newly borns and infants up to six months of age)	2.5–4.0 mm
Pediatric (for children 6 months–10 years of age)	3.5–5.5 mm
Adult (for children over 10 years of age)	5.5–10 mm

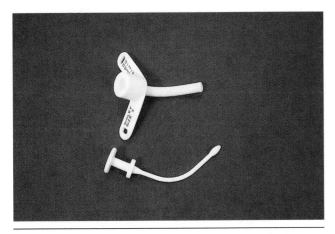

FIGURE 8-4 Single lumen, uncuffed tracheostomy tubes are most commonly used in infants and children.

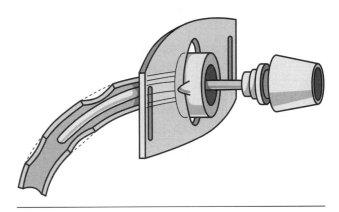

FIGURE 8-6 A fenestrated tracheostomy tube allows the child to speak.

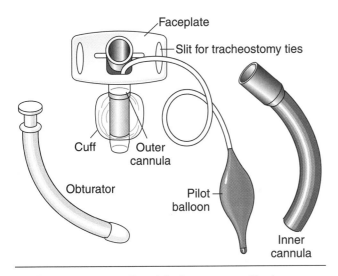

FIGURE 8-5 Double lumen, cuffed tracheostomy tubes are also used.

in the trachea during that removal. These tubes may also be cuffed or uncuffed.

Fenestrated Double Lumen

Fenestrations or holes are present along the length of these tubes so air can move up through the larynx and mouth when the child exhales (Figure 8-6). This action allows the child to practice regular breathing and also to speak. The removable inner cannula without holes must be in place for mechanical ventilation or ventilation with a bag-valve device. See Table 8-2 for a comparison of tubes.

TABLE 8-2
Types of Tracheostomy Tubes

Type of Tracheostomy Tube	Description
Single	• For all newly borns • Most pediatric tubes • Single passage for airflow and suctioning • Use an obturator for insertion
Double	• Sizes 4–8 • Removable inner cannula • Outer cannula keeps stoma open when inner cannula is removed for cleaning
Fenestrated	• Teaches child to breathe naturally • Allows child to talk • Inner cannula must be in place for effective ventilation

Assessment

Obstruction may occur in the tracheostomy tube or the child's airway. Look for these causes as the assessment progresses:

1. Difficulty clearing secretions
2. Foreign bodies
3. Improper positioning
4. Problems with the tube itself (e.g., kink in the tube)
5. Incorrect insertion of the tracheostomy tube

   Signs and symptoms of an obstruction include:

   - Signs and symptoms of hypoxia
     —Change in level of consciousness
     —Cyanosis
     —Tachypnea
     —Tachycardia
     —Use of intercostal muscles
   - Restlessness or other signs of altered level of consciousness
   - Sternal retractions
   - Increase in respiratory effort and rate
   - Absent or decreased breath sounds
   - Lack of chest rise with assisted ventilation
   - Diaphoresis

 Tricks of the Trade

Change in level of consciousness is an important early warning of respiratory distress! Ask the parents or caregivers if the child's current level of consciousness is typical. Respiratory distress should be immediately suspected if there is any change in the child's mental status.

Management

Treatment of airway or breathing compromise must begin as soon as a problem is suspected. Any delay may be fatal.

If there are secretions around the opening of the tube, disconnect the child from the ventilator and suction them out. Do NOT use a bag-valve device on the child before suctioning as any ventilations will force those secretions down the trachea and into the lungs. Provide extra ventilations once the airway is clear before reconnecting the ventilator.

In the event the tracheostomy tube is out of the stoma and cannot be replaced, an endotracheal tube may be inserted into the stoma as a temporary measure by an advanced life support provider trained in this procedure. If there is no upper airway blockage, oral or nasal endotracheal intubation may also be attempted.

Examine the tracheostomy tube to verify that it is correctly in place in the stoma. Make sure the obturator has been removed. In addition, place a rolled towel under the child's shoulders to help keep the airway open and make ongoing assessment easier.

If the child uses a ventilator, disconnect the ventilator from the tracheostomy tube and connect a bag-valve device. Attempt to ventilate the tracheostomy tube. If there is no chest rise and an obstruction is still suspected, immediately prepare to irrigate and suction the tube (see Appendix C—Suctioning a Child with a Tracheostomy).

There are several methods to provide oxygen: blow-by technique, direct ventilation of the tracheostomy tube, mask to tracheostomy tube or stoma, and mask to mouth (and nose if the child is small enough). See Appendix C—Assisting Ventilations in the Child with a Tracheostomy.

In some situations, the tracheostomy tube may need to be changed (e.g., obstruction in tube that cannot be removed). If the tube has been dislodged, inspect it for damage or obstruction. Reinsert the tube directly into the stoma as long as it is open or can be cleared after suctioning. See Appendix C—Changing a Tracheostomy Tube.

Transport

Use caution when moving the child onto the stretcher and into the ambulance so as not to dislodge the tracheostomy tube. If the child is being ventilated by a bag-valve device, be careful not to pull on the tracheostomy

 Safety Tip

- Use extra caution when moving the child with a tracheostomy. If the child is being ventilated by a bag-valve device, be careful not to pull on the tracheostomy tube during the transfer onto and off the stretcher and into the ambulance or hospital.

tube during the transfer. Continue ventilations throughout transport, or use a portable mechanical ventilator if available. Notify personnel at the receiving hospital that the child has a tracheostomy. Some institutions prefer to have members of the anesthesiology team available upon arrival.

MECHANICAL VENTILATORS

Children with tracheostomies may require ongoing assisted ventilations using a mechanical ventilator (Figure 8-7). Some may require full-time support, and others may only need assistance while sleeping.

Etiology

Conditions requiring ongoing support may include:

- Bronchopulmonary dysplasia (BPD) causing chronic lung disease
- Muscular dystrophy which results in weakened respiratory muscles
- Spinal cord injury in the cervical region which has severed the nerve impulses responsible for breathing
- Head injury causing decreased level of consciousness and inadequate respiratory drive
- Progressive hypoxia despite oxygen therapy

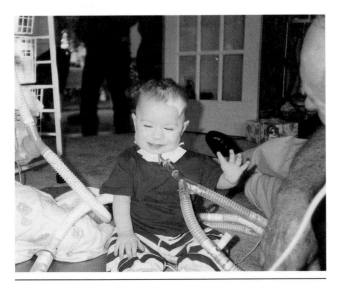

FIGURE 8-7 This child has a tracheostomy and uses a portable mechanical ventilator to breathe.

- Medication toxicity or side effects (i.e., large doses of morphine sulfate for pain control)
- Excessive work of breathing demonstrated by retractions, tachypnea, and abnormal respiratory patterns

Equipment Overview

Mechanical ventilation is designed to replace the function of the diaphragm and the thoracic chest wall muscles. Inflation of the lungs is caused by either positive or negative pressure.

Ventilators have different settings prescribed by the child's physician. There may be documentation beside the ventilator that reads: FiO_2 0.5, V_T 300, R 24, PEEP 5 cm. Interpretation of these settings is as follows:

- $FiO_2 \rightarrow$ fraction of inspired oxygen; reflects the percent of oxygen delivered by the machine (i.e., 50% in the example provided—remember that room air is 0.21 or 21% oxygen)
- Tidal volume (V_T) $\rightarrow$ reflects the amount of air delivered by the machine with each breath (i.e., 300 cc with each breath)
- Rate (R) $\rightarrow$ reflects the number of breaths per minute delivered by the machine (i.e., 24 breaths/minute)
- Positive end-expiratory pressure (PEEP) $\rightarrow$ reflects the amount of air pressure remaining in the lungs to keep the air passages slightly inflated during exhalation (i.e., 5 cm. of H_2O pressure; usually ranges from 2.5 to 15 cm of H_2O)

Pressure-Cycled Ventilators

These devices inflate the lungs using positive or negative pressure. With **positive-pressure ventilation**, the tidal volume is related to the pressure setting. The ventilator "pushes in" each breath at a certain tidal volume and pressure. This type of ventilator is most commonly used in the hospital and home settings.

Negative-pressure ventilation requires the use of a hard shell or body suit that fits over the child's chest and abdomen. A vacuum or negative pressure is created in the shell or suit which then causes air to enter the lungs. An "iron lung" uses this same concept except that the patient's entire body is in the chamber. These devices are not routinely used outside of the hospital setting.

Volume-Cycled Ventilators

These machines deliver ventilation using a preset tidal volume. Once that volume is reached in the lungs, the machine ends the breath. The lungs' compliance and resistance will change the pressure needed to deliver the preset volume.

Intermittent Mechanical Ventilation (IMV)

This mode of ventilation allows the child to breathe on his or her own as much as possible. The machine provides a breath in between those breaths initiated by the child. For instance, if the child takes 10 breaths per minute and the machine is set at an IMV of 24, the machine will deliver 14 breaths during that minute to make sure the child's rate stays at 24. If the child breathes 26 times in one minute, the machine will not trigger during that minute. If the child does not initiate any ventilations during that minute, the machine will provide all 24 breaths.

Continuous Mechanical Ventilation (CMV)

This mode of ventilation provides all breaths at a set rate. It does not adjust for any breaths initiated by the child. This method is used primarily for a child who makes no effort to breathe unassisted. In fact, a child who is trying to breathe on his or her own may become very frustrated if the machine continues to force breaths at a preset rate.

Assessment

Depending on the etiology, ventilation may be required 24 hours per day or only at certain times (i.e., at night while sleeping or during times of illness). Talk with the family and/or caregivers to determine when the child requires full ventilatory support. Ask them if there has been a change in the child's usual condition (i.e., illness, new medication, increase in seizures, decrease in level of consciousness, etc.).

After assessing the child, also look at the equipment. How long ago was the tracheostomy tube changed?

 Tricks of the Trade

Connection to a mechanical ventilator does not ensure the child is being properly ventilated. If the child is using a ventilator yet appears cyanotic and in respiratory distress, suspect a problem with the machine. Remove the child from the machine and provide several ventilations with a bag-valve device and high concentration oxygen. If the child's respiratory distress improves, the ventilator may be faulty.

If the tube was recently changed, was there a problem with the ventilator before the change? Has the ventilator been functioning properly? Is there adequate oxygen in the tank? Is there some type of obstruction in the ventilator tubing (e.g., the tubing is kinked under the child's shirt) or in the tracheostomy tube? Check the ventilator settings on the machine. Do they match what has been prescribed? Is the ventilator receiving power either by being plugged in at the wall or using some auxiliary power supply such as a battery? Is the battery properly charged?

Management

Suctioning and ventilations with a bag-valve device may be required to ensure adequate oxygenation. See Appendix C for a review of suctioning and ventilation skills.

If the machine is not adequately oxygenating the child, the child should be manually ventilated until the machine can be fixed or replaced. If there is going to be a significant delay in getting a working ventilator, the child may need to be transported to the hospital.

Transport

If the child needs to be seen at the hospital yet the ventilator is working properly and there are no signs of respiratory distress, transport the child without disconnecting the ventilator if it is portable and convenient for the family. Work with the parents or caregivers to properly transport the machine with the child. Using the ventilator may seem unnecessary and cumbersome, yet the child may be most comfortable when ventilated in this manner. In addition, one provider will not have to manually ventilate the child during the entire transport (which could be an hour or more in some rural areas of the country).

CONTINUOUS POSITIVE AIRWAY PRESSURE (CPAP)

Children with respiratory complications may not always need full ventilatory support with an artificial airway. Intubation or a tracheostomy are not necessary yet the underlying problem must still be treated.

Etiology

Some children have weak respiratory effort or recurrent problems with partial airway obstruction. The child may have a disorder that affects the ability of the muscles to keep the airway open or some anatomical obstruction of the airway (see Chapter 7—Children with Special Health Care Needs).

Equipment Overview

In an effort to keep the airway open, positive airway pressure is constantly maintained with a special device that provides **continuous positive airway pressure (CPAP)**. This device fits closely over the mouth and nose of the child so that constant airway pressure is applied as the child inhales and exhales. Like the mechanical ventilator, some children may require this equipment all the time while others may only use it at certain times (e.g., at night when airway obstruction is most likely to occur).

Assessment

Some children may have a higher risk for partial or total airway obstruction when they are sick or experience some type of trauma. Ask the parents or caregivers about the child's baseline respiratory status. How often does the child routinely use CPAP? Has the child been ill, had a medication change, had a change in his or her usual routine, or been under unusual stress at school or with the family? Does the current level of discomfort exceed what the child usually tolerates?

Management

Remove the CPAP device to see if the child's respiratory distress improves. It is possible that there may be a problem with the equipment. If the child's status gets worse, reapply the CPAP device and prepare for transport.

The device may also be removed if it significantly interferes with the assessment and treatment process. The child may tire easily yet will still be able to breathe. Reapply the device if there is any significant decline in the child's respiratory status, and be prepared to manually assist ventilations or intubate if necessary.

Transport

Continue use of the CPAP device during transport. Notify the personnel at the receiving hospital so they can have additional equipment available.

CENTRAL VENOUS ACCESS DEVICES (VADS)

Children requiring frequent blood testing or intravenous therapy may have extended access to a vein without the need for a continuous infusion or repeated venipunctures. An indwelling catheter may be inserted depending on the child's diagnosis, length of time therapy is required, risk of insertion, and availability of resources to help the family maintain the catheter at home and at school as applicable. The tip of the catheter rests in the superior vena cava or the right atrium of the heart regardless of the insertion site (Figure 8-8).

Etiology

Reasons for a central venous access device include:

- Repeated blood sampling
- Administration of blood products
- Central venous pressure monitoring
- Administration of large concentrations and/or quantities of fluids
- Administration of medications (e.g., chemotherapy)
- Administration of drugs that given peripherally cause damage to small veins (e.g., potassium, some chemotherapy drugs, etc.)
- Total parenteral nutrition (TPN)

Equipment Overview

There are three categories of central venous access devices.

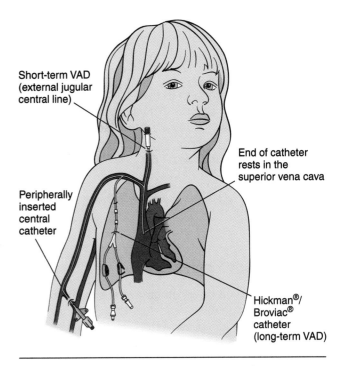

Short-term VAD (external jugular central line)

Peripherally inserted central catheter

End of catheter rests in the superior vena cava

Hickman®/ Broviac® catheter (long-term VAD)

FIGURE 8-8 Central venous access devices (VADs) may be inserted in the arm, neck, chest, or groin of the child.

Short-term or Nontunneled Catheters

These catheters are made of polyurethane and are most commonly used in emergency situations (Figure 8-8). They are placed in large veins such as the jugular, femoral, or subclavian veins. A chest x-ray is taken at the hospital to confirm correct placement.

Peripherally Inserted Central Catheters (PICC)

These catheters are made of silicone or polymer material and are used for therapy that is short to moderate in duration. The antecubital vein is the most common insertion site. There are less complications associated with this catheter so it is ideal for pediatric patients. It also is the least costly.

Long-Term Central VADs

These catheters may have one, two, or three lumens and include tunneled and implanted infusion ports (see Figure 8-9 a and b). Those with more than one lumen are called **multilumen** catheters. Administration of incompatible drugs or fluids through two sites at the same time is a good reason to use a multilumen catheter. See Table 8-3 for a comparison of long-term central VADs.

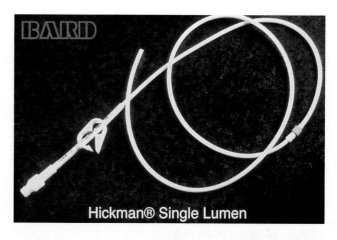

Hickman® Single Lumen

a.

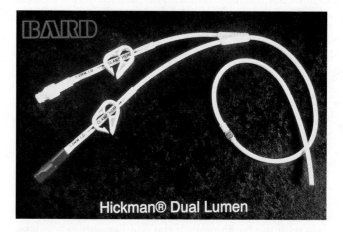

Hickman® Dual Lumen

b.

FIGURE 8-9 a. A Hickman catheter requires daily heparin flushes and the site must be kept dry. Photo provided by Bard Access Systems. Hickman is a registered trademark of Bard Access Systems. **b.** A Port-A-Cath® requires a special needle for access. Courtesy of SIMS Deltec, Inc., St. Paul, Minnesota.

Safety Tip

- Pay special attention to the PICC catheter and the security of the dressing. Most PICC catheters are not sutured in place and may become dislodged during treatment if the child is moving around forcefully.

Assessment

Inspect the catheter and the insertion site. Is the site clean and well maintained? Are there any signs of infection? Sepsis can occur if the infection has entered the bloodstream. Signs and symptoms of infection include:

- Redness, swelling, and tenderness at the insertion site
- Purulent drainage from the insertion site
- High fever and chills (seen with sepsis)
- Circulatory compromise (seen with sepsis)

TABLE 8-3
Long-Term Central Venous Access Devices (VADs)

Type of Catheter	Benefits	Maintenance Considerations
Tunneled catheter • Hickman® • Broviac®	• Easy to use for self-administered infusions	• Daily heparin flushes required • Must be clamped or have clamp ready at all times • Site must be kept dry • Risk of infection • Protrudes from body —Susceptible to damage —May be pulled out —May alter body image of child
Implanted ports • Port-A-Cath® • Infus-A-Port® • Mediport®	• Reduced risk of infection • Only slight bulge on chest; completely under skin • Increased safety (under skin and no maintenance care) • Reduced cost for family • Regular physical activity (including swimming) not restricted • Heparinized monthly and after each infusion	• Must pierce skin to access port • Pain associated with needle insertion (may use local anesthetic like EMLA cream) • Special needle (Huber) required to access port • Must prepare skin before injection • Catheter may dislodge from port especially if child "plays" with site • Generally not allowed to engage in vigorous contact sports • Difficult for self-administered infusions

Wong, D. (1999). *Whaley and Wong's nursing care of infants and children* (6th ed.). St. Louis, MO: Mosby Year-Book.

Abbreviations: EMLA, eutectic mixture of local anesthetics.

Do fluids flow adequately through the catheter? Is the catheter intact? If the catheter is dislodged or broken, is bleeding present? Is there any bleeding at the insertion site? Are there any signs of allergic reaction from the medication being infused?

If the child is receiving nutritional fluid and that fluid it is not prepared properly (e.g., too much water or too little water is used to mix the formula), the child may have an abnormal heart rhythm or abnormal blood pressure due to the incorrect amount of electrolytes. For children receiving narcotics for pain, respiratory depression may be present if the concentration of the mixture or rate of administration are wrong.

If the catheter is not well maintained and flushed as directed, blood clots can form. These clots adhere to the inside of the catheter, break off, and lodge in another area, potentially blocking blood flow to significant organs. If a clot has dislodged, the child may exhibit an altered level of consciousness (blood clot in the brain) or respiratory distress (blood clot in the lungs).

Air can also get into the catheter, enter the bloodstream, and cause an **air embolism** (blockage of a blood vessel with air). The child may begin coughing, have pain in the chest, experience shortness of breath, and become cyanotic.

In some children, the distal end of the catheter moves from its original position in the superior vena cava. If the catheter moves further into the heart, dysrhythmias may occur.

Management

If a short-term catheter or PICC line has become dislodged or completely pulled out, control bleeding with a sterile dressing and direct pressure to the site. If the catheter itself is damaged, place a clamp closest to the skin before the damaged area or at the exposed end of the tube. If a plastic clamp is not available, use hemostats without teeth or hemostats over a piece of gauze so that the tube is not damaged. Be especially careful not to let air enter the catheter.

Assess breath sounds, and estimate the amount of blood lost. Treat respiratory distress or shock as appropriate and provide rapid transport if the child is in distress.

If an air embolism or blood clot is suspected, clamp the catheter. Administer high-concentration oxygen, and place the child on his or her left side with the head down (Trendelenberg position) so that no air floats to a blood vessel in the brain via gravity. Initiate rapid transport to the hospital.

Traditionally, most prehospital providers have not had the opportunity to access central venous catheters. However, in a life-threatening situation, short-term and PICC lines may be considered for use especially when those lines may be the only opportunity for fluid resuscitation. Follow local protocols and/or contact the medical control physician for direction.

With Hickman® or Broviac® catheters, medication may be given directly through the injection cap (see Appendix C for Administration of Fluid/Medications through a Hickman® catheter). Implanted devices, such as the Port-A-Cath®, Infus-A-Port®, and Mediport® must only be accessed using a special noncoring Huber needle since the device can be permanently damaged by other needles, necessitating surgery to repair or replace the device. Be aware that this needle is not traditionally used in the prehospital setting.

If the catheter is not damaged and the child depends on the infusion of nutrition or glucose through the central line, transport while continuing the infusion. Ask the parents or caregivers to assist in transporting the equipment and maintaining the infusion.

 Tricks of the Trade

If an air embolism or blood clot is suspected, place the child on his or her left side with the head down (Trendelenberg position) so that no air floats to a blood vessel in the brain via gravity.

Transport

If you need to discontinue an infusion that contains glucose, assess the child's glucose at least once during transport or more often if the transport is prolonged. Depending on local policies, procedures, and protocols, consider asking the parent or caregiver to ride in the patient compartment to assist with care during transport.

If the child requires continuation of an infusion and/or medication not approved for administration by prehospital personnel in that state, contact the medical control physician for direction. In some children, discontinuation of the fluid or medication can be life threatening.

ARTIFICIAL PACEMAKERS

Many children with congenital heart disease or other cardiac irregularities have an artificial pacemaker implanted. This pacemaker then enables them to participate in child care programs, school, sports, and other regular events within their own communities.

Etiology

Some children may have an unusually slow or irregular heart rhythm that cannot be controlled by the intrinsic pacemaker of the heart. These situations are common in children with congenital heart disease who may have had surgical corrections (e.g., atrioventricular block after repair of a ventricular septal defect). The pacemaker either assists or completely takes over for the conduction system of the heart.

Equipment Overview

Pacemakers are quite sophisticated and can be programmed to do many things. For instance, heart rate can be controlled based on the child's respirations, cardiac output, and activity.

The pacemaker consists of two parts: the **pulse generator** and the **lead**. The pulse generator contains the electronic circuitry and the battery. It produces electrical impulses and responds to signals from the heart. The lead is a flexible, insulated wire that conducts the impulses between the heart and the pulse generator. The lead is either inserted into a vein (**transvenous**) or directly attached to the outside layer of the heart (**epicardial**). Most parents will know which type of lead has been implanted in their child.

The pacemaker is surgically implanted sometimes as an outpatient depending on the child's overall med-

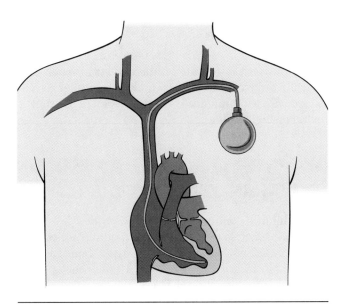

FIGURE 8-10 In this example, pacemaker leads are threaded through a vein (transvenous).

ical status. The pulse generator is placed in the abdominal cavity or right under the skin of the chest wall (Figure 8-10).

There are three types of pacemakers (Table 8-4). The child's particular heart problem will define what type of pacemaker is used.

Assessment

Parents are usually taught how to transmit electrocardiogram readings through the telephone. The child's physician can evaluate electrocardiogram (EKG) strips and also check on the battery life and overall pacemaker function. Ask the parent or caregiver about the last time they sent a transmission over the telephone. Were there any problems at that time? Was the child's rhythm regular, fast, or slow? Did the physician make any changes to the pacemaker settings?

Upon cardiac monitoring, the EKG strip may have wide QRS complexes and look like the child is in ventricular tachycardia. If the child is awake, appropriately responsive, has a good pulse, and is maintaining an adequate blood pressure, the complexes are more than likely the pacemaker waveforms. Include a strip with the routine documentation.

Parents may have an identification card for the child that lists the specific pacemaker settings. Review this card and document the settings in the written report. In addition, the child may have an identification

TABLE 8-4
Types of Artificial Pacemakers

Type	Characteristics
Demand	• Senses the heart's natural rhythm • Set at a certain rate • Only fires (provides impulse) "on demand" when child's heart rate falls below the preset rate
Constant	• Fires at a preset rate • Maintains a constant heart rate • Some models can sense when the heart rate should be increased and adjust on their own
Antiarrhythmia	• Senses the heart's natural rhythm • "Overrides" the natural rhythm when an unusually fast or slow heart rate is sensed

 Tricks of the Trade

The heart rate on the cardiac monitor may appear to be regular yet the child does not have a regular pulse or an adequate blood pressure. In this instance, the pacemaker may not be "capturing," meaning that the pacemaker impulses may not be initiating muscle contractions in the heart. Compare the pulse rate palpated with the heart rate seen on the monitor. If there is a substantial difference, the pacemaker is not functioning properly; and the child must be evaluated at the hospital. If there is no pulse palpable, auscultate the chest to see if heart sounds are present.

bracelet or other documentation describing the heart condition and the pacemaker settings (see Chapter 7—Children with Special Health Care Needs—Emergency Information Form). Use these items as references.

In children with minimal to no underlying heart rhythm, pacemaker malfunction or failure can be fatal. The child's heart rate may be too fast, too slow, or absent. Perfusion will not be adequate, and the child will immediately deteriorate.

Management

In children with artificial pacemakers, shock can occur quickly and progress rapidly. In early stages of shock, the heart rate usually increases. Because the preset pacemaker rate does not allow the heart rate to compensate naturally, no increase occurs. In that instance, shock progresses rapidly. Treat for shock, provide cardiopulmonary resuscitation as appropriate, and rapidly transport the child to the closest hospital.

When a child is traumatically injured, the pacemaker leads may become dislodged or break. The child may display signs and symptoms of shock or the underlying heart problem that required the pacemaker in the first place. Treat for shock and rapidly transport the child.

If the pacemaker is malfunctioning yet the child still has an underlying heart rhythm, the pacemaker may fire during a regular cardiac cycle. If the firing occurs on the T wave, the child may go into ventricular fibrillation. Any random pacemaker impulses should be evaluated immediately at the hospital.

One unusual complication occurs when the pacemaker lead makes contact with the child's diaphragm instead of the heart. Once dislodged, the lead will cause the diaphragm to contract each time the pacemaker fires; and the child will hiccup. This condition may not be critical from a cardiovascular standpoint but can be very annoying or disturbing to the child. The condition may become critical if the child's heart needs the pacemaker yet the leads are not in the proper position to stimulate the heart muscle. In either case, the child should be evaluated by his or her physician.

Exploring the Web

● Look at the Web site for the American Heart Association for information related to pacemaker use in children.

Transport

Monitor the child and continue to reassess vital signs. Rapid transport is indicated if the child is in shock or is critically bradycardic due to a faulty pacemaker or dislodged wire. Communicate all information to the staff at the receiving hospital.

VAGUS NERVE STIMULATORS

Many children continue to have **intractable** (not easily managed) seizures despite surgery, multiple antiepileptic drugs (AEDs), and special diets. After about 10 years of research, on July 16, 1997, the United States Food and Drug Administration (FDA) approved a new device called the **vagus nerve stimulator (VNS)**. This device is sometimes referred to as a "pacemaker for the brain" and is heralded as the first new approach to treating epilepsy in the last 100 years. It is being used primarily as an additional treatment for adults and adolescents greater than 12 years of age with partial-onset seizures (Schachter & Saper, 1998). Studies are continuing to look at other age groups and other types of seizures that might be more successfully treated with the VNS.

Etiology

The actual mechanism of action of this stimulation is unknown. During an epileptic seizure, the electrical activity of the brain is disturbed when hundreds of thousands of neurons fire in a rhythmic pattern. It is believed that the vagus nerve stimulator sends its own impulses intended to stop the electrical impulses from the seizure. The left vagus nerve is used as it is less likely to produce cardiac effects.

The VNS is not a cure for epilepsy. Instead, it significantly decreases the number and severity of seizures. In turn, quality of life for those children can be significantly enhanced because of their new ability to increase their activities, self-confidence, and overall well being when their brains are not so overwhelmed with frequent seizures. The rate of success differs from child to child.

Equipment Overview

A programmable signal generator called the neurocybernetic prosthesis (NCP) is surgically implanted in the patient's upper left chest cavity (Figure 8-11). Stimulating electrodes are then carefully wrapped around the left vagus nerve. These electrodes transport the electrical signal from the generator to the nerve.

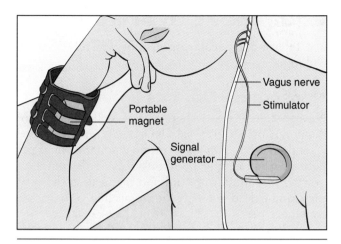

FIGURE 8-11 The vagus nerve stimulator is implanted in the left upper chest under the child's skin. Stimulating electrodes wrap around the left vagus nerve.

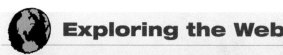

Exploring the Web

Learn more about new treatments for epilepsy at the Epilepsy Foundation of America Web site.

The amperage of the seizure-blocking signals is programmed to regulate the impulses sent to the brain through the vagus nerve. A magnet can also be used by the child to activate the generator as he or she feels a seizure starting. In the child who is significantly developmentally delayed, a parent or other caregiver can use a magnet to activate the generator when a seizure is observed. The battery controlling the activity lasts approximately four years before it must be replaced.

Assessment

When assessing the chest, a raised area can be palpated in the left upper chest where the pulse generator was implanted. There will also be a scar on the left side of the neck where the left vagus nerve was exposed during surgery.

Some children may carry a magnet or wear a special wristband that contains a magnet. Parents or other caregivers may have a separate magnet used to trigger the VNS when they see the child begin to have a seizure.

Children with a VNS may also have hoarseness, cough, throat pain, or dyspnea related to the device, depending on the degree of stimulation of the vagus nerve. If the child has had recent surgery, look for any signs of infection around the incision areas.

Management

As with an artificial pacemaker, the electrodes wrapped around the vagus nerve may become dislodged during significant trauma or movement of the neck. The child may have seizure activity that was previously controlled by the VNS.

Manage the seizure activity with an intravenous line and medication as per protocol or direct physician order. Monitor the child's airway and breathing after any medications, and treat any complications that may occur (e.g., ventilate the child if the breathing rate decreases).

Transport

Rapid transport is needed if the child is having prolonged seizure activity or needs advanced airway intervention. In other instances, make sure the personnel at the receiving hospital know that the VNS is in place. They may choose to have a neurologist standing by when the patient arrives.

FEEDING TUBES

Some infants and children are not able to eat by mouth and require an artificial access for nutritional support. Tubes or catheters may be inserted through the mouth or nose or surgically implanted through the abdomen. Liquid nutrition and medications are then delivered directly into the stomach or small intestine (Figure 8-12).

Etiology

A **stoma**, derived from the Latin word meaning "mouth," is an opening from the gastrointestinal or urinary tract to the outside of the body. A **gastrostomy** is a surgically created stoma whereby the stomach is brought to the level of the skin. This artificial opening into the stomach through the abdominal wall is used most typically in children who are unable to take adequate oral nourishment for a prolonged period of time. The inability to tolerate sufficient oral feedings can be related to a number of conditions (see Chapter 7—Children with Special Health Care Needs—Chronic Conditions).

Feeding via gastrostomy tubes has become more common in recent years. Therefore, prehospital

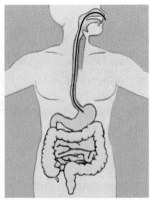
Nasogastric Route

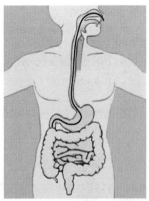
Nasoduodenal Route

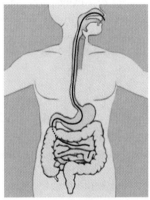
Nasojejunal Route

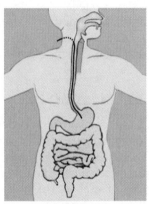
Esophagostomy Route

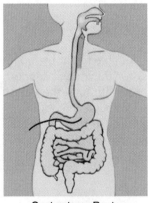
Gastrostomy Route

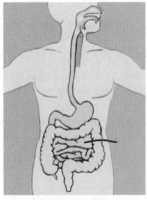
Jejunostomy Route

FIGURE 8-12 Feeding tubes may be placed nonsurgically through the mouth or nose or surgically through the abdomen into the stomach or small intestine.

personnel should become familiar with the various types of gastrostomy or "G-tubes," the supporting types of apparatus, and the complications inherent in the usage of these lifesaving feeding devices.

Equipment Overview

See Table 8-5 for a comparison of feeding tubes used in children.

Nonsurgical Devices

Nasogastric or **orogastric** tubes may be inserted for temporary use. Nutritional supplements may be infused via a pump that delivers a certain amount of fluid per hour or given at specific intervals using the pump or gravity. In addition to fluid and medication delivery, they can be used to empty the stomach of air or gastric contents.

Nasojejunal or **orojejunal** tubes may also be used. Fluid and medications are delivered directly into the **jejunum** or small intestine.

Surgical Devices

There are several types of gastrostomy tubes. These devices vary in their length, the number of ports, the type of catheter tip, the number of **lumens** or openings, and the manner of securing them to the patient's skin. Nutritional supplements may be infused via a pump that delivers a certain amount of fluid per hour or given at specific intervals using a pump or gravity. In addition to fluid and medication delivery, they can be used to empty the stomach of air or gastric contents.

Gastrostomy Tube

The *mushroom* types have soft, flexible tips that require an obturator or stylet to stretch the tip. These devices have a single lumen (Figure 8-13a & b). The *collapsible wings* tube is not as available but functions in a similar manner. The *balloon tip devices* have become very popular and have begun to replace the mushroom tip and collapsible wings devices. The inflatable balloon is located at the tip, similar to a urinary Foley catheter. They are easy to secure and do not dislodge as easily.

Jejunostomy Tube

These tubes are very similar to gastrostomy tubes. However, they are inserted directly into the jejunum or small intestine. From the surface of the abdomen, they look the same. The parent or caregiver will need to tell you if it is a J-tube versus a G-tube.

Percutaneous Endoscopic Gastrostomy (PEG) or Button

The most recent advance in gastrostomy tubes is the introduction of the low-profile G-tube at skin level, commonly referred to as a *button* (see Figure 8-14). The advantage of this type of device is that there is no long piece of tubing arising from the stoma. Replacement

TABLE 8-5
Feeding Tubes Used in Children

Type of Tube	Location	Special Considerations
Nasogastric tube (NGT) • Nonsurgical • Also called NG tube	Placed through nose into the stomach	• Temporary device • Commonly becomes dislodged • May be replaced by parents or caregivers at home • Check nose for signs of skin irritation or infection
Orogastric tube (OGT) • Nonsurgical	Placed through mouth into the stomach	• Temporary device • Used when nasal tube not feasible • Commonly becomes dislodged • May be replaced by parents or caregivers at home • Check mouth for signs of skin irritation or infection
Nasojejunal tube (NJT) • Nonsurgical	Placed through nose into the small intestine (jejunum)	• Temporary device → may be used for several weeks • Less risk of aspiration than NG tube • May become dislodged • Check nose for signs of skin irritation or infection
Orojejunal tube (OJT) • Nonsurgical	Placed through mouth into the small intestine (jejunum)	• Temporary device → may be used for several weeks • Used when nasal tube not feasible • May become dislodged • Check mouth for signs of skin irritation or infection
Gastrostomy tube (GT) • Surgical insertion • Also called G-tube	Surgically implanted through abdominal wall directly into the stomach	• Used to provide long-term nutritional support • Tube protrudes from skin in left upper quadrant of abdomen • Check insertion site for signs of leakage, bleeding, skin irritation, or infection
Jejunostomy tube (JT) • Surgical insertion • Also called J-tube	Surgically implanted through abdominal wall directly into the small intestine (jejunum)	• Used to provide long-term nutritional support • Tube protrudes from skin in left upper quadrant of abdomen • Check insertion site for signs of leakage, bleeding, skin irritation, or infection
Percutaneous endoscopic gastrostomy (PEG) • Surgical insertion • Also called a "button"	Similar to gastrostomy tube; cap and valve used instead of tube	• Used to provide long-term nutritional support • No tube protruding from skin • Small cap with valve located in left upper quadrant of abdomen • Routinely changed by parents and caregivers • Check insertion site for signs of leakage, bleeding, skin irritation, or infection

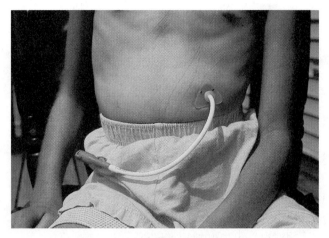

a.

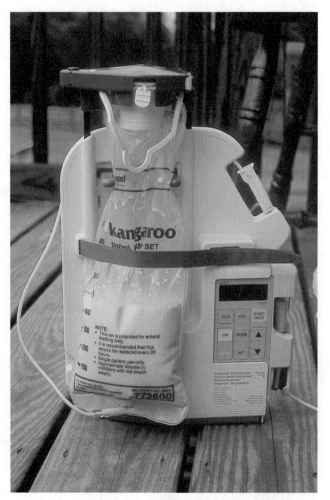

b.

FIGURE 8-13   a. The gastrostomy tube is inserted through the abdomen into the stomach. Extra care must be taken not to pull on the tube hanging from the abdomen. **b.** Portable pumps can be used with the gastrostomy tube.

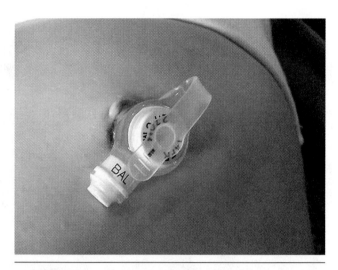

FIGURE 8-14 The PEG or "button" has a small cap with a valve for access. No tube hangs from the stomach.

devices need to be matched for both the size of the stoma (the external diameter of the tube) and the length of the stoma tract.

Assessment

Children with feeding tubes who present with symptoms that seem to be related to the tube require a full evaluation. If the problem is directly related to the feeding tube, prehospital personnel will be able to offer efficient evaluation and therapy only if familiar with potential complications. Complications are divided into *tube-related problems* and *stomal problems*.

Tube-Related Problems

Dislodgement is one of the most common complications. This problem can occur due to a traumatic event, inadvertent balloon deflation, or rupture of the internal balloon.

When nasogastric or orogastric tube dislodgement occurs, parents or caregivers may be trained to reinsert the tube. They may have already tried reinsertion and were not successful before they requested the ambulance.

For surgically implanted tubes, many parents or caregivers will either remember the size of the tube or have another one available. It is equally important to know the interval since *initial* placement of the tube. Postoperative displacement is treated differently and more urgently than dislodgement of a mature stomal tube. An older tube that has dislodged should be replaced quickly with the same size and type of tube to avoid narrowing of the stoma.

Clogging or obstruction of the lumen of the feeding tube can occur due to dried, solidified formula, or twisting or kinking of the tube. Tube blockage is usually noted when the caregivers cannot infuse fluids.

Leaking can occur directly from the lumen of the surgically implanted tube or from the area around the stoma. Leaking from the stoma often indicates that the stoma has widened and now exceeds the size of the tube. If there is purulent drainage from the stoma, an infection is likely. If formula is leaking from the lumen of the tube, the tube position or balloon inflation may be inadequate. It is also possible that the stoma has become disrupted and therefore may require surgical evaluation.

Gastric irritation leading to ulceration may occur as a complication of a gastrostomy. If the tip of the gastrostomy tube is too long, it may abrade the opposite surface of the stomach mucosa, resulting in traumatic ulceration. Similarly, the balloon may accidentally become overinflated and thereby cause friction, especially when the stomach is empty.

A child with a gastric ulcer due to mechanical trauma will present with similar symptoms as other patients with ulcers. Common findings include:

- Abdominal pain
- Irritability
- Bright red blood in the emesis
- Coffee-ground gastric drainage from the G-tube lumen
- Tarry stools

The child may be unable to verbalize pain (i.e., nonverbal due to the underlying condition). Look for other signs such as an increase in pulse and/or respirations, discomfort with light abdominal palpation, and decreased activity because movement increases the pain.

Stomal Problems

The area surrounding the stoma may become irritated or infected. Skin irritation around the stoma may result from chronic leakage of gastric fluid around the tube. If the stoma widens, the leakage may become excessive resulting in more significant dermatitis.

Granulation occurs when extra tissue grows around the stomal site (Figure 8-15). These lesions are harmless but occasionally become infected. If the overgrowth is significant, it may cause occlusion of the stoma.

When skin surrounding the G-tube is irritated by recurrent or intermittent exposure to drainage, cellulitis (acute infection of the skin) may occur. The infection may begin as a superficial skin irritation or contact **dermatitis** (inflammation of the skin) and then evolve into a deeper infection. Symptoms include:

- Red, warm, tender, swollen area around the stoma
- Discomfort associated with manipulation of the tube or button
- Resistance to continued feedings due to discomfort

Recurrent moisture due to gastric leakage in the stomal area can predispose the patient to **fungal infection**. The most common etiologic organism is *Candida albicans*, which will appear as fiery, red plaques at the stoma site.

Management

If the child is vomiting blood or blood is leaking from the tube or button, monitor the child's vital signs and level of consciousness. Rapid transport and intravenous fluid replacement may be necessary if signs and symptoms of shock are present (see Chapter 3—The Critically Ill Child).

If any signs of infection are present, the child should be evaluated by a physician. Some parents may have already spoken to the pediatrician or surgeon by telephone and made arrangements for a direct admission to the hospital.

Nonsurgical tubes may need to be replaced to continue delivery of fluid nutrition. If the parent or caregiver cannot replace the tube, transport to the hospital may be required. This situation is usually not urgent.

Tube replacement is required for dislodgement of surgically implanted tubes. If the tube size is unknown or another device is not available, the most common temporary method of replacement is insertion of a Foley catheter, a skill which is not traditionally performed by

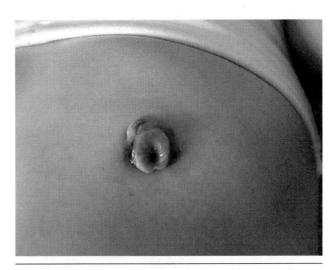

FIGURE 8-15 This stoma has healthy granulation tissue around it.

emergency providers. It is crucial to determine the length of time of dislodgement and relay that information to the personnel at the hospital. If hours have elapsed, the stoma may be smaller and require insertion of a smaller replacement tube. Caution is necessary when reinserting a G-tube because extreme force can lead to tube insertion into the peritoneal cavity.

When ventilating children who also have a gastric feeding tube in place, these tubes may be used to decompress the stomach. Decompression (removal of air or stomach contents) will relieve pressure on the diaphragm, allowing the ventilations to be more effective, and reduce the risk of aspiration of stomach contents.

If the feeding tube is clogged, it needs to be aspirated and flushed with warm water. Parents and caregivers are taught how to irrigate the tube. If their irrigation has not been successful, the tube may need to be repositioned or replaced at the hospital.

Transport

Provide comfort measures and transport the child to the hospital for further evaluation and management. Parents may prefer to have the child taken to the hospital at which the tube was inserted.

If the child is being transported for a condition NOT related to the feeding tube, the tube may be clamped or the infusion stopped for transport. In the case of continuous feedings, ask the parent or caregiver if the child will tolerate an interruption in the nutritional support.

SHUNTS

Cerebrospinal fluid (CSF) or the fluid surrounding the brain and spinal cord accumulates in the ventricles of the brain. When there is too much fluid present, pressure increases in the skull and causes damage to the brain (see Chapter 7—Children with Special Health Care Needs).

Etiology

In order to drain the excess fluid, a **shunt** or special catheter is surgically inserted from the brain to either the chest or abdomen. Infants with a shunt in place should not be held in the head-down position for long periods as the CSF will not be able to drain properly.

A **ventriculoperitoneal (VP) shunt** starts in the ventricle of the brain and ends in the peritoneum (Figure 8-16). It is the preferred treatment for neonates and young infants. Extra tubing can be used which decreases the number of revisions needed as the child grows.

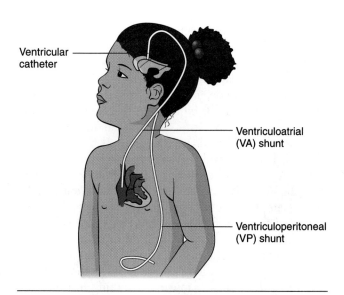

FIGURE 8-16   A ventriculoperitoneal shunt drains cerebrospinal fluid from the ventricle of the brain to the peritoneum. A ventriculoatrial shunt drains cerebrospinal fluid from the ventricle of the brain into the right atrium of the heart.

A **ventriculoatrial (VA) shunt** starts in the ventricle of the brain and ends in the right atrium of the heart. This option is used in older children or those with any pathology in the abdomen. It is not used if the child has any preexisting cardiopulmonary disease.

Complications can develop related to the shunt such as infection or malfunction. Malfunction is most often due to obstruction of the catheter from CSF, a blood clot, or displacement as a result of the child's growth.

Infection is the most serious complication and can occur at any time. The child is most susceptible to infection during the first one to two months after placement of the catheter. Infections include wound infection, bacterial endocarditis, meningitis, ventriculitis, peritonitis, abdominal abscess, and septicemia.

Equipment Overview

The shunt system includes a ventricular catheter, a flush pump, a flow valve to make sure the fluid only goes in one direction (i.e., out of the ventricle), and a distal catheter. The valves open when the intraventricular pressure reaches a certain level and then close when the pressure falls below that same level so that no CSF goes back into the ventricles.

Assessment

The catheter lies under the skin and can be palpated. It will feel like IV tubing under the skin on the head and down the side of the neck.

Malfunction of the shunt will present as signs and symptoms of increasing **intracranial pressure (ICP)**. These include:

- Change in level of consciousness
  - —Irritability
  - —Unusual sleepiness
  - —Lethargy
  - —Coma
- Headache
- Nausea and/or vomiting
- Bulging fontanelles in infant
- Difficulty walking
- Periods without breathing
- Seizures

Parents and other caregivers are usually taught to recognize signs and symptoms of shunt malfunction. They may tell the responding provider that the child needs to go to the hospital because of problems with the shunt.

Infections may cause some of the same signs of increased ICP in addition to fever and general malaise. The child may stop eating or drastically reduce his or her intake.

Management

Support airway, breathing, and circulation as best as possible. Make special note of any changes in the child's level of consciousness, ongoing seizure activity, etc. Keep the head elevated whenever possible to decrease intracranial pressure.

Transport

In the infant or child with a shunt who demonstrates an altered mental status or level of consciousness, transport should be rapid and to a facility capable of providing pediatric neurosurgical support. The parent or caregiver may have contacted the child's physician before EMS arrival and should decide where the child will be taken whenever possible.

If the child lives in a rural area without access to a tertiary facility, consider air transport to the tertiary facility or transport to the local hospital with notification that this child may need to be transferred for definitive

treatment. Reassess vitals frequently and update the receiving facility with any significant changes.

OSTOMIES

Some children may have a stoma for elimination of urine and feces. Some conditions that interfere with regular elimination include but are not limited to:

- Necrotizing enterocolitis in the infant
- Imperforate anus in the infant
- Crohn's disease (inflammatory bowel disease) in older children
- Distal ureter or bladder defects
- Spinal cord anomalies or injury
- Cancer
- Severe abdominal wound

Etiology

A **colostomy** or **ileostomy** is a surgically created opening that brings a portion of the small or large intestine to the surface of the abdomen. A **urostomy** is the same type of surgically created opening that is used for elimination of urine (Figure 8-17).

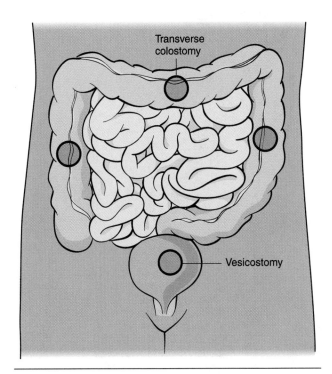

FIGURE 8-17 An ostomy is named for the area in which it originates.

EQUIPMENT OVERVIEW

Feces or urine drain from the stoma into a closed pouch or appliance attached to the skin (Figure 8-18). These devices are then emptied and changed periodically. They can be worn under clothing, and there are tablets available to put into the pouch to decrease odor.

Assessment

Inspect the ostomy site. Are there signs of infection, irritation, or unusual drainage such as pus or blood? Does the area seem more tender than usual?

In a traumatic event, look for blood in the pouch. There may be internal bleeding that drains into the pouch that may be a clue to intra-abdominal trauma. Remember that blood can still be present in the stool even though it may not be obvious to the observer.

These children are at risk for dehydration. Check skin turgor and mucous membranes. Ask the child, parent, or caregiver if there have been any episodes of diarrhea or any decrease in the child's usual oral intake.

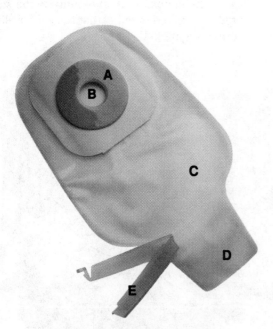

A. Adhesive ring seals around stoma to prevent leakage
B. Opening placed over stoma
C. Collection pouch
D. Drainage end of pouch
E. Secures drainage end of pouch to prevent leakage

FIGURE 8-18 An example of an ostomy pouch.

Management

If an infection is suspected, a physician should evaluate the child. Monitor vital signs, and make the child as comfortable as possible.

Treat for dehydration if present. Insertion of an intravenous line should be determined by local protocol.

If the pouch or appliance over the stoma has broken or is leaking, talk with the parent or caregiver about replacing it. Any fecal matter or urine should be removed from the skin to prevent irritation. If a replacement is not available, apply moist gauze on the stoma with a large, bulky dressing to absorb the drainage until a proper substitute is available.

Transport

Monitor vital signs during transport, and notify personnel at the receiving hospital. Continue to evaluate any increase in bleeding or draining from the stoma. Make every effort to minimize the amount of feces or urine that stays in contact with the child's skin.

SUMMARY

Multiple technological devices are available to support the child with special health care needs in the community. Incorporate these devices into routine assessment and treatment modalities. See Table 8-6 for a summary of devices, common findings, and treatment necessary.

Utilize the family and caregivers as much as possible for assistance. In most cases, they are well versed in the operation of the specific equipment.

 Exploring the Web

- What sites can you find related to children assisted by technology?

- Check the Emergency Medical Services for Children (EMSC) Web site. What information does this government site offer?

- Review sites that pertain to specific disabilities and conditions (see Appendix D).

- What professional journals could you search for information on children assisted by technology?

TABLE 8-6
Children Assisted by Technology—Common Findings and Treatment Necessary

Device	Problem	Treatments
Tracheostomy	Obstruction	• Attempt to assist ventilations with high-concentration oxygen • Attempt to suction • Change tracheostomy tube • Ventilate through stoma • Transport
Tracheostomy	Dislodgement	• Replace tracheostomy tube • Assist ventilations with high-concentration oxygen through stoma • Transport
Mechanical ventilator	Respiratory distress	• Assess tracheostomy for obstruction • Check with parents/caregivers to see if ventilator is working correctly • Assist in ventilator adjustment • Remove child from ventilator and assist ventilations
Central intravenous catheters	Dislodged or damaged	• Apply direct pressure to stop bleeding • Clamp or tie exposed catheter to prevent further blood loss • Assess and treat patient for hemothorax and shock • Transport
Central intravenous catheters	Signs of infection at site	• Assess vitals • Assess and treat for shock if present • Transport
Pacemakers	Failure	• Assess heart rate and perfusion • Treat for shock • Provide urgent transport
Feeding tubes (surgically placed)	Dislodged	• Apply direct pressure to stop bleeding if present • Transport promptly
Shunts	Failure	• Assess level of consciousness • Assist ventilations if necessary • Transport promptly
Ostomies	Bleeding around stoma Infection around stoma	• Apply direct pressure to stop bleeding if present • Monitor for signs of septic shock • Transport promptly

Center for Pediatric Emergency Medicine (CPEM). (1998). *Teaching resource for instructors in prehospital pediatrics (TRIPP)*, Version 2.0. New York: Center for Pediatric Emergency Medicine.

Management of the Case Scenario

Your partner gets information from the school nurse while you start the assessment. There is mucus gurgling at the tracheostomy site, and the child is struggling to breathe through the obstruction. He is breathing at about 32 times per minute, and auscultation of the chest reveals rales in both upper lung fields. His lips are cyanotic, he is diaphoretic, and his skin is very warm to the touch.

You speak to the child while your partner sets up the suction equipment. You then disconnect the child from the ventilator and suction the trach tube. You then assist ventilations with a bag-valve device and repeat suctioning as needed. Once the airway has been sufficiently cleared, you connect him back to the ventilator.

After suctioning and bagging the child, the cyanosis disappears. His respiratory rate is now down to 22 times per minute. Rales are still present in his upper lung fields, and his skin is still very warm. Vitals are stable, and the remainder of the exam is unremarkable.

You prepare the child for transport and make arrangements to leave the wheelchair with the school nurse. You are not able to take the ventilator with you as it is secured to the wheelchair. You must bag the child during the 20-minute trip to the hospital. All of these things are explained to the child, and he nods his head to indicate that he understands what you have said. The parents have been contacted and will meet their child at the hospital.

During transport your partner calls the hospital to provide a report. You find out that the child's medical history includes frequent pulmonary infections. He has been trached since he had bronchopulmonary dysplasia as a premature infant.

▶ REVIEW QUESTIONS

1. Define tracheostomy, stoma, and obturator.

2. Which of the following are indications for a tracheostomy in an infant or child?
   a. Need for long-term ventilator support
   b. Muscular disease
   c. Neurological disease
   d. All of the above

3. List three causes of tracheostomy obstruction.

4. Change in level of consciousness is an important early warning sign of respiratory distress. True or False?

5. Examine the tracheostomy tube to:
   a. Verify correct placement
   b. Determine manufacturer
   c. Make sure the obturator has been removed
   d. a and c only

6. Intermittent mechanical ventilation (IMV) refers to the mode of ventilation that:
   a. Provides all breaths at a set rate
   b. Delivers ventilation at a preset tidal volume
   c. Allows the child to breathe on his or her own
   d. None of the above

7. List three questions to use during the assessment of a child using a mechanical ventilator.

8. List three reasons for a central venous access device in children.

9. Match the following central venous access devices used in children to their types.
   a. Tunnelled
   b. Implanted
   c. Peripheral insertion
   d. None of the above

   _____ Broviac®   _____Mediport®
   _____IVAC   _____Hickman®
   _____Port-A-Cath®   _____Infus-A-Port®
   _____PICC

10. Implanted central venous access devices can be accessed by prehospital personnel with a regular needle through the injection cap. True or False?

11. Name the two components of an artificial pacemaker.

12. A demand pacemaker senses the heart's natural rhythm. True or False?

13. A vagus nerve stimulator is used for children with intractable seizures. True or False?

14. On assessment, the child with a vagus nerve stimulator (VNS) will have a magnet placed under the skin on the left side of the chest. True or False?

15. List two types of feeding tubes used in children, the location, and their special considerations.

16. What should be done for a dislodged feeding tube that was originally surgically implanted?

17. List three signs and symptoms in a child with a malfunctioning shunt.

18. Define colostomy and urostomy.

REFERENCES

Schachter, S., & Saper, C. (1998). Progress in epilepsy research—vagus nerve stimulation. *Epilepsia, 39*(7).

Wong, D. (1998). *Whaley and Wong's nursing care of infants and children* (6th ed.). St. Louis, MO: Mosby-Year Book.

BIBLIOGRAPHY

Anderson, K. N., et al. (1998). *Mosby's medical, nursing, & allied health dictionary.* St. Louis, MO: Mosby-Year Book.

Christian, S. (1998). Stimulating degree of hope—implant aids battle against epilepsy. *The Chicago Tribune.*

Estes, M. E. Z. (1998). *Health assessment and physical examination.* Albany, NY: Delmar Thomson Learning.

Graneto, J. W. (1997). *Textbook of pediatric emergency medicine procedures* (pp. 915–920). Baltimore, MD: Williams & Wilkins.

Kazi, S., Gunasekaran, T. S., Berman, J. H., Kavin, H., & Kraut, J. (1997). Gastric mucosal injuries in children from inflatable low-profile gastrostomy tubes. *Journal of Pediatric Gastroenterology and Nutrition, 24,* 75–79.

Krajicek, M. J. (1998). *Instructor guide for the care of infants, toddlers, and young children with disabilities and chronic conditions.* Austin, TX: PRO-ED.

Rushton, D. B., & Witte, M. (1998). *Children with special health care needs—technology assisted children.* Salt Lake City, Utah: Primary Children's Medical Center.

Salinsky, M., Uthman, B., Ristanovic, R., Wernicke, J., & Tarver, W. (1996). Vagus nerve stimulation for the treatment of medically intractable seizures. *Archives of Neurology, 53.*

Tsarouhas, N. (1997). Tube replacement. In *Illustrated textbook of pediatric emergency and critical care procedures* (pp. 366–369). St. Louis, MO: Mosby-Year Book.

Vessey, J. A., & Jackson, P. L. (1996). *Primary care of the child with a chronic condition.* St. Louis, MO: Mosby-Year Book.

Virginia Office of EMS, Division of Educational Development. (1994). *Children with special needs: High tech kids videotape.* Roanoke, VA: Virginia Office of EMS.

Wallace, H. Biehl, R., MacQueen, J. & Blackman, J. (1997). *Mosby's resource guide to children with disabilities and chronic illness.* St. Louis, MO: Mosby-Year Book.

Wertz, E. (1997). The patient with special needs. *The Basic EMT—comprehensive prehospital patient care.* St. Louis, MO: Mosby-Year Book.

Wertz, E. (1997). Pediatric emergencies. *Mosby's EMT—intermediate textbook.* St. Louis, MO: Mosby-Year Book.

Wertz, E. (1993). Special needs pediatric patient. *Emergency Medical Services, 22*(3), 40–49.

Head and Spinal Trauma

OBJECTIVES

Upon completion of this chapter, the student should be able to:

- Compare and contrast the major differences between adult and pediatric head injury.
- Compare and contrast the major differences between adult and pediatric spinal injury.
- Describe the assessment and prehospital care of the pediatric patient with a suspected head injury.
- Describe the assessment and prehospital care of the pediatric patient with a suspected spinal injury.

KEY TERMS

ataxic respirations
central neurogenic hyperventilation
Cheyne-Stokes respirations

primary injury
secondary injury
subluxation

Case Scenario

You are dispatched to a motor vehicle accident involving two patients. You note that one vehicle has rear-ended another vehicle. You are assigned to care for the four-year-old boy who is found lying face forward across the console of the front seat with his torso and legs in the back seat. His mother is responsive and tells you that the boy was playing with his toys in the back seat and was not restrained. The child is awake and crying softly but does not appear to be moving. How would you manage this child?

INTRODUCTION

The differences between head injury and spinal cord/column injury in the pediatric and adult age groups are major and significant. Head injury is the most common cause of death in the pediatric age group and is a significant cause of morbidity (National Association of Emergency Medical Technicians [NAEMT], 1999). Spinal cord/column injury is relatively uncommon in children; but when it occurs, it represents a significant morbidity.

The National Pediatric Trauma Registry (NPTR) records a frequency of 1.9 percent of all hospitalized injured children have either head or spinal injuries. However, more than 50 percent of children with spinal injuries have accompanying head injuries.

This chapter focuses on head injuries and spinal cord/column injuries in infants and children. It describes the findings and prehospital management necessary to deliver the child with a potential head and/or spinal cord/column injury to the trauma center in the best possible condition.

HEAD INJURY

Up to the age of approximately four years, a child's head is larger and heavier in proportion to the rest of the body. This statement means that the head is not only a large target but also acts as the lead point when the child falls or otherwise becomes airborne.

Etiology

Several anatomical characteristics make the child's head a magnet for injury. The thin, soft skull of the infant or child offers only minimal protection. It is more easily dented by an injuring force. This force is transmitted to the structure underlying the bone, in this case, the brain. Skull fractures are less common in infants and children as compared to adults; but when they occur, there is usually evidence that a significant force has been transmitted to the underlying brain.

Because the size of a child's head is so large and the scalp is so vascular, a significant volume of blood goes to the head and brain. Children can bleed significantly from any external and internal head injuries with the resultant development of shock.

Even though brain injury is the most common cause of death in pediatric injury, the fact remains that a child with a given degree of injury severity has a better outcome than an adult with a similar degree of injury severity (Tepas, DiScala, & Ramenofsky, 1990). Furthermore, multiple system injury is more common in children than adults. Adults who die of head injury do so due to the head injury. Children most often suffer multiple system injuries. In effect, the other systems that are injured have the potential for making the brain injury worse. That is, the combination of central nervous system (CNS) injury plus any other organ system injury sets the stage for death from the CNS injury. Secondary head injury in children resulting from hypovolemia and/or hypoxia is the major cause of death in the child with a head injury (NAEMT, 1999).

The majority of children who succumb to injury do so as a result of increased intracranial pressure (ICP). While some injuries do such immediate and massive damage to the brain that death is nearly instantaneous, the majority of children die from progressive intracranial hypertension.

Increased intracranial pressure results from a combination of factors. It was assumed for years that the usual cause of death from brain injury was hypoxia. A study from the University of Vermont evaluated the factors leading to death from injury in children suffering significant central nervous system injury (Lui, Lee, & Wong, 1996). In this study, children with brain injury were classified as having died due to hypoxia, hypovolemia, both hypoxia and hypovolemia, or neither. The study clearly identified hypovolemia as the single most common element resulting in death from brain injury, much more common than hypoxia but less common than death from both hypovolemia and hypoxia.

It is important to differentiate primary from secondary CNS injury. **Primary injury** is the injury that occurs due to the injuring force. **Secondary injury** is the brain injury that occurs as a result of problems due to other organ system injuries (e.g., hypovolemia and/or hypoxia).

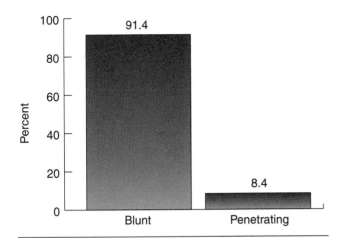

FIGURE 9-1 Mechanism of injury. NPTR 1998; *n* = 74,541.

Mechanism of Injury

The majority of children who suffer trauma receive their injuries as a result of blunt mechanisms (Figure 9-1). Although penetrating injuries have increased, this mechanism is somewhat limited to large urban areas. Data from the National Pediatric Trauma Registry (NPTR) has clearly shown that blunt mechanisms account for 90+% of injuries.

Motor vehicle crashes (MVC) represent the single most lethal element in the child's environment (Figure 9-2). Falls from a height are also a significant mechanism of injury (25.8%); yet, falls account for a mortality rate of

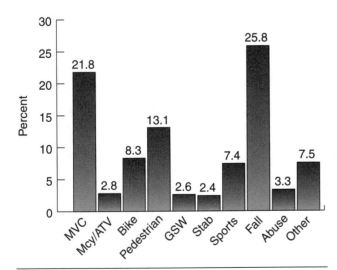

FIGURE 9-2 Specific mechanism of injury in pediatrics NPTR 1998; *n* = 74,541.

Abbreviations: MVC, motor vehicle crashes; Mcy, motorcycle; ATV, all-terrain vehicle; GSW, gunshot wound.

only 0.4% as compared to motor-vehicle-related deaths of 20.6 percent. The second most common mechanism of injury resulting in mortality is beating, accounting for 10.9 percent of deaths in the pediatric age group. Gunshot wounds (GSW) result in death 8.3 percent of the time in childhood.

Signs and Symptoms

The signs and symptoms of increased intracranial pressure in children are the same as in the adult. These can include:

- A loss or changing level of consciousness
- Nausea and vomiting
- History of seizure
- Severe headache
- Increased blood pressure with accompanying decrease in pulse rate and changing respiratory patterns
  - **Cheyne-Stokes respirations** (respiration pattern with periods of shallow, slow breathing increasing to rapid, deep breathing, then returning to shallow, slow breathing followed by a short period of apnea; commonly associated with increased intracranial pressure)
  - **Central neurogenic hyperventilation** (pattern of breathing with rapid and regular ventilations at approximately 25 per minute; the increasing regularity indicates an increasing depth of coma)
  - **Ataxic breathing** (breathing pattern due to a lesion in the medullary respiratory center; characterized by a series of inspirations and expirations)
- Changes in size and reactivity of pupils
- Posturing

It is important to remember that these signs and symptoms may not be as dramatic in infants because the skull sutures are not fused. The anterior fontanelle allows for expansion of the skull to accommodate the injured tissue. This situation is particularly true in children under eight years of age.

Along with the head injury, the pediatric age group often has a femur fracture and a splenic injury. Both the spleen and orthopedic injuries have the potential for causing hypovolemia.

The signs of hypovolemia in the child are often misunderstood because of the child's vital signs. The heart rate of a child decreases with age. The younger the child, the higher the heart rate. This difference is due to the fact that the heart rate is the primary regulator of a child's cardiac output. Thus, a newly born child may have a normal heart rate of 160 beats/minute and, although this would be distinctly abnormal for a 20-year-old adult, it is normal for an infant. The blood pressure is lower in a child than an adult. The systolic blood pressure of a four-year-old child is normally 80 mm Hg. This number would be considered quite low for a 20-year-old adult. Thus, knowledge of normal vital signs based on age is extremely helpful. Knowing the age-based vital signs in addition to other signs of hypovolemia are key to the identification of hemorrhagic shock (for an in-depth discussion on shock, see Chapter 3—The Critically Ill Child).

As blood loss increases, CNS perfusion decreases resulting in a changing status in the level of consciousness. (Table 9-1). A blood loss of less than 25% results in a patient whose level of consciousness may be lethargic, irritable, combative, and/or confused. With up to 45% blood volume loss, the level of consciousness decreases to the point at which there is a dulled response to pain. A child suffering this percent of volume loss generally does not react to painful stimuli. At a blood loss of greater than 45%, the child is comatose.

Assessment

Airway, breathing, and circulation must be fully evaluated. If the child's level of consciousness is altered, airway and breathing may be compromised. It is crucial to determine the child's neurological status. Using the AVPU mnemonic (A for alert, V for responsive to verbal stimuli, P for responsive to painful stimuli, and U for unresponsive) or the Glasgow Coma Scale combined with the patient's pupil evaluation (e.g., equal/unequal, responsive, slowed, dilated, or pinpoint), the level of consciousness and hence neurological status can quickly be defined.

Management

In the field, management of the child with a head injury should focus on careful attention on the ABCs. The lack of a patent airway kills the quickest, followed by the inability to breathe. If the child has an adequate ventilatory rate and tidal volume, give high-concentration oxygen via a nonrebreather mask. If the child's airway and/or breathing is compromised in any way, an oral airway, ventilations using a bag-valve mask with high-concentration oxygen, and endotracheal intubation using cervical spine precautions must be immediately instituted.

Management of the child with a head injury and increased intracranial pressure is aimed at improving cerebral perfusion. Although controversial in many areas, hyperventilation using 100 percent oxygen with either a bag-valve-mask device or an endotracheal tube at a rate of 20–24 breaths/minute is still the recommended field approach. The goal of hyperventilation is to decrease the pCO_2, subsequently dilating cerebral vessels and increasing blood flow. The rate of hyperventilation must be controlled to prevent too much elimination of carbon dioxide. A pCO_2 of 15–20 mm Hg can cause cerebral ischemia.

TABLE 9-1
Major Organ Responses to Blood Volume Loss

System	<25% Volume Loss	25%–45% Volume Loss	>45% Volume Loss
Cardiac	Weak, thready pulse Increasing heart rate	Tachycardia Hypotension	Hypotension Tachycardia → bradycardia
CNS	Lethargic Irritable Combative Confused	Dulled response to pain	Comatose
Skin	Pale Cool Clammy	Cyanotic Decreased capillary refill Cold extremities	Pale Cold

Once airway and breathing have been treated, the next priority is the circulation or the child's blood volume. If shock is suspected, the treatment should be aimed at restoring circulating blood volume.

Starting an IV or doing any other manipulation is very difficult in a child who is irritable, combative, and/or confused from the decreased perfusion of the brain. If a significant blood loss has occurred (e.g., 25 to 45 percent), the child's response to pain will be dulled, and starting an IV will be easier. It is this second group, however, in which time should not be wasted at the scene with multiple attempts to start an IV. It should be started en route so that time at the scene is minimal.

Attempt to establish venous or intraosseous access en route. Infuse a physiologic crystalloid solution such as normal saline or Ringer's lactate solution. The resuscitation volume should be directed at restoring 25 percent of the blood volume. Thus, the solution should be administered as a bolus of 20 cc/kg. Remember that not all of this crystalloid fluid will remain in the intravascular space; thus, if transport is delayed or prolonged, additional boluses of 20 cc/kg of the same fluid should be infused. Local protocol or contact with a medical command physician should determine the number of additional boluses in the field.

Once fluid resuscitation has been started, assessment of the effectiveness of treatment should be ongoing. If the treatment is successful, the pulse rate should decrease, the blood pressure should increase, the level of consciousness should improve, and perfusion of the skin should reveal more normal color and warmth.

Transport

The child with a serious head injury should be transported to a pediatric trauma center with the capability of neurosurgical intervention. By delivering the child to the appropriate tertiary facility, he or she will have the best opportunity for a favorable outcome.

Exploring the Web

● Search for Web sites related to head trauma. Are there any specific to prehospital care? Are there any specific to pediatric care? Are there any sites that would be helpful in supporting the families of victims of head trauma? Create flash cards specifying mechanism of injury, assessment, and management of the victim of head trauma.

SPINAL CORD/COLUMN INJURY

Spinal cord/column injuries (SCCI) are thought to be a very uncommon occurrence in the pediatric age group (National Pediatric Trauma Registry, 1998). The spinal column offers good protection to the underlying spinal cord.

Etiology

There are major anatomical differences in the spinal column of a child. The vertebrae are narrower and wedge-shaped, with the narrow part of the wedge located at the anterior border of the spinal column (Figure 9-3). Facet joints are flat rather than cupped as in the adult spinal column, and the spinal ligaments are flexible. All of these factors allow for posterior to anterior movement of individual spinal vertebral bodies.

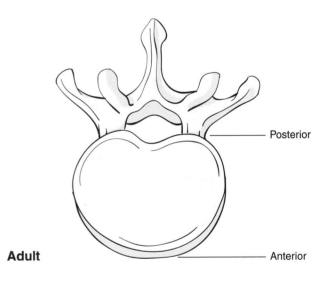

Adult — Posterior — Anterior

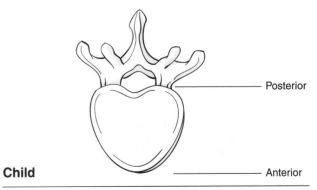

Child — Posterior — Anterior

FIGURE 9-3 The pediatric vertebrae are narrower and wedge-shaped, with the narrow part of the wedge located at the anterior border of the spinal column.

A child, lying supine, naturally has slight flexion of the head. In this situation, the second cervical vertebrae tends to slip forward on the third cervical vertebral body giving the appearance of a **subluxation** (a partial abnormal separation of the articular surfaces of a joint) of C-2. Although this situation can neither be diagnosed nor identified in the prehospital setting, appropriate positioning and immobilization using towels to pad under the shoulders to maintain the head in the "sniffing" position avoids this misleading finding and keeps the spinal cord and column in neutral alignment.

A common concept in pediatric spinal injury is that most injuries occur above the C4 level (Lui, Lee, & Wong, 1996). This assumption stems from the anatomical fact that a child's head size and weakness of the neck muscles results in the fulcrum of neck motion occurring around C2 to C3.

The notion that cervical spine injuries in children are rare has been recently challenged by a study done at the Children's Hospital of Alabama where they found 34 such injuries in a 36-month period. The group also challenged the dogma that most cervical spine injuries in childhood occur above the C4 level as 50 percent of their patients had lesions below C4.

Mechanism of Injury

The mechanism of injury is invaluable in alerting the prehospital provider to the possibility of spinal cord/column injuries. Specific mechanisms that should raise the index of suspicion for SCCI include:

- Landing on the feet following a fall from a height
- Motor vehicle crash involving no or improperly applied restraints accompanied by complaints of abdominal pain (with or without a "seat belt" sign)
- Any injury above the clavicles, blunt or penetrating
- Acceleration/deceleration motor vehicle injuries
- Gunshot injuries, including those of low caliber and low velocity

The number of spinal injuries in childhood does appear to be increasing. Since most pediatric cervical spinal injuries have a motor vehicle crash or a fall as the primary cause of the injury, this increase in incidence may be related to the raising of maximum allowable speed limits. Lack of or inappropriately applied child restraints and unfastened window guards are additional factors in the mechanism of injury.

The bulk of the vertebral bodies and the disks between the vertebrae are relatively resistant to fracturing forces. However, as in skull fractures, the presence of a spinal column fracture indicates a significant injuring force.

If a child lands on his or her feet following a fall from a height, forces are transmitted toward the head along the vertical axis of the spinal column. These forces may result in compression fractures anywhere along the spinal column.

SCCI commonly seen in children and their causes include the following:

- Atlanto-occipital dissociation—acute flexion or extension of the head on the neck
- High cervical spinal injuries (above C4)—flexion injury
- Low cervical spinal injuries (below C4)—flexion injury (50 percent of injuries)
- Lumbar spinal injury—inappropriate seat belt use
- Majority of spinal injuries caused by motor vehicles

Other types of injuries occurring with apparently increasing frequency are lower thoracic or lumbar spinal column injuries resulting from the inappropriate use of seat belts. The use of a lap belt, rather than the safer three- or four-point restraint, results in rapid flexion of the lumbar or lower thoracic spine (Figure 9-4). However, if a three-point restraint does not fit properly, the child is able to slip out from under the belts, which also results in flexion injuries. The "seat belt" sign is a bruise or abrasion starting at the point of the restraint buckle insertion and progressing across the abdomen at the angle of the belt. This finding should raise the prehospital provider's index of suspicion that a lumbar spine or abdominal injury may be present.

Assessment

Precise diagnosis of a specific injury is the ideal in terms of care. However, precise diagnosis, as a general rule, is not achievable in the prehospital setting. At a minimum, the prehospital provider must consider the possibility of a spinal cord/column injury based on the data gathered through the history and limited physical examination.

The field assessment should be a focused examination rather than a complete neurological assessment. There are a number of things that can be accomplished in a minimal amount of time. Level of consciousness should be evaluated using either AVPU or the Glasgow Coma Score. A rapid motor and sensory examination, including observation for spontaneous and purposeful movement of extremities, should be conducted. The spinal column should be palpated, without moving the patient, to check for hematoma, swelling, step-off, pain, and/or tenderness. At least one of these is generally present with a spinal column injury. A quick, limited assessment of the patient's abdomen should be con-

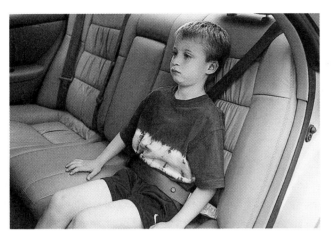 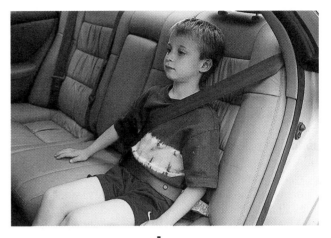

a.   **b.**

FIGURE 9-4   a. Use of a lap belt only can result in rapid flexion of the lumbar or lower thoracic spine. **b.** The three-point restraint is the proper method of using the seat belt and avoiding injury.

ducted to determine the presence of tenderness and/or a "seat belt" sign.

Management

Even in the absence of positive findings, a significant mechanism of injury requires that the child be immobilized. When in doubt, the child should be immobilized. Pediatric spinal immobilization is not easy but can and must be done properly.

Although the principles of immobilization are the same as for the adult, methods of immobilization do vary. Remember that the occipital area of children less than eight years of age is larger than that of the adult. When a child is placed supine on a hard surface, the neck will flex, resulting in flexion of the cervical spine

 Exploring the Web

● Search for Web sites related to spinal trauma. Are there any specific to prehospital care? Are there any specific to pediatric care? Are there any sites that would be helpful in supporting the families of spinal trauma victims? Create flash cards specifying mechanism of injury, assessment, and management of the victim of spinal trauma.

and possibly obstruction of the airway. In order to maintain in-line support and alignment, the head should be brought into the "sniffing" position and the shoulders and trunk padded to make the chest-to-backboard and cranial depths approximately the same. Do not allow the head and neck to move independently from the remainder of the torso.

There are also a variety of commercially available types of pediatric immobilizers available. See Appendix C for pediatric spinal immobilization.

SUMMARY

Head and spinal cord/column injuries frequently coexist. Usually, the presence of a head and/or spinal cord/column injury can only be suspected based on the mechanism of injury, the limited physical examination, and findings that may be evident.

The mainstay of treatment for the pediatric patient with a head injury is the appropriate management of the ABCs. The lack of an airway is a serious matter and must be dealt with in a rapid, appropriate fashion. The greatest threat to life in the child with a head injury is blood volume loss. Once the airway and breathing are controlled, focus should shift to supporting the circulatory system.

The optimum field management of the child with a head injury involves:

• Appropriate and rapid assessment and treatment of the child's airway, breathing, circulation, and neurological status

- Rapid volume resuscitation, if shock is present, without spending undue time trying to initiate IV or IO access

Spinal cord/column injuries are relatively rare in children but should always be suspected in the child suffering head injury. In addition to the mechanism of injury, a rapid and limited neurological assessment should create a high index of suspicion for spinal injuries. Complete immobilization of the child for transport, following the guidelines discussed in the chapter, is critical to avoid making the existing injury worse.

The goal is to deliver the child to the appropriate medical facility with the ABCs adequately controlled and the neurological status determined and documented. The overall care for head and spinal cord/column injuries should accomplish the following:

- Identify potential and actual injuries
- Provide initial treatment for those injuries
- Package and transport the patient to the appropriate medical facility in the best possible condition, without adding to or making worse the injuries the patient may have sustained

Exploring the Web

- Search for articles in professional journals or research related to care and outcomes of victims with head or spinal trauma.

Management of Case Scenario

The mechanism of injury creates a high index of suspicion for both head and spinal injuries. The fact that the child is not moving increases that suspicion even more. The position of the child indicates an acceleration/deceleration force with the head being the lead point of impact. The mechanism also raises suspicion of a potential abdominal injury from blunt force of striking the console.

The initial priority is to secure the airway and immobilize the child. The child must first be removed from the vehicle to a spine board while maintaining manual spinal immobilization. Manual immobilization must be maintained while assessing the airway, respiratory effectiveness, skin appearance, and heart rate. Level of consciousness should be assessed using AVPU or the Glasgow Coma Scale. A limited neurological examination should be conducted to determine pupil size and equality as well as motor and sensory response. The entire spinal column should be palpated to determine the presence or absence of hematoma, swelling, step-off, pain, and/or tenderness.

The child requires total immobilization. Main-

tain in-line support and alignment. Bring the head into the sniffing position and pad the shoulders and trunk to make the chest-to-backboard and cranial depths approximately the same.

High-concentration oxygen should be started immediately if the child has an altered level of consciousness or signs of shock. If the child exhibits signs of shock, vascular access should be established and fluid resuscitation begun at 20 cc/kg. However, under no circumstances should transport be delayed to establish venous access. Rapid transport to definitive care at the appropriate medical facility is imperative to give the child the greatest chance for a positive outcome.

Level of consciousness must be continually reassessed to monitor for changes that might indicate the development of increased intracranial pressure as well as effectiveness of fluid resuscitation if shock is present. Respiratory status must also be constantly monitored. A cervical injury may result in edema of the cord that affects the phrenic nerve and compromises an initially effective respiratory effort.

▶ REVIEW QUESTIONS

1. What is the major difference in outcome between children and adults suffering from head injuries?

2. What is the major difference in cause of death between children and adults suffering from head injuries?

3. Your five-year-old patient responds to voice with agitation and irritability.

a. What Glasgow Coma Scale score would you give him for "verbal response"?

b. What overall Glasgow Coma Scale score would you give him?

4. Describe the "seat belt" sign and list the potential injuries it may indicate.

5. Describe the potential complications that can occur if cervical alignment is not achieved when immobilizing a child to a spine board. Explain the underlying cause(s) of these complications.

6. Describe the method for achieving cervical alignment when immobilizing a child on a spine board.

REFERENCES

Lui, T. N., Lee, S. T., & Wong, C. W. (1996). C1-C2 fracture-dislocations in children and adolescents. *Journal of Trauma*, 40(3), 408–411.

National Association of Emergency Medical Technicians. (1999). *Prehospital trauma life support*. 4th ed. St. Louis, MO: Mosby-Year Book.

National Pediatric Trauma Registry. (1998). Rehabilitation and Research Training Center, Tufts University School of Medicine. Boston, MA: Author.

Tepas, J. J., DiScala, C., & Ramenofsky, M. L. (1990). Mortality and head injury: The pediatric perspective. *Journal of Pediatric Surgery*, 25, 92–96.

BIBLIOGRAPHY

Givens, T. G., Polley, K. A., Smith, G. F. (1996). Pediatric cervical spine injury: a three-year experience. *Journal of Trauma*, 41(2), 310–314.

Pugula, F. A., Wald, S. L., & Shackford, S. R. (1993). The effect of hypotension and hypoxia on children with severe head injuries. *Journal of Pediatric Surgery*, 28(3), 310–316.

Chapter 10 — Thoracic and Abdominal Trauma

OBJECTIVES

Upon completion of this chapter, the student should be able to:

- Identify the predominant mode of injury in children.
- Identify the second leading cause of death from accidental injury.
- List the main reason for less severe blunt thoracic trauma in children.
- Define the following:

    —Pneumothorax
    —Tension pneumothorax
    —Open pneumothorax
    —Hemothorax
    —Pericardial tamponade
    —Cardiac contusion
    —Flail chest
    —Paradoxical respirations

- List signs and symptoms for the following:

    —Pneumothorax
    —Tension pneumothorax
    —Open pneumothorax
    —Hemothorax
    —Pericardial tamponade
    —Cardiac contusion
    —Flail chest

- Identify the major cause of serious abdominal injuries in children.
- List the four most commonly injured intra-abdominal organs in children.
- Differentiate between the signs and symptoms of splenic and liver injuries.

KEY TERMS

cardiac contusion	pericardial tamponade
flail chest	pericardiocentesis
hemothorax	peritonitis
open pneumothorax	simple pneumothorax
paradoxical respirations	tension pneumothorax

Case Scenario

You are called to the local community park for a boy hit by a ball. You arrive to see a large crowd in the middle of the baseball field. A man in a referee uniform comes up to you and explains that the pitcher was a 10-year-old boy who was hit in the chest after a boy on the other team hit a line drive. The pitcher never had a chance to move out of the way. The child was knocked to the ground and did not move for several seconds. The child is crying and struggling to breathe. The mother comes forward and identifies herself as a critical care nurse. How would you manage this situation?

INTRODUCTION

Blunt trauma is the predominant mode of injury in children (Stylianos, 1995). This fact is especially true when discussing thoracic and abdominal trauma. Penetrating injuries to the chest and to the abdomen in children are rare; however, there has been an increase in this mechanism over the past decade (Cooper, 1994). The incidence of penetrating injuries to the chest in children results from fractured ribs and fractured clavicles and not from extrinsic sources such as bullets or knives.

THORACIC TRAUMA

In the United States, thoracic injury is second to head injury as the leading cause of death from accidental injury (National Association of Emergency Medical Technicians, 1998). Children may have significant injury to the organs or blood vessels in the thorax despite the absence of any injury to the rib cage.

Blunt thoracic trauma in children is generally less severe than that which is seen in the adult population due to the following reasons:

- Blunt thoracic trauma seen in adults is usually the result of high-speed motor vehicle accidents
- Blunt thoracic trauma seen in children is usually the result of the child being struck by a car at a fairly low speed or riding unrestrained in a motor vehicle
- Compliance of the thorax in a child is unique in that the thoracic structures in children are flexible
- Although a child may suffer major internal injury from compression of the thorax, the ribs are rarely broken.

Injuries to the thorax may result in hypoxic events or hypotension, which do not allow for long periods of time, thought, or prehospital treatment. Often the physical examination in children who have suffered from thoracic injuries is unreliable. Only prehospital providers who are appropriately trained in pediatric trauma management are capable of the quick intervention that must take place.

Thoracic injuries in children carry a mortality of about 15 percent, and many fatalities occur after the child reaches the hospital. In many cases, the child is stable with no outward signs of injury. These children can deteriorate rapidly. Once the child becomes hypoxic and hypotensive, rapid treatment and transport are critical.

Remember that when there is a major thoracic injury, there most likely will be an injury to some other organ system. These other injuries occur in over 50 percent of cases of thoracic trauma.

Simple Pneumothorax

A **simple pneumothorax** is a collection of air in the pleural space that causes the lung to collapse. In blunt trauma, there is a tear in the visceral pleura, and air rushes out of the lung, causing it to collapse (Figure 10-1). Rupture of the bronchi or trachea may also cause a pneumothorax.

Mechanism of Injury

A simple pneumothorax can be caused by any trauma to the thoracic cavity strong enough to rupture the lung. Examples include a motor vehicle accident in which the child is not restrained, a child hit by a car while riding a bicycle, or an object striking the child's chest (e.g., baseball, baseball bat, fist, etc.).

Signs and Symptoms

Signs and symptoms of a simple pneumothorax include:

- Absent or decreased breath sounds on the side of the injury

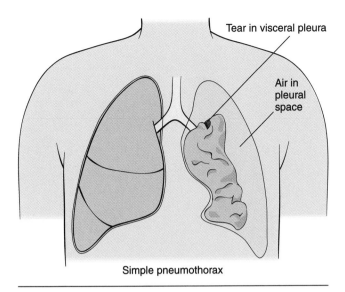

FIGURE 10-1 A closed pneumothorax occurs when the visceral pleura tears and air rushes out of the lung, causing it to collapse.

- Respiratory distress
- Tachycardia
- Cyanosis (late sign)

Assessment

Pay close attention to the child's respiratory status. Continually evaluate the respiratory rate and the child's ability to speak. As the dyspnea gets worse, the child will have difficulty speaking in complete sentences. Look for other associated injuries depending on the mechanism of injury.

Assess the skin color and lips for cyanosis. Cyanosis is a late sign and may indicate the child is rapidly decompensating.

Management

Treatment includes high-concentration oxygen, ventilation, endotracheal intubation if necessary, rapid transport, and frequent reassessment. Remember that aggressive positive pressure ventilation may cause a pneumothorax to progress to a tension pneumothorax as discussed below.

Transport

If the child is having significant respiratory distress, initiate rapid transport. Continue to monitor vital signs and the child's ability to breathe. Transport the child in a sitting position to maximize respiratory effort unless immobilization is indicated. In that case, elevate the top of the long backboard to decrease the child's anxiety and promote the best exchange of oxygen.

Tension Pneumothorax

A simple pneumothorax may lead to a **tension pneumothorax**. If not treated, a tension pneumothorax can be fatal.

Mechanism of Injury

The initial injury creates a one-way valve that allows air to enter but not leave the pleural space. If untreated, enough pressure accumulates to shift the mediastinum, compromise venous return, and decrease cardiac output (Figure 10-2). This condition is known as a tension pneumothorax.

Signs and Symptoms

Signs and symptoms of a tension pneumothorax include:

- Severe dyspnea
- Tachycardia
- Cyanosis
- Decreased or no breath sounds on side of injury

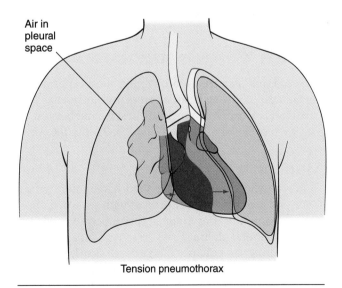

FIGURE 10-2 A tension pneumothorax occurs as pressure accumulates in the pleural cavity, leading to compression of the heart and uninjured lung. The mediastinum shifts AWAY from the injured lung.

- Hypotension leading to shock
- Subcutaneous emphysema (not always present)
- Tracheal shift away from injured lung (late finding—may not be visible in young children with short, chubby necks)
- Distended neck veins (may not be present in child who is hypotensive; difficult to see in young children with short, chubby necks)
- Hyperresonance to percussion (may be difficult to hear in the prehospital setting)

Assessment

The degree of signs, symptoms, and respiratory difficulty depends on how much air has built up in the child's chest. As the pressure and dyspnea increase, the child will become very agitated and not listen to directions. Continual reassessment is necessary.

Management

Advanced life support providers may perform a needle thoracentesis to relieve the pressure from a tension pneumothorax. See Appendix C for a skills review of needle thoracentesis in pediatric patients. Reassess frequently in case the condition reoccurs. A second procedure may be necessary.

Transport

Rapid transport is necessary for the child with a tension pneumothorax. Needle thoracentesis is a temporary measure to provide some relief. More definitive treatment is needed at the hospital as quickly as possible.

Open Pneumothorax

A wound that penetrates through the chest can produce the collapse of a lung or an **open pneumothorax**. This condition is also called a sucking chest wound because of the sound of air moving in and out of the hole in the chest.

Mechanism of Injury

Children who are stabbed or who have fallen onto a fence and are impaled may present with a sucking chest wound. In penetrating trauma, disruption of the chest wall and parietal pleura allows air to rush in, again causing the lung to collapse (Figure 10-3). Less air is brought down through the trachea than through the open wound. This action occurs because the dynamic of gases is to select the path of least resistance. By virtue of its volume, an open pneumothorax is a far less resistant area for air to travel through than the volume-limited larynx.

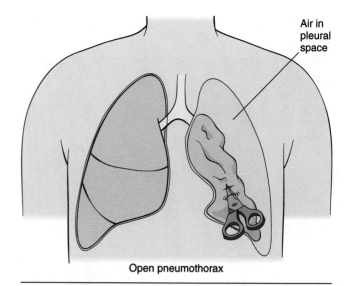

Air in pleural space

Open pneumothorax

FIGURE 10-3 An open pneumothorax occurs from disruption of the chest wall and the parietal pleura, allowing air to rush into the pleural space and causing the lung to collapse.

Signs and Symptoms

In addition to the signs and symptoms of a simple pneumothorax, the child may present with pain at the site of injury. In addition, there may be a moist bubbling sound coming from the chest as air moves in and out of the pleural space through the hole in the chest.

Assessment

Monitor the child's respiratory status and the amount of air being released from the chest wall defect. Assess for bleeding from the wound itself.

Management

If an open chest wound is present, apply an occlusive dressing that is taped on three sides. This "flutter-valve" effect will allow air to release from the pleural space through the untaped fourth side of the dressing yet occlude the opening so no additional air can move into the pleural space (Figure 10-4).

Provide high-concentration oxygen, and assist ventilations as necessary. Treat for hypovolemia if there is the potential for blood loss.

Transport

A child with an open pneumothorax usually requires rapid transport. The destination should be a pediatric

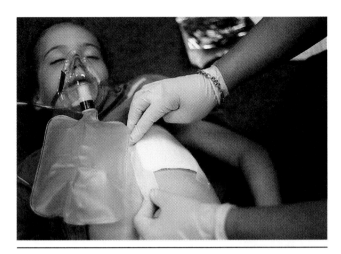

FIGURE 10-4 An occlusive dressing is applied to an open chest wound. It is taped on three sides to create a "flutter valve" effect.

trauma center whenever possible. Reassess the adequacy of the dressing on the defect to make sure air is not getting sucked into the wound. Continue to monitor for progression to a tension pneumothorax.

Hemothorax

A **hemothorax** is the collection of blood in the pleural space. It can occur at the same time as a simple or open pneumothorax if there is any injury to blood vessels in the chest.

Mechanism of Injury

Hypovolemia occurs as blood moves from a ruptured blood vessel into the pleural space. It can have the same physiologic consequences as air. Enough blood in the pleural space can shift the mediastinum and delay central venous return.

Signs and Symptoms

Breath sounds will be decreased with hyporesonance or a dull sound upon percussion on the side of the injury. It is difficult to find this sign in the prehospital setting.

Assessment

Assessment is similar to a pneumothorax except that the symptoms are more related to the loss of blood. Hypotension will occur quickly if the blood loss is significant.

In addition, the side of the hemothorax will be dull upon percussion because of the accumulation of fluid.

Management

Treatment includes high-concentration oxygen, ventilation and/or endotracheal intubation if necessary, rapid transport, and frequent reassessment. Lactated Ringer's or normal saline solution can be infused en route through a large-bore intravenous or intraosseous line.

Transport

A child with a hemothorax should be rapidly transported to a pediatric trauma center capable of performing pediatric cardiovascular surgery. Vital signs and respiratory status should be meticulously monitored en route.

Pericardial Tamponade

Between the heart and the pericardium is a potential space that can fill with blood. Accumulation of blood within that space is called a **pericardial tamponade** (Figure 10-5).

Mechanism of Injury

Blunt or penetrating trauma can cause this condition. It is most frequently associated with stab wounds. A gunshot wound usually creates a hole big enough for blood to leave the pericardial space.

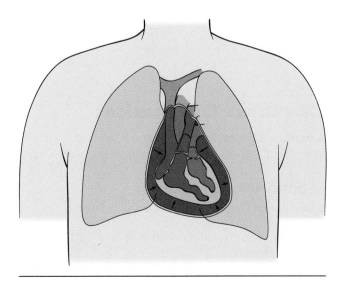

FIGURE 10-5 A pericardial tamponade occurs when blood collects in the space between the heart and the pericardium.

As blood leaks from the wound in the wall of the heart, if fills up the pericardial sac and exerts pressure. This pressure on the heart decreases its ability to expand with blood and pump it out to the rest of the body with each contraction of the ventricles. The result is decreased blood return to the heart and decreased cardiac output.

Signs and Symptoms

Signs and symptoms include a weak pulse, narrowing pulse pressure (i.e., the difference between the systolic and diastolic pressures), hypotension, diminished heart sounds, and jugular venous distention. Again, jugular venous distention is difficult to see in a young child with a short, chubby neck.

Assessment

Assess for specific chest injuries and signs of shock, which may progressively worsen. The remainder of the exam may be negative.

Management

Treatment includes high-concentration oxygen, ventilation, endotracheal intubation if necessary, cardiac monitoring, and frequent reassessment. Definitive treatment is **pericardiocentesis** or aspirating the fluid from the pericardial space with a needle. It is usually done by a physician with surgical training and experience and is not commonly available in the prehospital setting.

Transport

Rapid transport is essential so that periocardiocentesis can be performed. Inform the receiving hospital of the child's status so they can have the necessary equipment available upon arrival of the child at the Emergency Department.

Cardiac Contusion

A **cardiac contusion** or bruising of the heart muscle is more commonly seen in older children and adolescents.

Mechanism of Injury

Three distinct injury patterns may be present:

1. The electrical conduction system of the heart may be disrupted.
2. The myocardial wall may be bruised by the impact of blunt trauma.
3. The actual myocardium (i.e., heart muscle) can rupture.

Mechanisms causing compression of the chest in a child include sports injuries, motor vehicle accidents, being struck by a motor vehicle, and violent attacks such as beatings. Any child who has sustained a blunt force to the chest should be suspected as having a cardiac contusion until proven otherwise.

Signs and Symptoms

Signs and symptoms may include:

- Chest pain and/or anterior chest tenderness
- Bruising to the anterior chest
- Bent steering wheel of an automobile or bent handlebars of a bicycle
- Dysrhythmias on the cardiac monitor
- Decreased blood pressure due to reduced cardiac output

Assessment

Use a cardiac monitor to evaluate the heart rate and regularity of the rhythm. Tachycardia without other reasons (e.g., hypovolemia) is common as are premature ventricular contractions (PVCs). Right bundle branch block may be present due to injury to the septum.

Management

High-concentration oxygen and cardiac monitoring are necessary. An intravenous line of lactated Ringer's or normal saline solution should be used instead of D5W since hypovolemia may occur requiring fluid resuscitation. Lidocaine may be given for ventricular dysrhythmias depending on local protocols.

Transport

Transport to the hospital for ongoing monitoring of the child's cardiac status. If any other traumatic injuries are suspected, a pediatric trauma center may be more appropriate.

Flail Chest

A **flail chest** occurs when multiple rib fractures are present causing instability of the chest. It is not commonly seen in young children.

Mechanism of Injury

Usually, two or more adjacent ribs are broken in two or more places causing a flail or independent segment (Figure 10-6). Flail chest generally occurs in children over the age of 12 years. The rib cage in younger children is usually too flexible to be broken.

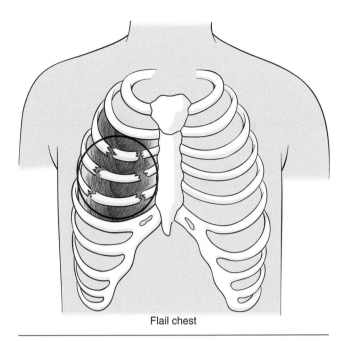

Flail chest

FIGURE 10-6 A flail chest occurs when two or more adjacent ribs break in two or more places.

Older children who have sustained some impact to the sternum or lateral side of the thoracic wall may have a flail chest. Examples include motor vehicle accidents, blunt objects to the chest, and auto/pedestrian collisions.

Signs and Symptoms

The child will not want to breathe deep as that activity causes more pain. Other signs and symptoms include:

- Dyspnea
- Sharp pain leading to splinting and decreased movement of air in and out of the lungs
- Short, shallow respirations
- Uneven chest expansion
- Decreased breath sounds on the side of the injury
- Tachycardia
- Cyanosis
- Crepitus

Assessment

The hallmark of a flail chest is **paradoxical respirations**. The flail segment moves inward on inspiration and outward on exhalation, opposite from the rest of the

ribs. A pulmonary contusion is usually present, which adds to the severity of the respiratory compromise.

Management

High-concentration oxygen should be administered. If the child is extremely dyspneic, he or she may resist a nonrebreather face mask because of the "smothering" feeling. Provide blow-by oxygen rather than make the child more agitated, causing a further increase in the level of respiratory distress. A bulky dressing may be applied to the flail segment to reduce the paradoxical movement. However, do not put anything heavy on the chest as has been previously recommended.

Transport

This child needs rapid transport to the hospital for stabilization of the flail segment and definitive pain control. Some children require prolonged intubation and ventilatory support for a severe injury.

ABDOMINAL TRAUMA

The most commonly injured intra-abdominal organs are the spleen, liver, pancreas, and intestine. It is the physical forces of crushing and deceleration that result in injury to the viscera when a child is struck in the abdomen.

Approximately 90 percent of serious abdominal injuries in children are the result of blunt mechanisms. Motor vehicle accidents are the leading cause followed by falls and child abuse (see Chapter 12—Child Abuse).

The crushing type of injury leads to splenic bursting and pancreatic hematoma and contusion. The physics of deceleration involved in blunt trauma injuries result in harm to organs that are fixed by attachments such as the liver by the hepatic veins.

Children are at a greater risk of serious injury than adults because of their poorly developed abdominal musculature and their small size. They are very vulnerable to being thrown long distances if struck by a motor vehicle or unrestrained within a motor vehicle. Life-threatening intra-abdominal trauma must be suspected in any child who has been struck by an automobile, has fallen from a considerable height, or appears to be unconscious.

In some instances, an intra-abdominal injury is complicated by the presence of coma from an associated head injury. It is important to remember that undiagnosed, uncontrolled bleeding must be presumed to be of intra-abdominal origin until ruled out. Any child who has hemodynamic instability must be considered a patient in shock from an injury to the abdomen (Wilson, 1997).

Splenic Injuries

The spleen is the organ most likely to be injured in a child. It can be bruised or ruptured, depending on the mechanism of injury.

Mechanism of Injury

Evidence of upper quadrant abrasions, tire marks, or other local trauma should alert prehospital personnel to the possibility of a splenic injury. One example of how this injury might occur is the child being run over by an automobile, dirt bike, farm tractor, or other equivalent machine. Other examples include skiing, sled riding, and beatings.

Signs and Symptoms

When the child is seen right after the injury or if the rate of blood loss is slow, the child may not have any signs or symptoms. Conversely, children with a major splenic injury may be in shock from rapid blood loss. Typical signs and symptoms include:

- Bruising or other marks on the abdomen
- Abdominal swelling, rigidity, or tenderness
- Respiratory distress in children under 8 years of age (as they tend to be "belly breathers")
- Unexplained levels of shock
- Left upper quadrant pain and tenderness
- Left shoulder pain

Assessment

In the conscious child, physical examination remains the primary method of evaluation. If the child is crying, abdominal examination may be difficult. Guarding and abdominal swelling may be missed if the child is upset.

If the child who has been crying and upset suddenly allows an abdominal exam, be concerned. This cooperativeness may be a sign that the level of consciousness is deteriorating because of the increasing hypovolemia due to abdominal bleeding.

Management

Definitive care for this child is surgical evaluation at a pediatric trauma center. Even if the child appears stable, do not waste any time in the field. Provide high-concentration oxygen, control any external bleeding, and prepare for transport.

Transport

Rapidly transport this child to a pediatric trauma center whenever possible. These children can decompensate very quickly to the point at which they cannot be resus-citated. Intravenous fluids of lactated Ringer's or normal saline solution can be administered en route anywhere from a KVO (keep vein open) rate to 20 cc/kg boluses as the child's condition warrants.

Liver Injuries

Rupture of the liver is responsible for more death and injury than any other abdominal organ. This organ is very vascular and bleeds easily even with minimal trauma.

Mechanism of Injury

The right lobe is involved four times more frequently than the left lobe. Blunt trauma usually results in a bursting injury, which may vary from a relatively minor capsular tear to destruction of an entire lobe. Suspect liver injury in any patient with severe abdominal impact, a direct blow, unexplained hypotension, or intraperitoneal bleeding.

Suspect liver injury if there is gross evidence of severe upper abdominal trauma. Tire marks, major abrasions, or ecchymosis in the right upper quadrant, massive intra-abdominal bleeding, and shock suggest injury to the liver. Great vessel injury can also cause hemorrhage, but it is much less common.

Signs and Symptoms

Again, signs and symptoms may be absent if the child is seen right after the injury or if the bleeding is slow or has stopped momentarily. Specific signs and symptoms include:

- Right upper quadrant pain
- Tenderness
- Right shoulder pain
- Tachycardia

Other injuries that commonly accompany liver rupture may complicate the evaluation of physical signs. Most common are injuries to the lower chest wall, pulmonary contusion, diaphragmatic rupture, hemothorax, and renal trauma.

Assessment

Assessment is the same as for splenic injuries. Be alert if the child becomes more cooperative as the hypovolemia increases.

Management

Management continues to be definitive care in the operating room. Control airway, breathing, and circulation while preparing for transport.

Transport

Rapidly transport this child to a pediatric trauma center. Provide advanced notice so that the trauma team can be activated.

Pancreatic Injuries

The pathophysiology of pancreatic injury involves release of highly irritating pancreatic enzymes, which produce a severe inflammatory reaction. The local inflammatory reaction subsequently causes a systemic inflammatory response.

Mechanism of Injury

The location of the pancreas overlying the vertebral column makes it a target for injury when a child is run over by a car's tire, falls on a handlebar of a bike, or is kicked in the upper abdomen. Always suspect pancreatic injury if there is significant upper abdominal trauma or peritoneal signs without evidence of bleeding.

Signs and Symptoms

The peritoneal contamination, which occurs with pancreatic injury, results in chemical **peritonitis**, or inflammation of the peritoneum, and severe abdominal pain. Rigidity of the abdominal wall may be a late sign. Children with pancreatic injury usually have other serious injuries at the same time.

Assessment

Use caution when palpating the child's abdomen. Palpate the abdomen last as any severe pain may cause the child to be uncooperative during the remainder of the exam.

Management

Management continues to be definitive care in the operating room. Control airway, breathing, and circulation while preparing for transport.

Transport

Rapidly transport this child to a pediatric trauma center. Provide advanced notice so that the trauma team can be activated.

Intestinal Injuries

The mobility of the intestine makes it less likely to be injured than the solid organs. However, once the intestines are injured, significant contamination of the abdominal cavity can occur.

Mechanism of Injury

Not surprisingly, intestinal injuries are most common in the segments that are fixed: the duodenum, the ascending colon, and the descending colon. In adults, penetrating trauma is the major cause of intestinal injuries; but in children, blunt trauma is the chief offender.

Duodenal injury results in an intramural hematoma, which is the most common intestinal injury in children as the duodenum is compressed against the spine. Such injuries are more common in children than adults because of a child's smaller size and weaker abdominal musculature, which holds true for injuries to the entire abdomen in children. Even mild blunt trauma such as a punch in the stomach may cause serious injury. Always suspect a duodenal injury in any child with focal blunt injury to the upper abdomen, such as a handlebar injury or kick.

Intestinal injuries of the remainder of the small bowel are uncommon after blunt trauma but common after penetrating trauma. Rectal trauma, stabbing, or a gunshot wound to the abdomen can cause injury to the colon. Always suspect intestinal injury in every child with penetrating injury to the abdomen.

Rectal injuries may result from penetrating injury through the anorectum or from a fractured pelvis. Suspect a rectal injury if the pelvis is fractured.

Signs and Symptoms

In addition to general signs and symptoms of abdominal trauma, Table 10-1 outlines specific organs and their related signs and symptoms.

Assessment

Use caution when palpating the child's abdomen. Palpate the abdomen last as any severe pain may cause the child to be uncooperative during the remainder of the exam.

Management

Management continues to be definitive care in the operating room. Control airway, breathing, and circulation while preparing for transport.

Transport

Rapidly transport this child to a pediatric trauma center. Provide advanced notice so that the trauma team can be activated.

TABLE 10-1
Signs and Symptoms of Intestinal Injuries

Type of Injury	Signs and Symptoms
Perforation of the intestine	• Prompt peritoneal contamination with intestinal contents • If it is the upper intestine that is perforated, the injury is largely chemical; and peritoneal irritation produces early symptoms
Duodenal	• Signs of obstruction • May not be evident for several days after the injury when bilious vomiting occurs
Small bowel	• Immediate peritonitis and distention
Rectum	• Rectal bleeding may be the only early sign

SUMMARY

Blunt trauma is the predominant mode of injury in children. Thoracic injury is second to head injury as the leading cause of death from accidental injury. Children can suffer serious thoracic trauma without any outward signs of bony injury because the child's rib cage is so flexible. Various types of thoracic trauma exist.

Abdominal trauma should always be suspected if unexplained hypotension is present. Children are at a greater risk of serious injury than adults because of their poorly developed abdominal musculature and their small size. Various types of abdominal trauma exist.

If trauma to the chest or abdomen is suspected, the child should be prepared for rapid transport to a tertiary facility capable of performing major surgery on a child. Time should not be wasted in the field even if the child appears to be stable.

Management of Case Scenario

The child is awake, crying, and taking shallow breaths. He states it hurts to take a deep breath. Auscultation of the chest reveals clear, shallow breath sounds in both lungs. The child is guarding the left chest, and there is a large reddened area in the left upper chest where the ball hit him. The area is tender to palpation, and no bruises or broken bones are found. Respiratory rate is 36 and shallow, heart rate is 144 and regular, and blood pressure is 128/74. His face is pale, and his lips are slightly cyanotic. Capillary refill is normal. Cardiac monitoring reveals sinus tachycardia with rare premature ventricular contractions (PVCs).

Treatment includes high-concentration oxygen with a nonrebreather face mask and continual cardiac monitoring. An intravenous line of normal saline or lactated ringers may be started in case he needs Lidocaine® for any increase in the PVCs. Allow the child to sit at a 45° angle during the transport to promote comfort and ease of breathing. Reassess vital signs and his respiratory and cardiac status frequently throughout transport.

Provide reassurance to the child and his family. Explain everything being done. Since his mother is a critical care nurse, allow her to see the cardiac monitor; and provide her with frequent updates regarding the reassessment and subsequent vital signs. Provide a report to the receiving facility so they may have adequate time to prepare for arrival of the child.

REVIEW QUESTIONS

1. What is the predominant mode of injury in children?
2. What is the second leading cause of death from accidental injury?
3. Severe blunt thoracic trauma is less likely in children because:
   a. Children are not hit as hard as adults.
   b. Children's rib cages are more flexible than adults.
   c. Children can withstand pain more than adults.
   d. None of the above.

4. Define the following terms:

 a. Pneumothorax

 b. Tension pneumothorax

 c. Open pneumothorax

 d. Hemothorax

 e. Pericardial tamponade

 f. Cardiac contusion

 g. Flail chest

 h. Paradoxical respirations

5. List signs/symptoms of a tension pneumothorax in a child.

6. What is the major cause of serious abdominal injuries in children?

7. List the four most commonly injured intra-abdominal organs in children.

8. The child will have left shoulder pain with a liver injury. True or False?

REFERENCES

Cooper, A., et al. (1994). Mortality and thoracoabdominal injury: The pediatric perspective. *Journal of Pediatric Surgery*, 29, 97.

Krige, J. E., et al. (1990). Severe juxtahepatic venous injury: Survival after prolonged hepatic vascular isolation without shunting. *HPB Surgery*, 3, 39.

National Association of Emergency Medical Technicians. (1998). *Prehospital trauma life support—basic and advanced*. 4th ed. St. Louis, MO: Mosby-Year Book.

Stylianos, S. (1995). Controversies in abdominal trauma. *Pediatric Surgery*, 4,116–119.

Wilson, E. F. (1997). Estimation of the ages of cutaneous contusions in child abuse. *Pediatrics*, 60, 75l.

BIBLIOGRAPHY

McSwain, N. E., White, R. D., Paturas, J. L., & Metcalf, W. R. (1997). *The Basic EMT—comprehensive prehospital patient care*. St. Louis, MO: Mosby-Year Book.

Trunkey, D. (1991). Initial treatment of patients with extensive trauma. *New England Journal of Medicine*, 324, 1259.

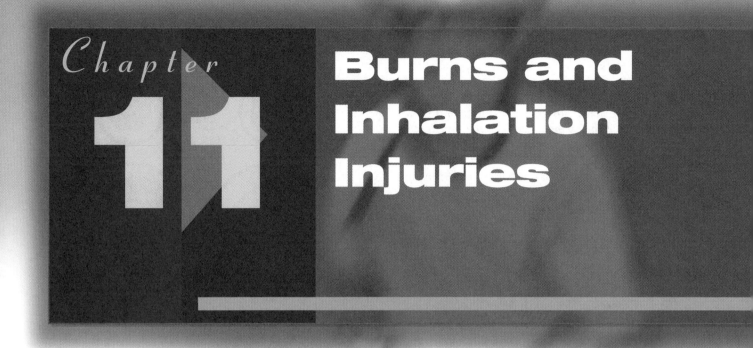

Chapter 11

Burns and Inhalation Injuries

OBJECTIVES

Upon completion of this chapter, the student should be able to:

- Explain the physiological differences between adults and children with respect to burn and inhalation injuries.
- Describe the most common causes of burns within each developmental age group.
- List the six components for determining burn severity.
- Outline the specific assessment and resuscitation procedures for burns in children.
- Explain the pathophysiology, assessment, and management of children suffering from airway injuries and carbon monoxide poisoning.

KEY TERMS

alternating current (AC)
bronchorrhea
carbonaceous
carboxyhemoglobin

compartment syndrome
direct current (DC)
entrance wound

escharotomy
exit wound
fasciotomy

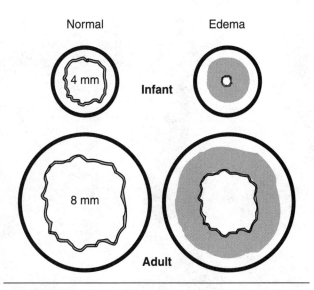

FIGURE 11-1 Effect of edema on airway resistance in the infant versus the adult.

Case Scenario

You are dispatched to a house fire to stand by for potential victims. Upon arrival, the firefighters bring a four-year-old child to you. They tell you he was inside the house hiding in a closet. He is crying and coughing. There is black soot around his mouth and nose. His clothes have a strong smell of smoke. What would you do?

INTRODUCTION

A child's physical and emotional immaturity make burns one of the most devastating forms of trauma that a child can suffer. A child who survives the initial burn often faces prolonged hospitalization associated with painful treatments, frequent operations, and multiple complications. In addition, the burn and continuing care may leave unsightly physical and deep emotional scars.

ANATOMICAL AND PHYSIOLOGICAL CONSIDERATIONS

Burns can cause a tremendous amount of anatomical and physiological changes in children. Prehospital providers should be concerned primarily with changes that affect the respiratory system, circulatory system, integumentary system, and immune system.

Respiratory System

Children are more vulnerable to respiratory complications than adults due to the size of their airways and the rate at which they breathe (see Chapter 2—Assessment of the Stable Child and Chapter 4—Respiratory Emergencies). The diameter of the pediatric airway is smaller than the adult's airway; therefore, minimal swelling may cause airway obstruction (Figure 11-1). Inhaled hot air and toxic fumes will cause the same degree of swelling in children and adults. However, the amount of swelling that will result in a decrease of 10 to 15 percent in an adult's airway diameter will result in a decrease of over 50 percent in a child's airway diameter.

Children breathe at a faster rate than adults. This increased rate can lead to two problems: (1) an increase in pulmonary fluid loss and (2) an increase in the uptake of toxic gases. Children involved in closed space fires usually die of the increased uptake of toxic gases rather than their burn injuries.

Circulatory System

The body's response to burns is to shift fluid from the intravascular space to the interstitial space (Figure 11-2). As a result, this third-space shifting causes increased edema at the burn site and a decrease in circulating volume. Children have less total circulating blood volume

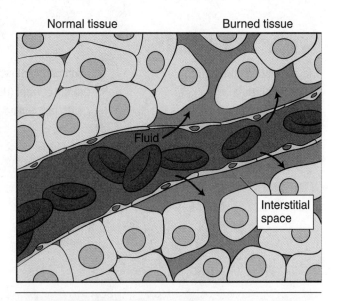

FIGURE 11-2 In a child with a burn, fluid shifts from the intravascular space to the interstitial space, causing hypovolemia.

than adults and are more susceptible to hypovolemia and shock. In addition, the child's blood vessels supplying the burned area are smaller. Therefore, injured cells may cause a vasoconstriction at the site of the injury. This condition leads to hypoxia and ischemia of tissue as well as tissue necrosis.

Integumentary System

The skin is the largest organ in the human body. It consists of two layers: the epidermis and the dermis (Figure 11-3). The epidermis acts primarily as the body's tough protective barrier against the invasion of infection from the external environment. The dermis contains the blood vessels, sweat glands, and nerves that act to provide protection against fluid and temperature loss as well as the ability to sense pain.

The skin of a child differs from that of an adult in terms of maturity, body surface area-to-weight ratio, and temperature regulation. A child has thinner skin than an adult, a greater body surface area in proportion to weight, and immature temperature control centers. These differences allow less heat to produce more serious burns in children. In addition, children will lose more heat and water faster.

Immune System

Burns disrupt the first protective barrier against infection—the skin. The immune system provides the human body with a second defense against infection. However, it is poorly developed in children, leaving the child more susceptible to infection following burn injury. It is important to remember that young infants and immuno-suppressed children are at an even greater risk for sepsis following burn injury.

DETERMINATION OF BURN SEVERITY

Burn severity is dependent upon age, depth of injury, body surface area affected, location, associated injuries, and general health. Each item is discussed briefly.

Age

Younger children are more at risk for serious burn complications because their bodies are still growing and their skin is thin and underdeveloped. Renal function and the immune system are immature. Infants do not

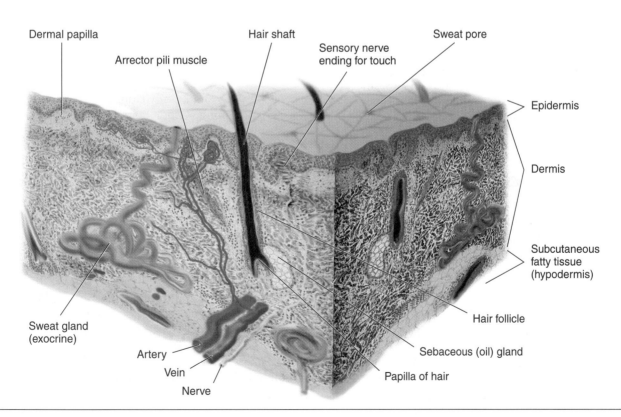

FIGURE 11-3 The epidermis protects the body while the dermis contains vital components.

store much protein, and what is available is quickly lost if burn shock is present. In addition, the small size of an infant's or young child's trachea leaves little room for edema in the event of an inhalation burn, quickly resulting in severe respiratory compromise. Children under two years of age, therefore, have a much higher mortality rate than an older child with the same type of burn.

Depth of Injury

A deeper burn is a much more serious burn. The longer the contact with the burning agent, the greater the destruction of tissue. Severe injuries may easily occur in very young children because of the thin nature of their skin (i.e., infants).

Body Surface Area Affected

In infants, the head makes up a much larger proportion of the body. As the baby grows, the head size decreases in relation to the remainder of the body. A modified "rule of nines" is used in children to account for these differences.

Location

Areas such as the hands, feet, genitals, and across the joints carry a higher risk of complications in children. Facial burns, for example, may involve the eye and contribute to ongoing vision and potential learning problems in the future. Burns to the perineum are easily infected, especially in those children who are still using diapers. To preserve maximum function, specialty care is usually necessary.

Associated Injuries

In many instances, the burn may be secondary to a traumatic injury. The child may have been involved in a motor vehicle accident in which the vehicle was on fire. The traumatic injuries take precedence over the burned skin.

General Health of the Child

The general health of the child provides important information in determining the severity of the burn injury. Any child with pre-existing illnesses such as asthma, diabetes, renal insufficiency, and/or cardiac problems may find recovery long and difficult.

CLASSIFICATION OF BURN SEVERITY

The determination of burn severity will help the prehospital provider classify burns into one of three categories: minor, moderate, or major. The appropriate treatment and transport of the burned child can be determined from this classification (Table 11-1).

Some burns that do not cover large body surface areas still require specialized care in a burn center. Examples include burns to the hands, feet, face and neck (i.e., raising the suspicion of inhalation injury), across joints, and genitalia. The burn injury and subsequent formation of scars have the potential to interfere with the child's future growth and development if not treated and managed appropriately. In addition, burns to the genitalia are prone to infection and may interfere with mobility and hygiene as the child recovers.

TYPES OF BURNS

There are several types of burns depending on the mechanism of injury. They are discussed in detail below.

Thermal Burns

Thermal burns are caused by direct contact with either hot liquid (e.g., water, coffee, or grease) or with a flame. Injuries depend on the exposure and length of contact with the substance or flame.

The most common early cause of death from thermal burns is smoke inhalation and carbon monoxide (CO) poisoning. Other complications include hypovolemia and shock.

Incidence

The most common burn injury in children under four years of age is a scald burn, and most of those children are actually between six months to two years of age (Wong, 1999). Scald burns are caused by direct contact with a hot liquid. Hot water followed by grease are the most common liquids (Figure 11-4). These burns are most common in children under the age of three years because of their inherent ability to explore. These "creepers, cruisers, and climbers" tend to get their burn injuries in the kitchen and bathroom.

The second most common thermal burn is caused by flame and represents 13 percent of all burns affecting children. Flame burns are most commonly seen in children over the age of four years. They are the result of the child playing with matches, flammable liquids, firecrackers, or open fires. Children less than four years of

TABLE 11-1
Classification of Burns

Type	Criteria	Treatment
Minor	• 15% or less of total body surface area • Face, hands, feet or perineum not involved • Inhalation injury, electrical burns, severe pre-existing medical problems, or complications not present	Supportive; brief admission (~1–2 days) or outpatient
Moderate	• 15%–25% of total body surface area • Face, hands, feet, or perineum not involved • Inhalation injury, electrical injury, severe pre-existing medical problems, or other related injury not present	Hospital admission required; burn center recommended
Major	• 25% or greater of total body surface area • Involvement of hands, feet, or perineum that significantly alters function • Inhalation or electrical injury • Related injury • Severe pre-existing medical problems	Admission to specialized burn center necessary

National Institute of General Medical Sciences, National Institutes of Health. (1999). *Trauma, burn, shock and injury: Facts and figures.* Bethesda, MD: The Institute.

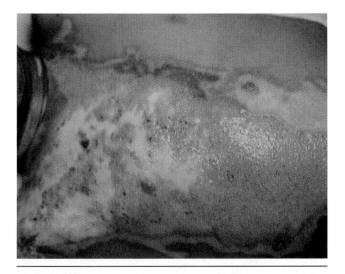

FIGURE 11-4 This child was burned when he pulled a pot of boiling water off of the stove. Courtesy of Dr. Robert Arensman, Chief of Pediatric Surgery, Children's Memorial Medical Center, Chicago, IL.

age tend to obtain the most severe flame burns from house fires (Wong, 1999).

Mechanism of Injury

The severity of a scald burn is, in part, dependent upon the contact time with the liquid and the temperature of the liquid. A child exposed to hot water tends to have a shorter contact time because water cools quickly and runs off. On the other hand, a child exposed to hot grease tends to have a greater contact time, thus allowing more heat to be transferred to the skin.

The temperature of the liquid and the age of the patient are major determinants in burn severity. According to the American Burn Association, an exposure to water temperatures above 130° Fahrenheit will result in a full-thickness burn in less than five seconds in young children. Exposure to the same water temperature by older children and adults will take 15 seconds to result in the same severity of burn.

The body areas most commonly burned are the face, neck, arms, and chest. Scalds tend to result in

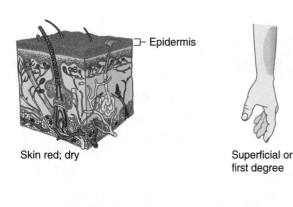

Skin red; dry

Superficial or first degree

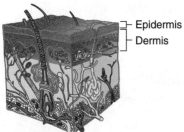
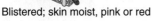
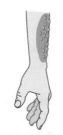

Blistered; skin moist, pink or red

Partial thickness or second degree

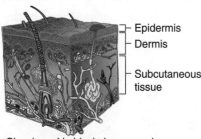
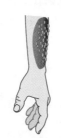

Charring; skin black, brown, red

Full thickness or third degree

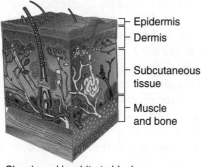
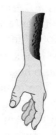

Charring; skin white to black with networks of thrombosed capillaries

Full thickness or fourth degree

FIGURE 11-5   Burn damage to the skin is classified as superficial, partial thickness, or full thickness.

burns with a sharp demarcation or outline of the burn site. In children who are abused, the abuser may drip scalding liquid on the surface of the skin causing a "drip" pattern at the burn site.

Flame burns can affect any part of a child's body, depending on the exposure to fire. Flame usually results in burns whose borders have an irregular pattern.

The depth of the thermal burn injury is generally classified as superficial (also known as first-degree), partial-thickness (or second-degree), or full-thickness (or third-degree). Refer to Figure 11-5 for a comparison of burn types. In superficial burns, the injury is to the epidermis. They result from either prolonged exposure to a low-intensity heat source, such as the sun, or short exposure to a high intensity heat source, such as a flame.

Partial-thickness burns involve injury to the epidermis and the dermis. Depending upon the amount of the dermis affected, these burns can further be classified as superficial or deep. Partial-thickness burns are generally the result of a deep sunburn, contact with hot liquids, or flash burns.

Full-thickness burns destroy the entire epidermis and dermis, including the regenerative properties and the peripheral nerve endings. Full-thickness burns are generally the result of fire, prolonged exposure to hot liquids, or electricity. These burns are also known as third or fourth degree.

Signs and Symptoms

The signs and symptoms of superficial burns include redness and dryness of the skin and pain (Figure 11-6). Superficial burns tend to heal in approximately one week.

The signs and symptoms of partial-thickness burns include a red, mottled appearance; blisters; edema; a weeping, wet skin surface; pain; and sensitivity to cold air (Figure 11-7). Partial-thickness burns tend to heal in approximately 10 to 14 days if not complicated by infection.

The signs and symptoms of full-thickness burns include a pale, white, leathery appearance to the skin (Figure 11-8). The skin surface is dry and does not blanch. The skin may be broken with fat exposed. Full-thickness burns are painless because of the destruction of nerve endings. However, the patient may complain of pain due to superficial or partial-thickness burn surrounding the full-thickness burn site These burns do not heal spontaneously, and the patient will require skin grafts.

Assessment

During the assessment of thermal burns, the following information should be gathered:

- When did the injury occur?

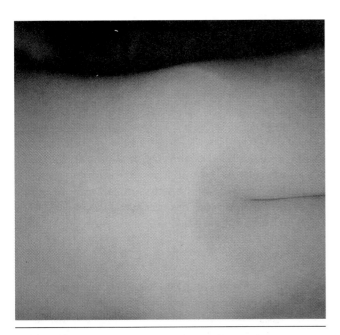

FIGURE 11-6 Example of superficial burn.
Courtesy of Dr. Robert Arensman, Chief of Pediatric
Surgery, Children's Memorial Medical Center, Chicago, IL.

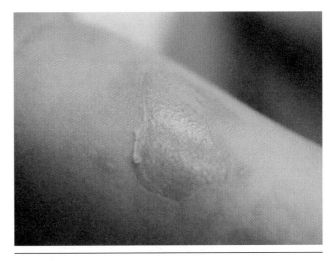

FIGURE 11-7 Example of partial-
thickness burn. Courtesy of Dr. Robert Arensman,
Chief of Pediatric Surgery, Children's Memorial Medical
Center, Chicago, IL.

- How did the injury occur?
- Was the child in a confined space with intense heat or smoke? If so, how long was the child in that environment?
- Was there any loss of consciousness? If so, how long was the child unconscious?
- Was any treatment given prior to the arrival of emergency medical services (EMS)?
- Were there any other mechanisms of injury? Is a cervical spine injury possible?
- Does the child have any history of chronic illnesses?

The body surface area (BSA) of the burn injury is used to determine the extent of the injury. In children less than ten years of age, the BSA can be determined by using the children's "rule of nines." In children over the age of ten years the Adult Rule of Nines is utilized (Figure 11-9).

Another method for estimating BSA is the use of the child's palm. The child's palm represents approximately 1 percent BSA. Remember it is the child's palm and not the provider's that is used to approximate the BSA involved. This method is also known as the "rule of palms."

The location of the injury also provides important information on the severity of the burn. Burns affecting the head, face, neck, and chest may indicate possible air-

way involvement. Burns of the hands and feet require extensive and meticulous care. Burns of the perineum may cause problems with elimination; but more importantly, the perineum has a high potential for infection.

Burns that are circumferential are dangerous because of the "tourniquet" effect they produce. The swelling of the burn creates pressure on the underlying structures and bones and will eventually constrict blood supply if not treated. This phenomenon is known as

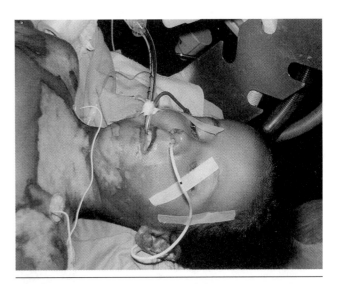

FIGURE 11-8 Example of full-thickness
burn. Courtesy of Dr. Robert Arensman, Chief of
Pediatric Surgery, Children's Memorial Medical Center,
Chicago, IL.

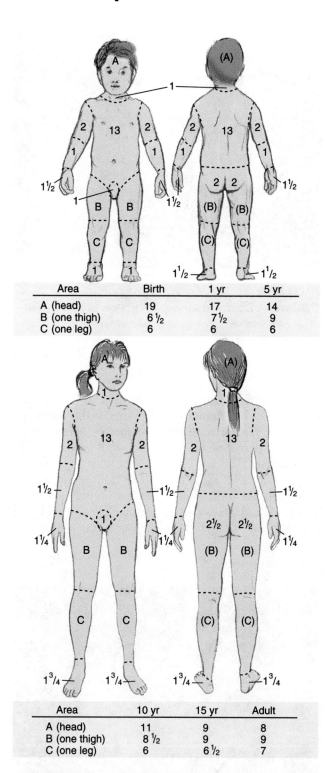

Area	Birth	1 yr	5 yr
A (head)	19	17	14
B (one thigh)	6 1/2	7 1/2	9
C (one leg)	6	6	6

Area	10 yr	15 yr	Adult
A (head)	11	9	8
B (one thigh)	8 1/2	9	9
C (one leg)	6	6 1/2	7

FIGURE 11-9 The extent of a burn is estimated using the body surface area (BSA) also commonly known as the "rule of nines."

compartment syndrome and will lead to loss of the limb if proper circulation is not restored. If the burned area is the chest and back, severe respiratory compromise will occur as the edema increases.

Associated injuries are another determinant of burn severity. Other major trauma, smoke inhalation, or CO and cyanide poisoning complicate the recovery process. Refer to the sections in this chapter on inhalation injuries and carbon monoxide poisoning, below.

Management

Once safety has been established, remove the child from the source of the burn and stop the burning process. Remove the child from the source of heat or flame *without becoming injured in the process*. If the child's clothing is on fire, extinguish the flames. Remove the burning or burned clothes as well as any constricting jewelry from the child's body.

Once life-threatening problems have been managed, turn your attention to managing the burn injury itself. The burn(s) should be covered with clean, dry sterile dressings. The dressings help decrease the possibility of infection, decrease pain by preventing exposure of the burn to air, and help maintain body temperature by preventing heat loss through the broken skin.

Remember that children are particularly susceptible to hypothermia. Wet dressings may be used but ONLY if less than 10 percent of the body surface area is involved (National Association of Emergency Medical Technicians [NAEMT], 1998).

Fluid resuscitation is only necessary for moderate and major burns. Intravenous access should be established with the largest possible catheter. When starting the IV, use a non-burned extremity whenever possible. The intravenous fluid of choice is Ringer's lactate, but normal saline is acceptable when Ringer's lactate is not available. Administer the fluid at 20 cc/kg over 20 to 30 minutes. If circulatory compromise is present, the fluid should be administered as a bolus.

Total fluid needs in the first 24 hours following the burn injury are determined using the Parkland formula (Figure 11-10). The goal of fluid resuscitation in the prehospital setting in a burn injury is to maintain adequate volume for perfusion of the child's vital organs. Monitor the child's vital signs, capillary refill, and level of consciousness during the infusion of fluids.

Management of pain should also be considered. Covering the burned area will help control pain. Local protocol will determine the type, if any, of analgesic that may be administered in the prehospital setting.

When a circumferential burn has occurred, some advanced life support personnel (i.e., paramedics and nurses affiliated with flight programs) are taught to do an **escharotomy**. This procedure is a surgical incision into the necrotic tissue of the burn. It expands the skin and prevents further ischemia until definitive care is available (Figure 11-11). An incision of the muscle sheath in an extremity, known as a **fasciotomy**, may be

Parkland Formula

4 ml of fluid

⬇

given in first 24 hours

⬇

for each one percent of partial-thickness and
full-thickness BSA burns

⬇

for each kg of weight

EXAMPLE:

4 ml of fluid × % of PT/FT BSA burns × kg = total fluid
replacement to be given in the first 24 hours

GIVE HALF OF THIS AMOUNT
IN THE FIRST EIGHT (8) HOURS

In children less than 30 kg, infuse fluids at 1 to 2 mL/kg.

FIGURE 11-10 Parkland Formula for
calculating fluid resuscitation.

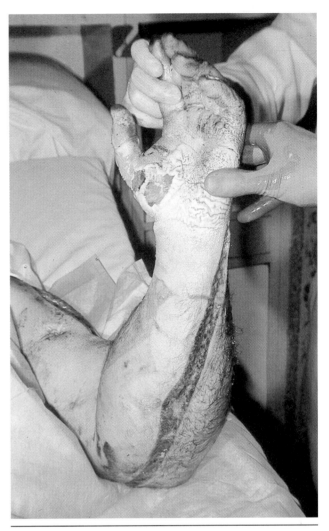

FIGURE 11-11 An escharotomy is
performed to expand the burned tissue and
prevent further ischemia until definitive care
is available. Courtesy of Dr. I. William Goldfarb,
Director, Burn/Trauma Center. Western Pennsylvania
Hospital, Pittsburgh, PA.

performed when an escharotomy is not successful in
restoring distal circulation. This last procedure is usually
done by a physician at the hospital. Check local protocols to determine if these procedures are available and
who is authorized to perform them.

Transport

DO NOT delay transport for the initiation of an intravenous line, especially in a child who is critically injured
or burned. Fluid resuscitation should be initiated while
enroute to the hospital.

Electrical Burns

Electrical burns may be deceiving because much of the
damage can be to internal organs and structures.
Injuries may occur all along the path traveled by the
electrical current.

Incidence

Electrical burns account for one percent of the burns
affecting children in the United States. However, children account for approximately one-third of the 1,300
fatalities each year.

The most common age groups affected by electrical injuries are toddlers and older school-aged children.
Toddlers may come in contact with electricity by playing

with electrical outlets in the home or by biting into electric cords. Older school-aged children may come in contact with electricity by playing near high-tension wires or
being struck by lightning.

Mechanism of Injury

Electrical burns result when the child comes in contact
with a high-tension wire, electrical cord, or electrical
outlet. Electricity causes not only external injuries but
also may affect the electrical conduction of the heart and
nervous system. The severity of electrical injuries
depends upon the voltage, path, type of current, the
resistance of the affected tissues, and the duration of
contact.

Alternating current (AC) is an electric current that reverses direction. **Direct current (DC)** is an electric current that flows only in one direction and is relatively constant. Injuries caused by household current (AC) account for the majority of electrical injuries in young children.

Electricity does not have any thermal properties when traveling unimpeded. Electrical burns are the result of the current meeting some resistance and transferring heat by conduction to the surrounding tissue.

Signs and Symptoms

Common signs and symptoms include:

- Burns at the side of the mouth (e.g., from chewing on an electrical cord)
- **Entrance wound** or site where electricity first strikes the body (e.g., necrotic area on hand from touching a high-tension wire or on top of the head from a lightning strike—Figure 11-12)
- **Exit wound** or site where electricity leaves the body (e.g., necrotic area on foot from a lightning strike)

Complications of electrical injury may include cardiorespiratory arrest, seizures, fractures, dislocations, amputations, and complications secondary to thermal injuries.

Assessment

Assess the child and try to get information about the following:

- What was the voltage?
- What type of current was involved (AC or DC)?
- What was the duration of contact?
- Are there any entry and/or exit wounds?
- Was there any loss of consciousness? If so, how long did the unconscious period last?
- Was any treatment given prior to arrival of EMS? Was any cardiopulmonary resuscitation (CPR) done?
- Were there any other mechanisms of injury? Is it possible that a spinal injury might exist?

Management

The first goal of management of an electrical burn is to remove the child from the source of electricity without compromising the safety of the rescuer. Exercise great care when working with electrical current; request additional help as necessary from the power company, fire department, or law enforcement. After safety is ensured, treat airway, breathing, and circulation. If the child is in

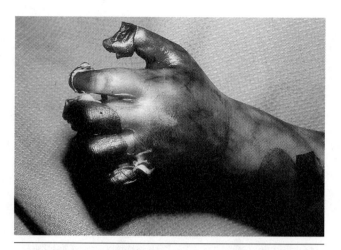

FIGURE 11-12 This child touched a high-tension wire. Courtesy of Dr. I. William Goldfarb, Director, Burn/Trauma Center. Western Pennsylvania Hospital, Pittsburgh, PA.

cardiac arrest, institute basic life support and pediatric advanced life support.

Transport

The child with an electrical burn, no matter how small the burn is, should be evaluated at a hospital. If the burns are extensive, transport the child to a burn center whenever possible. Continue to monitor the child's airway, breathing, and cardiac status throughout transport.

Chemical Burns

Chemical burns can cause extensive injury to pediatric patients. Curious toddlers easily become injured youngsters during routine exploration if injury prevention is not maintained. The type of agent and the duration of contact contribute to the severity of these types of burns.

Incidence

Chemical burns account for one percent of burns affecting children. Harmful chemicals that injure children are often found in the home or recreational areas.

The most common age groups affected by chemical burns are toddlers, preschoolers, school-aged children, and adolescents. Toddlers and preschoolers are more susceptible to accidental ingestions. School-aged children and adolescents may come in contact with harmful chemicals through actions such as chemistry set use, intentional ingestion for the purpose of committing suicide, or efforts to "get high."

Mechanism of Injury

Chemical burns are caused by exposure to any variety of caustic substances that can burn the eyes, skin, mucous membranes, or internal organs. The severity of a chemical burn is dependent upon the duration of contact, concentration or strength of the agent, and the amount of tissue affected. Exposure to chemicals can come from inhalation, skin contact, eye contact, or ingestion.

The most common causes of chemical burns in children are alkalis and acids. Chapter 6, Medical Emergencies, provides examples and further information on alkalis and acids.

Assessment

Collect as much of the following information as possible during the assessment:

- What is the name of the substance?
- What was the duration of contact?
- What was the concentration or strength of the chemical?
- Where was the child exposed? What amount of tissue was exposed?
- Did the child vomit?
- Was there any attempt made to decontaminate the child?

Complications associated with chemical burns include oropharyngeal swelling and airway obstruction. Also, permanent eye damage can result from exposure to a chemical agent.

Management

For chemical burns, *use protective gloves and eye protection*. For wet chemicals, immediately flush the affected area with large amounts of water while removing the child's clothing. In the case of a dry chemical, the toxin should be brushed from the skin; and all affected clothing should be removed. Be careful not to rinse or brush the chemical onto any part of anyone else's body. Establish a decontamination area whenever possible so that other rescuers, injured patients, bystanders, or family members are not exposed to the chemical.

Irrigate chemical burns to the eyes with large amounts of saline for approximately 20 minutes. Application of some type of topical anesthetic on the eye, if available and per local protocol, will help to decrease pain and eye movement.

Transport

In the event of a chemical burn, it is important to notify the receiving hospital of the incident, spill, or hazardous material situation. They may need to activate their hazardous materials team or prepare for decontamination. Provide as much advanced notice as possible.

Exploring the Web

- Search for information on each type of burn injury on the web. What information can you find relevant to the pediatric patient? Do they provide guidelines for prehospital care?

INHALATION INJURIES

Inhalation injuries can accompany different types of burns if the child has inhaled any toxic gases or heated air. Suspect inhalation injuries frequently if there is *any* index of suspicion.

Incidence

Inhalation injuries occur in approximately 19 to 26 percent of burn patients. Usually, patients with a body surface area burn greater than 20 percent also have an inhalation injury (Ramse, Barret, and Herndon, 1999).

Mechanism of Injury

The major cause of burn morbidity and mortality in children occurs in burns associated with pulmonary complications. Therefore, any child with a history of being in a heavy, smoke-filled environment should be treated for an inhalation injury. In addition, this type of injury should be suspected any time a child has been in an enclosed space where flames were present, even if the child was not burned. Inhalation injuries may result from exposure to hot air as well as toxic gases such as carbon monoxide and cyanide.

Airway injury results from exposure to heat or irritating gases. The upper airway is most commonly injured by heat. The nasopharynx and upper airway have the ability to dissipate a tremendous amount of heat. However, with the dissipation of heat comes edema and the possibility for airway obstruction.

The lower airway is rarely injured by heat. Lower airway injury usually results from inhalation of irritating gases such as chlorine, hydrochloric acid, or cyanide. These gases can cause inflammation, impaired ciliary activity, and ulceration of the bronchial mucosa as well as hypersecretion and edema leading to **bronchorrhea** (discharge of fluid in the bronchi) or bronchospasm. In addition, cyanide toxicity causes asphyxiation at the cellular level.

Signs and Symptoms

Signs and symptoms of inhalation injuries include:

- Burns about the face
- Singed nasal hairs and/or eyebrows
- Soot on the tongue or in the pharynx
- **Carbonaceous** (containing carbon) sputum
- Excessive coughing
- Stridor or hoarseness
- Dysphagia
- Severe wheezing and/or rales.

Assessment

In gathering the history of a child with potential airway injury, the following questions should be asked:

- Was the child in an enclosed space? If so, how long was the child inside?
- Was there an explosion? If so, was the child thrown any distance?
- Was there any loss of consciousness? If so, how long was the child unconsciousness?
- Was there any exposure to products of combustion?

Management

The management of airway injuries should include high-concentration oxygen via a nonrebreather face mask. The oxygen should be humidified whenever possible. If edema of the airway is present (e.g., stridor or hoarseness), early endotracheal intubation may be necessary to ensure a patent airway throughout transport. If bronchospasm is present, bronchodilators may help to relieve the child's discomfort and optimize breathing (see Chapter 4—Respiratory Emergencies).

Transport

If the child is critically injured or burned, transport to a burn or burn/trauma center for definitive care. If the child's airway cannot be properly managed, transport to the closest hospital for initial stabilization is appropriate.

Maintenance of a patent airway, adequate breathing, and optimum oxygen exchange remain the priorities during transport. If time permits, other associated burns and trauma should be managed.

CARBON MONOXIDE POISONING

Carbon monoxide (CO) is a colorless, odorless gas that has 200 to 250 times more affinity for hemoglobin than does oxygen (Wong, 1999). This affinity results in the CO binding to the hemoglobin instead of oxygen creating **carboxyhemoglobin**.

Two specific problems occur. First, unbound oxygen is not transported by red blood cells. Second, bound oxygen becomes even more tightly bound to hemoglobin and then is *not* released to the tissues.

Incidence

It is unknown how prevalent CO poisoning is. It is estimated that one third of all cases go undiagnosed (Varon and Marik, 1997).

Mechanism of Injury

The production of CO occurs due to incomplete combustion of carbon or items containing carbon such as wood or charcoal. These fumes are inhaled and compete with oxygen for binding on the hemoglobin. Examples include:

- Fumes from space heaters that are not ventilated
- Smoke during a structural fire
- Gas lamps or stoves that are operated improperly
- Charcoal grills or hibatchis operated in areas without appropriate ventilation
- Poorly ventilated recreational vehicles
- Faulty home furnaces

Signs and Symptoms

Findings indicative of CO poisoning include:

- Headache
- Dyspnea
- Irritability
- Nausea and vomiting
- Dizziness

 Exploring the Web

- Search the Web for information on inhalation injuries in children. Can you find information in guidelines for care in the prehospital environment?

- Fatigue
- Blurred vision
- Syncope
- Tachycardia
- Seizures
- Dysrhythmias
- Confusion or hallucinations
- Ataxia
- Unconsciousness

Cherry-red lips and skin are not observed quite as often as it is described. In most instances, the child will be pale or cyanotic from hypoxemia.

Prehospital personnel must also be cognizant of the effect CO poisoning has on pulse oximetry readings. Pulse oximetry does not measure the amount of oxygen that attaches to hemoglobin. Instead, it measures the amount of "free" oxygen in the system. As a result, a false pulse oximetry reading can result causing a false sense of security that the child is adequately oxygenated.

Tricks of the Trade

Be aware that a pulse oximetry reading may not be what is seems. Pulse oximeters measure the amount of "free" oxygen in the system. A high reading may indicate that the child is being adequately oxygenated when the opposite is actually true.

Assessment

In gathering the history of a child with potential CO poisoning, the following questions should be asked:

- Was the child in an enclosed space? If so, how long was the child inside?
- Did the child have to be removed from a burning building?
- Was there any loss of consciousness? If so, how long was the child unconscious?
- Was the child exposed to automobile exhaust or poorly ventilated heating devices?

Management

Management of potential CO poisoning is aimed at increasing the amount of oxygen dissolved in the blood

and decreasing the half-life of carboxyhemoglobin (red blood cells carrying CO). Increasing the amount of oxygen dissolved in the blood allows more oxygen to get to the tissues since oxygen follows a gradient. Decreasing the half-life of carboxyhemoglobin allows the hemoglobin to bind more oxygen and release it to the tissues of the body. Therefore, high-concentration oxygen via a nonrebreather face mask or endotracheal intubation is the treatment of choice in the prehospital setting.

Transport

Transport to a hospital with a hyperbaric chamber, if feasible, should be considered for those children presenting with severe signs and symptoms such as soot around the nose or mouth, severe respiratory distress, decreased level of consciousness, or seizures. Also, the environment in which the child was found may provide an indication for the potential need for a hyperbaric chamber, especially if the child has been in an enclosed place for an extended period of time.

Exploring the Web

- Search for sites that contain information on carbon monoxide poisoning. Can you find information related specifically to pediatric patients? What guidelines are available for prehospital care? Carbon monoxide poisoning is difficult to identify; can you find any tips that will aid you in increasing your awareness and ability to identify this disorder?

OVERALL SAFETY CONSIDERATIONS

The first step in burn management is to quickly assess the situation and ensure safety of the rescuer. Are prehospital personnel and the patient safe from toxic fumes, flames, heat, lack of oxygen, debris, etc.? Does the patient need to be immediately moved to a safer location? Can the patient be moved without risking injury or death to the prehospital personnel? Are additional personnel available to assist in the extrication?

Do not be tempted to compromise safety when the life of a child is at stake. Remember that individual protection remains the first priority. If prehospital personnel succumb to injury, they will not be of any value to that child.

GENERAL ASSESSMENT GUIDELINES

Once safety has been established, begin the initial assessment. As with other forms of trauma, this assessment consists of an evaluation of Airway, Breathing, Circulation, Disability, Exposure and Status (ABCDES). It is important to remember that the purpose of the initial assessment is to get a general impression of the patient, locate life-threatening injuries, and identify priority patients who need immediate care and transport. The burn itself is usually not life threatening. Therefore, burn care in the prehospital setting should be limited to those injuries that affect a child's airway, breathing, and circulation. For example, if shock is apparent within the first thirty minutes of a burn injury, the prehospital provider should assess for other possible causes of the shock. Refer to Chapter 2—Assessment of the Stable Child—to review the components of the initial assessment.

GENERAL MANAGEMENT GUIDELINES

Once the child has been removed from the source and the burning process stopped, perform an initial assessment to identify and correct any life-threatening problems. Remember that the potential for airway compromise is an ever-present problem with any significant burn. If there is any potential for airway involvement, high-concentration oxygen should be administered via a nonrebreather face mask, bag-valve-mask device, or endotracheal tube. Any sign of impending airway obstruction indicates the need for rapid intubation of the child. Use humidified oxygen whenever possible.

Any circulatory compromise may require the implementation of basic life support (BLS), advanced life support (ALS) protocols, and/or intravenous fluids. These protocols should be initiated immediately, while intravenous therapy can wait until transport has begun.

The potential for spinal injury should also be considered. Any mechanism of injury suggestive of the possibility of spinal injury should be treated with spinal immobilization.

GENERAL TRANSPORT GUIDELINES

The child suffering a burn injury should be transported to the appropriate medical facility. The following list,

developed by the American Burn Association, describes those burn injuries that require transport to a regional burn center.

1. Partial- and full-thickness burns that together cover more than 10% body surface area in patients below ten years of age

2. Partial- and full-thickness burns that together cover more than 20% body surface area

3. Partial- and full-thickness burns of the hands, feet, genitalia (due to potential loss of function and inability to care for self), or skin overlying major joints

4. Full-thickness burns of more than five percent of the body

5. Inhalation injury

6. Significant chemical burns

7. Significant electrical burns to include lightning injury

8. Burns with other associated injuries (e.g., fractures, head injury, etc.) that may be initially treated in a trauma center

9. Burns in patients with serious preexisting conditions that might affect mortality, complicate management, or prolong recovery

10. Children with burns that are initially treated at hospitals that do not have qualified personnel or equipment for burn care

11. Children with burn injuries who need long-term rehabilitation or special social and emotional care (includes cases of suspected child neglect and abuse)

SUMMARY

Morbidity and mortality in children suffering from burn injuries are more highly associated with inhalation injuries than shock or sepsis. The burn itself is rarely life threatening. Assessment and treatment should concentrate on identifying potential life-threatening problems related to the airway and cardiovascular systems. Treatment of the burn should never take precedence over treatment of more potentially lethal injuries. To assist in assuring the most favorable outcome for a child suffering from a burn injury, it is imperative to transport to an appropriate treatment facility.

Management of Case Study

The presence of soot around the mouth or nose is a tell-tale sign of a possible inhalation injury. The child was in a closet during an active fire, which constitutes a closed space. Upon questioning, the firefighters tell you that the house was full of thick smoke when they found him crying. There were no other signs of trauma in the house (e.g., no explosion or no fall down the steps).

Move the child into the ambulance, and speak to him in a soft, reassuring voice. Ask your partner to try to get more information about his family. If a family member or other adult he knows is available, have that person sit in the ambulance with him.

While he is crying, it indicates that his airway is patent and that he is moving air. He is also conscious enough to be crying. As you quickly feel for a pulse, you note a strong radial pulse of 132. Capillary refill is normal. His skin is warm, diaphoretic, and pale.

Listen for breath sounds if he stops crying. You hear rales throughout all lung fields. He continues to cough and is spitting out black saliva.

Quickly examine him for any other life-threatening injuries. You do not find any other problems. His clothes and some of his skin are blackened, but no burned areas are noted.

Administer cool, humidified oxygen via a non-rebreather face mask. Restrain the child in a child safety seat secured to the stretcher, and prepare for rapid transport.

This child is at a high risk for edema of the trachea due to the heat and smoke he breathed in while inside the house. Continue to monitor his vitals, level of consciousness, and respiratory status. Provide a report to the hospital, and update them if any signs of stridor or hoarseness develop.

▶ REVIEW QUESTIONS

1. Children are more vulnerable to respiratory complications than adults due to _____ and _____.

2. A child's increased respiratory rate can cause two problems. Name them.

3. Children involved in closed space fires actually die from:
   a. Burn injuries
   b. Organ failure due to hypotension
   c. Increased uptake of toxic gases
   d. Traumatic injuries

4. Children have less total circulating blood volume than adults and are more susceptible to _____ and _____.

5. The _____ is the largest organ in the body.

6. List the six components for determining burn severity.

7. List the three classifications of burns and give examples of each.

8. List three areas of burns that should be treated in a burn center.

9. List two causes of thermal burns.

10. The most common burn injury in children under four years of age is a scald burn. True or False?

11. The _____ and _____ are major determinants in burn severity.

12. List three types of burns, the areas affected, and examples of each.

13. Define compartment syndrome.

14. Cover the thermal burn with clean, wet dressings. True or False?

15. Electrical burns occur when the child comes in contact with a _____, _____, or _____.

16. Describe the first goal of management of electrical burns.

17. The severity of a chemical burn is dependent upon three factors. Name them.

18. Any child with a history of being in a heavy smoke-filled environment should be treated for an inhalation injury. True or False?

19. List four signs and symptoms of an inhalation injury.

20. Explain why endotracheal intubation may be necessary for an inhalation injury.

21. Define carboxyhemoglobin.

22. List four signs and symptoms of carbon monoxide poisoning.

23. Cherry-red lips and skin are very common in children. True or False?

24. List four burn injuries that require transport to a regional burn center according to the American Burn Association.

▶ REFERENCES

National Association of Emergency Medical Technicians. (1998). *Prehospital trauma life support—basic and advanced.* 4th ed. St. Louis, MO: Mosby-Year Book.

National Institute of General Medical Sciences, National Institutes of Health. (1999). *Trauma, burn, shock, and injury: Facts and figures.* Bethesda, MD: The Institute.

Ramsey, P. I., Barret, J. P., & Herndon, D. N. 1999. Environmental emergencies. *Critical Care Clinics,* 15(2).

Varon, J., & Marik, P. E. (1997). Carbon monoxide poisoning. *Internet Journal of Emergency and Intensive Care Medicine,* [On-line serial], 2(1). Available E-mail: http://www.ispub.com/journals/JCICM/Vol1N21CO.htm.

Wong, D. 1999. *Whaley & Wong's Nursing care of infants and children* (6th ed.). St. Louis, MO: Mosby-Year Book.

Chapter 12

Child Abuse or Neglect

OBJECTIVES

Upon completion of this chapter, the student should be able to:

- Define maltreatment, neglect, abuse, sexual abuse, and emotional abuse.
- Identify specific injuries that are suggestive of child abuse/neglect.
- Discuss the history-gathering process specific to suspected child abuse/neglect.
- Discuss the importance of unbiased documentation and its role in future legal action.
- List examples of bruises, burns, and head injuries found in children who may be abused.

KEY TERMS

abuse
alopecia
battered child syndrome
child maltreatment

emotional abuse
frenulum
Munchausen syndrome by proxy
neglect

physical abuse
sexual abuse
shaken baby syndrome

Case Scenario

You and your partner are called to the scene for a "child unconscious." You arrive at the house in an affluent, suburban part of town. As you enter the residence, a woman comes running to you with a "laundry list" of problems for which her child is being treated. She leads you upstairs to the bedroom where an 18-month-old little girl is sitting in her crib. She is alert and playing with some toys. How would you handle this situation?

INTRODUCTION

Child maltreatment is a term used to broadly describe intentional physical and emotional abuse or neglect of children as well as sexual abuse of children. It usually is inflicted by adults and represents one of the most significant social problems that affect children. It is present at all educational, social, and economic levels. Table 12-1 reviews the four major types of child maltreatment.

INCIDENCE

For infants and toddlers, child abuse continues to be a serious cause of mortality and morbidity. In the 10 years between 1988 and the end of 1997, child abuse accounted for 10.6 percent of all blunt trauma occurring in children younger than five years of age (DiScala et al., 2000). For those children injured and hospitalized for blunt trauma, injuries to the abused child were more severe than for those children with unintentional injuries. In addition, children who had been abused used more medical services and had worse survival and functional outcomes than those children who sustained unintentional injuries (DiScala et al., 2000). See Table 12-2 for a comparison of children injured by abuse and those with unintentional injuries.

Exploring the Web

- Research the statistics of child morbidity and mortality in your state. What percentage was the result of child abuse or neglect?

TABLE 12-1
Major Types of Child Maltreatment

Physical abuse	Infliction of physical injury through: • Beating • Punching • Biting • Burning • Shaking • Kicking • Otherwise injuring a child
Child neglect	Failure to provide for the child's basic needs: • Physical • Educational • Emotional
Sexual abuse	May include: • Fondling a child's genitalia • Intercourse • Rape • Incest • Sodomy • Exhibitionism • Prostitution • Production of pornographic materials
Emotional abuse	Acts or failure to act that cause serious disorders such as: • Behavioral • Cognitive • Emotional • Mental

National Center on Child Abuse and Neglect, 1996.

TYPES OF NEGLECT

The most common form of maltreatment is child neglect. **Neglect** is defined as the condition that exists when a parent or guardian fails to provide minimal physical and emotional care for the child. Contributing factors

TABLE 12-2
Comparison of Child Abuse and Unintentional Injuries

Child Abuse	Child Abuse	Unintentional Injuries
Median age	12.8 months	25.5 months
Incidence of preinjury medical history	53% of cases	14.1% of cases
Presence of retinal hemorrhages	27.8%	0.06%
Mainly injured by:	• Battering (53%) • Shaking (10.3%)	• Falls (58.4%) • Motor vehicle-related events (37.1%)
Incidence of injuries:	• Intracranial (42.2%) • Thoracic (12.5%) • Abdominal (11.4%) • Very severe (22.6%) • Admitted to ICU (42.5%) • Received Child Protective Services (82.3%) • Received social services (72.9%) • Mean length of stay in the hospital → 9.3 days • Developed extensive functional limitations (8.7%) • Discharged to custodial/foster/child protective services care (56.6%)	• Intracranial (14.1%) • Thoracic (4.5%) • Abdominal (6.8%) • Very severe (6.3%) • Admitted to ICU (26.9%) • Received Child Protective Services (8%) • Received social services (27.6%) • Mean length of stay in the hospital → 3.8 days • Developed extensive functional limitations (2.7%) • Discharged to home (96.1%)

National Pediatric Trauma Registry between January 1, 1988, and December 31, 1997.

Abbreviations: ICU, intensive care unit.

include poor parenting skills, lack of resources, ignorance of the child's needs, and the failure to recognize that emotional nurturing is essential to the growth and development of children.

Physical Neglect

An infant or child has various physical needs depending on the age. Things like food, shelter, and clothing are basic necessities. Medical care for illness and well-child care (i.e., routine immunizations) are important to keeping the child healthy and monitoring for potential problems during growth and development. Other items such

as education, ongoing medical care, and general supervision are also needed as the child grows older. When any of these physical needs are not being met by the parent or guardian, the child is suffering from physical neglect.

Emotional Neglect

In addition to physical requirements, children need affection, attention, and emotional nurturing to reach their potential and grow to become productive adults. Emotional neglect occurs when the parent, guardian, or other caregiver fails to provide that crucial nurturing.

The parent or guardian may also promote inappropriate behavior by ignoring substance abuse or delinquent acts by the child as he or she strives to get attention.

TYPES OF ABUSE

The term **abuse** means to "physically or verbally attack or injure." In children, abuse can be emotional, physical, and sexual in nature. There are many forms of physical abuse that have become so prevalent in our society that they have been named specifically, such as battered child syndrome, Munchausen syndrome by proxy (MSBP), and shaken baby syndrome (SBS).

Emotional Abuse

Emotional abuse encompasses any activity that attempts to destroy or significantly impair a child's self-esteem or competence. This form of abuse can be quite difficult to identify and define. The child may be rejected, isolated, or ignored by the parent or caregiver. Other parental behaviors that may result in emotional abuse include terrorizing, corrupting, verbally assaulting, or overpressuring the child.

PHYSICAL ABUSE

Any time physical injury is deliberately inflicted on a child, **physical abuse** occurs. It is usually administered by the child's routine caregiver such as a parent, foster parent, or babysitter. Major physical abuse may cause death, yet more cases of minor physical injury are reported (Wong, 1999). The abuse may range from minor cuts and bruises to severe neurologic injury and death.

Unfortunately, minor and major physical abuse are not universally defined. In the United States, each state has its own definition of abuse outlined in its individual reporting laws.

There are several risk factors present when a child is physically abused. In most cases, a single factor does not predict the likelihood of abuse. Instead, there are interactions between these factors that precipitate the abuse (Table 12-3). The more factors that exist in a family, the greater the chance for physical abuse.

TABLE 12-3
Predisposing Factors for Physical Abuse

Affected Group	Characteristic	Examples
Parents	• Severe punishment as child	Parents think their own treatment as a child was unfair and severe → has negative relationship with own parents
	• Violence between parents	Abused spouse may also abuse the children
	• Social isolation and loneliness • Fewer supportive relationships	Children of teenage mothers → presence of several stressors cause mother to strike child to release increasing frustration and anxiety
	Low self-esteem	Parent feels inadequate and may blame child
	Less adequate maternal functioning (inadequate knowledge)	Parent or caregiver may not know what child needs or how to properly care for the child
Child	Temperament	"Easy" child less abused than one who adds to parental stress by being "difficult" Key is parent's ability to deal with child's behavioral style

(continues)

TABLE 12-3
(Continued)

Affected Group	Characteristic	Examples
Child	• Position in family	Usually only one child is victim → when that child is gone (old enough to move out or placed in foster care), next oldest child may be the focus for abuse
	• Additional needs related to disability or chronic illness	Child with mental retardation may not understand parent's requests and attempts at behavior management → further increasing parent's frustration Parent may not accept child's diagnosis or the long-term prognosis Failure of parent-child bonding during early infancy (e.g., premature infant)
	• Similarities	Child may remind parent of someone he or she dislikes (e.g., younger brother or sister who received a great deal of attention)
Environment	• Chronic stress	Poverty Divorce Unemployment Frequent relocation Alcoholism Drug abuse
	• Increased exposure between child and parent	Crowded living conditions
	• Concealed crises	Unplanned pregnancy Wealthy family → unable to spend much time with child → alternate caregivers may abuse child(ren) Any major life change (i.e., death, job change, divorce, etc.)

Wong, D. (1999). *Whaley & Wong's nursing care of infants and children* (6th ed.). St. Louis: Mosby-Year Book.

Battered Child Syndrome

Some children who are abused routinely may be said to have **battered child syndrome**. This syndrome is a clinical condition in young children that results from serious physical abuse usually at the hand of a parent or foster parent. Clues to the presence of this syndrome may lie in the child's behavior. Children who are subject to frequent abuse may exhibit emotional and angry outbursts, little control over impulse, poor judgment, and manipulative behavior. As they get older they may become withdrawn, exhibit signs of drug or alcohol abuse, and perform poorly in school.

Munchausen Syndrome by Proxy (MSBP)

Munchausen syndrome by proxy is a rare type of child abuse in which one person (usually the parent) fabricates or induces illness in another person (usually the child). Although the prehospital provider will rarely be able to identify this syndrome as a potential problem due to the subtleties of presentation, it is worth addressing briefly to increase awareness.

The parent or caregiver either makes up or produces symptoms of an illness in a child. Examples include presenting a medical history that is not true, chronic poisoning of the child to produce symptoms, or suffocating the child to cause apnea and seizures. This process is usually repeated several times, resulting in multiple trips to the hospital and numerous tests, procedures, and possible surgeries. It may even result in the death of the child.

This syndrome may involve more than one child in a family and is usually initiated by the mother. Often the parent or caregiver that produces the symptoms has a health background.

The child will actually be ill and need evaluation at the hospital. The most common presentations are bleeding, seizures, central nervous system depression, apnea, vomiting and diarrhea, fever, and rashes. History may reveal that the child has had recurrent illnesses and numerous hospitalizations. If this pattern is revealed in the history, it is important that it be documented and passed on to personnel at the receiving hospital.

Shaken Baby Syndrome (SBS)

Shaken baby syndrome occurs when children are shaken violently. With this form of abuse, obvious signs and symptoms may not be evident. In fact, fatal intracranial trauma can occur without any signs of external head injury especially in infants less than six months of age.

Shaking may occur when the parent or caregiver tries to wake the infant or burp the infant. It may also occur when the parent or caregiver feels angry or tense, such as when the baby continues to cry despite feeding, a clean diaper, and warm clothes. Even tossing the infant in the air as a playful act can cause damage to the infant's brain.

Emergency assistance may be requested when the infant cannot be awakened from a nap. Signs and symptoms of increased intracranial pressure may be present.

Sexual Abuse

Sexual abuse is defined in the Child Abuse and Prevention Act (Public Law 104-235) as "the use, persuasion, or coercion of any child to engage in sexually explicit conduct (or any simulation of such conduct) for producing any visual depiction of such conduct, or rape, molestation, prostitution, or incest with children." Nontouching as well as touching offenses such as an adult exposing himself or herself to children or exposing children to pornography as well as fondling or engaging the child in a sexual act are included (Table 12-4).

If the activity is committed by a person who is responsible for the child's care, it is considered child abuse. If the activity is committed by a stranger, it is considered sexual assault. In the second instance, the police and criminal courts must address the situation.

TABLE 12-4
Types of Sexual Abuse

Term	Definition
Child pornography	• Depiction of erotic behavior involving children intended to cause sexual excitement • May be in pictures, writing, or any other media • Children may be involved alone, with adults, or with animals • Consent of child's legal guardian does not condone behavior • May include distribution of any material with or without profit
Child prostitution	• Children involved in sex acts for profit • Usually with changing partners
Exhibitionism	• Indecent exposure • Most commonly occurs when adult male exposes genitalia to children or adult females
Incest	• Any physical sexual activity between family members • Members do not have to be related by blood • Can include stepparents, unrelated siblings, grandparents, boyfriend or girlfriend of spouse, uncles, or aunts
Molestation	• Includes touching, fondling, kissing, and/or oral-genital contact • May include single or mutual masturbation
Pedophilia	• Means "love of child" • Adult prefers prepubescent children to achieve sexual excitement

Wong, D. (1999). *Whaley & Wong's nursing care of infants and children* (6th ed.). St. Louis: Mosby-Year Book.

Assessment Considerations

Injury to the genital area may be the result of an accident or sexual abuse. Obvious trauma to the genital area must be examined in light of the history given. Falls or straddle injuries from monkey bars or the bar on a boy's bicycle may result in bleeding and bruising to the genital area.

Sexual abuse may present with no physical signs. However, specific physical indicators that raise the index of suspicion include:

- Torn or stained underwear
- Trauma or bleeding from the rectum or vagina
- Discharge from the vagina or penis that might indicate a sexually transmitted disease
- Foreign bodies in the vagina, urethra, or rectum

Behavioral indicators of sexual abuse are usually regressive in nature. The child exhibits more infantile behavior such as thumb sucking, excessive crying, or bedwetting. He or she may appear preoccupied with sexual matters, be either obviously withdrawn, or act out in an aggressive or disruptive manner. The child who is a victim of sexual abuse may also exhibit self-mutilating behavior.

Treatment Considerations

If the child is stable and presents with discharge from the vagina or rectum suggestive of rape or sodomy, it is important that the provider not disturb potential evidence by cleaning the genital area. This procedure should be followed with any allegations of molestation that have occurred within 48 hours prior to the time the provider makes contact with the child.

The child should be supported emotionally and all clothing transported to the hospital. Ideally, a person experienced in sexual abuse cases should interview the child who is a possible victim of sexual abuse or incest. It is in the best interest of the child that the prehospital provider refrain from probing questions regarding the incident. However, it is important to document exactly what the child might volunteer.

PROFILE OF AN ABUSED CHILD

The abused child may be one who is illegitimate, unwanted, uncommunicative, or perhaps disabled with specific emotional or psychological needs. Young children are abused more frequently than older children. In 1995, child protective services reported that 56 percent of confirmed cases of abuse occurred in children less than four years of age (Wong, 1999). Of the 996 children who died as a result of abuse or neglect in 1995, most of them were three years of age or younger (Wong, 1999).

If the child has a disability or is suffering from a chronic illness, the incidence of abuse is higher. Boys tend to suffer more physical abuse than girls. However, girls tend to have a higher incidence of sexual abuse than do boys.

Most states legally define a child as one under the age of 18. Although it is common to think of abuse affecting only younger children, abuse must still be considered in the adolescent as well.

PROFILE OF AN ABUSER

Characteristics more frequently found in the abuser include marital/relationship stress, single parent situations, or financial stress. Often the abuser sets unrealistic expectations for the child, or the child may be used as a means of meeting the adult's own needs for comfort or satisfaction. Most abusers feel there is no one to turn to for help or support. One of the most common assumptions is that the abuser was abused as a child yet few studies support this theory (Wong, 1999).

EFFECTS OF ABUSE

Effects of child abuse are long reaching. Abused and neglected children frequently show drops in IQ as well as an increase in learning disabilities and depression. Suicide, violence, delinquency, drug and alcohol abuse, and other forms of criminal behavior are frequently related to child abuse. Studies regarding elder abuse have also revealed that a common characteristic of the abused elder is the fact that he or she was an abusing parent.

Although child abuse crosses all boundaries of racial, ethnic, cultural, and socioeconomic groups, minority children enter the child protection system in disproportionately large numbers. It has been suggested that this incidence reflects the high rate of poverty among ethnic minorities. However, this fact must be tempered with the question of whether occurrence rates in minority children are really significantly higher or whether the report rates in minority children are higher. Many consider abuse is more likely to be reported if the child comes from a poverty background.

HISTORY RELATED TO CHILD ABUSE

A thorough history is an integral part of determining the potential for child abuse. It involves not only what the parent or caregiver tells you but also what the child does or does not say.

Most of the history is usually obtained from the parent or caregiver. The history should be as complete as possible. For instance, if the parent states that the child rolled off the couch, ask how far was the drop to the floor and on what type of surface did the child impact (carpet versus hardwood). One clue to raise the index of suspicion is the caregiver denying any knowledge of how the injury occurred.

It is important to note inconsistencies between what is found on the physical exam and the presented history. Is it likely that this injury resulted from the given mechanism? As an example, a fractured femur in an infant does not usually occur from a fall off a couch onto a carpeted floor. Consider the developmental age of the child. Is the infant old enough developmentally to roll over on his or her own to fall off the couch?

It is important to note if there was a delay in calling for medical help following the injury. It is also important to note if the child has a history of other questionable injuries. Has anyone other than the parent cared for the child recently? Usually parents and caregivers are cooperative in the history-taking phase.

When talking with the child privately, use carefully phrased questions. It is not the role of the prehospital provider to bluntly ask if the parent or caregiver inflicted the injury. Ask how the injury occurred, and follow up with more specific questions as to the details. This method may bring forth inconsistencies in the child's version of the incident.

The child may verbally defend the abuse in the hopes of pleasing the abuser, may feel the punishment is deserved, or refuse to discuss the event out of fear, belief it is a family affair, or to avoid further punishment. If the child refuses to discuss the event, this refusal should be noted in the documentation. If the child does discuss the event, it is important to quote what is said exactly. One must take care in the communication process not to "put words in the child's mouth." Do not suggest possible answers. Rather, listen and quote what the child volunteers.

PHYSICAL EXAMINATION AND TREATMENT

Depending on the extent of injury, the prehospital provider may only be able to perform an initial assessment. The child's well being is the highest priority and should not be forsaken to do an in-depth history or physical to support any suspicions.

If the child's condition permits, complete a thorough exam. Note behaviors and reactions that would normally be considered inappropriate for the child's age.

Does the child appear frightened of the parent or caregiver? Does the child appear withdrawn and fail to react or cry when an IV or other painful procedure is initiated? Document these types of behaviors.

General Considerations

Be aware of physical findings that are inconsistent with the history obtained. If the child appears malnourished, has poor hygiene, or has what appear to be longstanding skin infections, consider these as important indicators of neglect. It is important for the prehospital provider to identify potential abusive situations as early as possible.

If at all possible, attempt to talk with the child alone. However, if the parent or caregiver is unwilling to allow the child out of his or her direct sight, do not force the issue. This fact should be noted in the documentation along with any observed inappropriate behavior associated with the refusal.

Bruises

Normal bruise areas for children include the bony prominences such as the knees, elbows, and forehead. Significant bruises found in areas other than these normal "bump" areas should raise the index of suspicion for potential abuse and be examined thoroughly.

The prehospital provider should look for multiple bruises in various stages of healing. The typical healing of a bruise takes approximately two weeks. During the first five days, the bruise is swollen and tender with color progressing from red to blue. After five to seven days, the bruised area takes on a greenish appearance. At seven to ten days, the color changes to yellow. From 10 to 14 days, the color becomes brownish, with the bruise clearing to normal skin color in about two weeks (Figure 12-1). Bruises in various stages of healing may be indicative of an ongoing pattern of injury that should be noted and reported to the receiving facility.

Bruises that result from physical abuse often have particular shapes that may indicate how the bruise was inflicted. Oval or round bruises may result from finger pressure as the child is grabbed and held by another person. These may be found on the upper arms or legs or on the chin and cheeks and may also indicate the pattern of finger location. Linear or parallel bruising may be indicative of slapping or the use of a belt or strap. Straps, belts, or cords may also leave a loop pattern if any were doubled over at the time the injury was inflicted (Figure 12-2). Injuries resulting from the bristles of a hairbrush usually present as multiple superficial puncture wounds accompanied by bruising.

Typical sites for bruises to be evident following abusive injury include the buttocks, lower back, upper arms, inner thighs, genital area, and earlobes. Earlobes

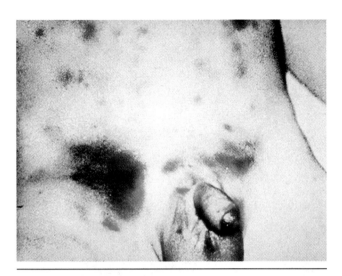

FIGURE 12-1 Bruises in various stages of healing may indicate a child is being abused. Photo courtesy of Emergency Medical Services for Children, NERA, Torrance, CA.

may exhibit bruising as the result of pinching and pulling as well as a direct blow. Marks at the corners of the mouth may be the result of being gagged (Figure 12-3). These marks may be quite obvious if the instrument used to gag the child was narrow and cinched around the head. Circumferential bruises around the ankles or wrists indicate the child has been tied with a rope or other object (Figure 12-4). Circumferential bruises around the neck indicate choking.

All bruising injuries may not be obvious. Attempts to force-feed an infant to stop him or her from crying may result in obvious swelling and/or bruising of the upper lip. However, bruising or tearing of the **frenulum** (the tissue between the upper lip and gum) will be noted only if the inside of the lip is examined.

Bite marks and pinch marks may be the result of injury from another sibling or playmate. The prehospital provider must be cautious in accepting this explanation at face value without carefully examining the injury. It is important to examine the size of the arch left by teeth

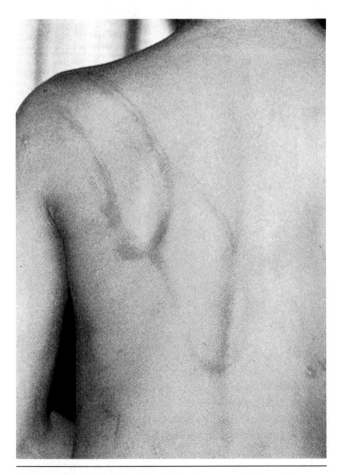

FIGURE 12-2 Bruising in specific patterns such as the loop of a strap often is an indicator of child abuse. Photo courtesy of Emergency Medical Services for Children, NERA, Torrance, CA.

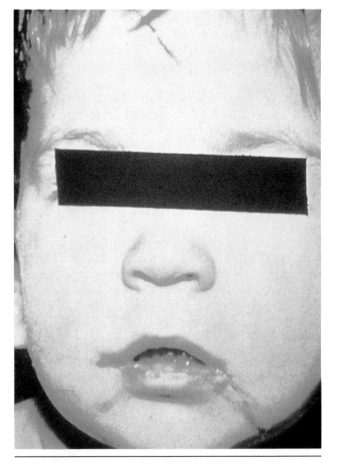

FIGURE 12-3 Bruising and marks around the mouth may indicate the child has been gagged. Photo courtesy of Emergency Medical Services for Children, NERA, Torrance, CA.

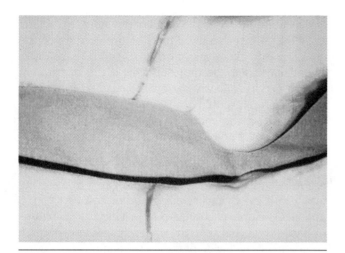

FIGURE 12-4 Bruises that encircle the extremities may indicate the child has been bound. Photo courtesy of Emergency Medical Services for Children, NERA, Torrance, CA.

marks to determine if the injury size would indicate that of a young child versus that of an adult. Also be aware of bizarre or questionable patterns. For instance, a parallel line of three or four puncture marks may be the result of fork tines.

One final note regarding bruising is worth including in this section. A folk medicine technique called coin rubbing is used within the Asian culture. This technique may result in what appears to be a non-accidental bruising pattern. Coin rubbing is used primarily to treat fever. Warm oil is rubbed on the skin and the edge of a coin is repeatedly rubbed in linear strokes across the oiled area. Because the capillaries are dilated and the coin creates repeated friction, bruising results. This process may be done on more than one area of the child's back, thus resulting in a distinct pattern of linear bruises. This procedure is not painful to the child. Rather, it feels much like a massage. It is not considered child abuse.

Burns

Burn injury in children may well be accidental. It is important to view burn injuries in children with a critical eye as to the potential mechanism of injury. Scald burns may be accidental if the child's caregiver is unaware of the actual temperature of the water. Examine the water line on the child and document the exact exposure areas.

Intentional scald burns in children often result from forced immersion. These burns may be evident on the buttocks and back of the legs. They may or may not include the feet, depending on how the child was held during the immersion (Figure 12-5a). A burn pattern

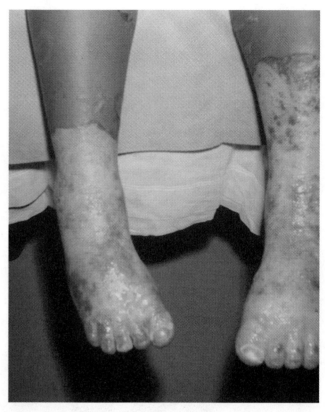

a.

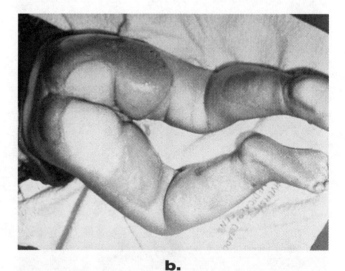

b.

FIGURE 12-5 **a.** Circumferential burns to the extremities may indicate the child was intentionally held in scalding water. Photo courtesy of Emergency Medical Services for Children, NERA. **b.** Likewise, burns to the buttocks and legs with an unburned area on the center of the buttocks may also indicate a child was intentionally held in scalding water. Photo courtesy of Emergency Medical Services for Children, NERA, Torrance, CA.

that involves the back of the legs and top of the buttocks with an unburned area in the center of the buttocks should raise suspicion that the buttocks were held forcefully against the bottom of the tub (Figure 12-5b). Forcing the buttocks against the bottom of the tub results in that particular portion of the skin avoiding prolonged contact with the scalding water.

Splash burns are the result of hot liquid being spilled, thrown, or poured over the child. They typically involve a relatively large area surrounded by smaller scattered burns that may be partial- or full-thickness burns. Splash burns may occur accidentally. Burn location and history are critical when determining the potential cause as abuse.

Cigarette burns may also occur accidentally. However, if a child inadvertently touches a burning cigarette, he or she normally pulls quickly away leaving an oval or incomplete burn pattern. Deliberately inflicted cigarette burns are often round as the result of the cigarette being held directly against the skin. Often, accidental cigarette burns are only partial thickness (second degree) due to the rapidity with which the child pulls away. Deliberate burns may be full thickness (third degree) due to the cigarette being held against the skin for a prolonged period. In addition, there are often multiple burn sites instead of a single, isolated site. Cigarette burns are often inflicted to the bottom of the feet or the palms of the hand (Figure 12-6).

"Branding" burns result from exposure to heated metals. This activity can include hot plates, radiators, heating grates, and electric stoves for example. Branding burns often leave distinct patterns (Figure 12-7). These patterns should be noted and described in detail along with the depth of the burn.

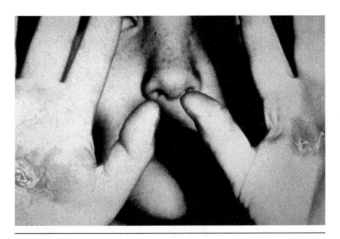

FIGURE 12-6 Cigarette burns often found on the hands that are full-thickness burns may indicate child abuse. Photo courtesy of Emergency Medical Services for Children, NERA, Torrance, CA.

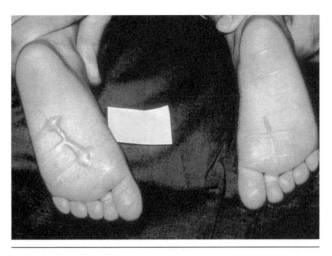

FIGURE 12-7 Burns that have specific shapes and patterns, called branding, may be an indicator of abuse. Photo courtesy of Emergency Medical Services for Children, NERA, Torrance, CA.

Head Injuries

Head injuries are the most common cause of death in children (see Chapter 9—Head and Spinal Trauma). Injuries to the head may include scalp injuries with resultant swelling and bruising, traumatic **alopecia** (loss of hair), skull fractures, and subdural hematomas. External swelling and bruising of the scalp may result from a fall or may be the result of a deliberate blow. It is important to note the location of the injury and the extent. Depending on the force involved, external scalp injuries may or may not be accompanied by an underlying skull fracture. Since there is not a way to determine the presence or absence of an underlying fracture in the prehospital environment, assessment and intervention must be centered on the obvious injury and the index of suspicion.

Traumatic alopecia may result from an infant or child's head being forcefully rubbed back and forth across a rough surface such as a chair, couch, or carpet. In some instances, the hair may be literally pulled out. Traumatic alopecia is usually accompanied by noticeable swelling of the scalp. If the pulling is severe, it may result in lifting the scalp up from the skull resulting in a hematoma under the scalp. It is important to be aware that alopecia may also result from other than traumatic causes, such as chemotherapy. Again, the extent of accompanying bruising, swelling, and history play a key role in raising the index of suspicion for the potential that an abusive injury exists.

Children presenting with black eyes must be assessed for the potential of the injury resulting from direct blows (either deliberate or accidental) versus the possibility of a basilar skull fracture. Care must be taken to rule out underlying injury to the eye itself if the mechanism is that of a direct blow. Examine the eye for signs of overt bleeding as indicated by blood in the sclera. Any visual change, such as blurring or double vision, should be determined. Assessment for signs of mastoid bruising (Battle's sign), traumatic blows to other parts of the head, and/or increased intracranial pressure is important in determining the possibility of a basilar skull fracture.

Subdural hematoma or intracranial bleeding as the result of shaken baby syndrome may be difficult to identify in the prehospital setting. Often the history given by the caregiver is one of a minor fall or seizure that has now resulted in the child being unresponsive or apneic. There are no overt signs of trauma to the head in this particular situation. Assessment for signs of increased intracranial pressure is critical. Examination may reveal an altered level of consciousness, fixed and/or dilated pupils, posturing, and decreased respiratory rate. One particularly helpful indicator of increased intracranial pressure in a neurologically depressed infant is a bulging anterior fontanelle.

Finger marks may be visible on the upper arms if that was where the infant was grasped and shaken. Instead of the arms, the infant may have been grasped around the thorax. Therefore, it is also important to look for finger marks on the back. Often marks from the thumb on the front of the thorax are not visible. Any infant or young child presenting with signs of increased intracranial pressure with the history of a minor fall should be considered suffering from an inflicted injury until it can be proven otherwise within the hospital setting.

Abdominal Injuries

Abdominal injuries are the second leading cause of death in children (see Chapter 10—Thoracic and Abdominal Trauma). It is often difficult, if not impossible, to determine the specific organ(s) involved in the prehospital setting. At this point, specific determination is not necessary. Recognize the potential for abdominal injury through history, overt signs of bruising to the abdomen, or abnormalities in the abdominal assessment (e.g., a distended, firm abdomen). Even in the absence of specific abdominal findings, unexplainable signs of shock should be identified as a potential abdominal injury. History and stated mechanism of injury are central to raising the index of suspicion for potential abuse.

DOCUMENTATION

If the incident proves to be one of abuse, it may be several months or longer before the case is ever presented in court. Because of the time delay, it is absolutely critical that documentation be complete to the point that any questions that might be raised can be answered by reviewing the patient encounter form. It is just as critical to the credibility of the report and possible testimony that the encounter form be objective. Several areas should be included in the encounter form documentation.

- Describe the scene if appropriate. Include cleanliness, numbers of other children present and their appearance in terms of cleanliness, and others' reactions to the situation. The prehospital provider may be the only person to see the child in the actual home environment at an unexpected time. If there are relevant observations related to that environment, they should be documented in an objective manner on the encounter form.

- Describe behavioral characteristics. Take care not to include any personal interpretation of the significance of those behaviors.

- Quote exactly what the parent, caregiver, and/or child states relative to a history. Never chart that the child was abused.

- Although the hospital medical records and law enforcement evidence routinely involve photographs, it is extremely important to describe injuries in detail. Include the size, color, location(s), and patterns of bruises and burns.

Remember that the prehospital patient encounter form, as well as hospital records, are examined and reviewed by both prosecutor and defense attorney in preparing for legal action. Because the documentation is detailed, it will probably require supplemental sheets. Do not condense or summarize the report in order to accommodate completion on one sheet. Once the documentation is completed, it is a good idea to number all of the sheets (i.e., 1 of 4, 2 of 4, etc.) and make sure they are attached together. This numbering will ensure that the entire document is present if retrieval is necessary (Figure 12-8).

The copy left with the hospital must be exactly the same as the copy retained by the service. If relevant information has been recalled after completing the original form, document that information as an addendum to the original encounter form. The addendum should contain the number of the original encounter form, the date, and the time it was completed. Be sure that the hospital receives a copy of the addendum to be added to the original encounter form left at the time the patient was delivered to the emergency department.

All states require suspected child abuse to be reported to law enforcement. However, who is obligated to report and to whom they must report varies. In some

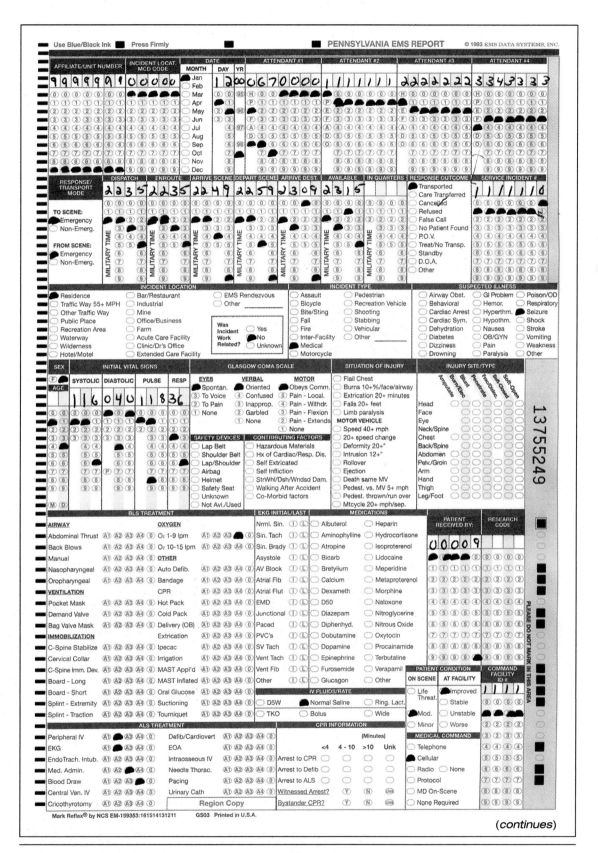

FIGURE 12-8 Sample documentation of suspicion of abuse.

(continues)

Use Blue/Black Ink - Press Firmly

| SERVICE NAME | | | SERVICE # 00000 | INCIDENT # 11111 | TODAY'S DATE 4/12/00 |

INCIDENT LOCATION

PATIENT INFO

PATIENT LAST NAME Doe	FIRST Johnny	M.I.	PHONE	AGE 11	DATE OF BIRTH	SEX M
STREET ADDRESS 111 Doe Street			SOCIAL SECURITY NUMBER		MEMBERSHIP (Y) Yes (N) No	
CITY Town ,	STATE PA	ZIP CODE 00000	INSURANCE CODE #		MILEAGE	
PRIVATE PHYSICIAN			MEDICAID #		OUT 55459	
○ BILL TO (COMPANY or NAME)		PHONE	MEDICARE #		SCENE 55459	
ADDRESS	STREET		GROUP INSURANCE #		DEST 55468	
CITY	STATE	ZIP CODE	OTHER INSURANCE #		IN 55472	

CHIEF COMPLAINT Pain

CURRENT MEDICATIONS ● NONE KNOWN

ALLERGIES (MEDS) ● NONE KNOWN

PAST MEDICAL HISTORY ○ MI ○ CHF ○ COPD ○ ↑ BP ○ DIABETES ○ CANCER ○ NONE KNOWN ○ OTHER

NARRATIVE

Patient was an 11 y/o male with CC of pain. Pt. condition on scene was moderate. An injury was sustained to the abdomen (blunt)

Pt was found crying and screaming on couch at home. Mother expressed HPI: He was knocked to the ground by a group of boys and kicked in the abdomen. He then ran home. No n/v, SOB, CP, or dizziness. Pt. had no signs of bruising, point tenderness or palpable masses. Pt. did have "guarding" over the mid-abdomen.

Pt. placed on stretcher - no other interventions necessary. Mother accompanied pt. in patient compartment of Ambulance.

No changes occured enroute.

○ Narrative 1 of _____

TIME	P	R	B/P	RHYTHM	TREATMENT	PROVIDER ID #	RESPONSE/COMMENTS
2256	118	36	116/40	NA	Assessment	#1	Normal
2258					Lung Assmt/Abd. Asses	#1	Normal
2259					Stretcher	#1/#2	

Crew Signatures:

Signature of Person Receiving Patient _____ Time _____

Command Physician _____ ID# _____

A#1 _____
A#2 _____
A#3 _____
A#4 _____

| Service Copy | 13755249 |

FIGURE 12-8 Continued

states, it is considered adequate for the prehospital provider to report suspicions to the receiving hospital personnel. It is then the hospital personnel who follow up with contacting law enforcement. In other states, the prehospital provider is legally bound to contact law enforcement directly. Be aware of the legal requirements and incorporate these regulations in the service's policies and procedures.

Express any concerns about abuse of a child to the emergency department medical personnel. If those individuals do not have the same concern, report the information to the appropriate law enforcement or child protective services agency.

Exploring the Web

● Search the Web site of your state EMS agency to determine the regulations regarding reporting of child abuse in your state.

PERSONAL BIASES

Most health care workers have strong personal emotions regarding child abuse and neglect. Be very aware of personal reactions and emotions, including body language in the situation where abuse is suspected. It is unacceptable to convey judgment or appear threatening. The prehospital provider's role is to give needed medical attention to the child, gather an objective history, and provide documentation of the incident.

PREVENTION ACTIVITIES

Prehospital personnel can be key to breaking the cycle of abuse and taking action to prevent future occurrences. Early identification of suspicious behavior and reporting of this information in an unbiased format to local authorities are the first steps in prevention.

Participating in continuing education programs aimed at recognizing the signs and symptoms of child abuse can be helpful. In these programs, prehospital providers can enhance their assessment abilities and learn techniques to interact with potential abusers.

Teaming with law enforcement agencies to present educational programs in the community is another way to help prevent child abuse. These programs can be aimed at children and adults alike. Visit the schools and teach children safety in terms of potential risk situations. Include handouts for the children to take home that outline methods for parents to protect and educate their children against possible sexual abuse.

Babysitting safety and "new parent" classes can help educate adults about proper care of children. Team up with local pediatricians and family practice physicians to present these programs and increase the ability of parents to adequately care for their children.

Exploring the Web

● Search the Web for child abuse prevention projects in your state or local area. Come up with a plan that will get your agency involved in prevention programs.

SUMMARY

Child abuse is a major concern in the welfare of children in our society today. The prehospital provider must be aware of significant history findings, behavioral characteristics, and physical signs and symptoms that would indicate the potential for physical abuse, neglect, sexual abuse, and emotional abuse. The priority of the prehospital provider in potential abuse is to provide medical interventions and to support the child's physical well being. However, also be knowledgeable of state law regarding obligation to report and be able to document all injuries, behaviors, and inconsistencies in a complete and objective manner to support future legal action.

Management of Case Scenario

Calmly talk with the mother and ask what happened today that prompted her to call for the ambulance. She tells you that her child stopped breathing and had a seizure. The mother is very calm and does not appear to be all that concerned. You notice a large pillow in the crib. Your examination reveals the following:

> *Neuro: Awake, active, and playful*
>
> *Airway: Patent*
>
> *Breathing: Nonlabored with respiratory rate of 26; breath sounds clear bilaterally*
>
> *Circulation: Strong, regular brachial pulse of 102; skin pink and warm*
>
> *The remainder of the exam is unremarkable.*
>
> *HPI: The child has not been ill, has not had a temperature, and has been eating regularly without any vomiting or diarrhea.*
>
> *PMH: Child has had seizures before but is not on any medication. All testing at the hospital has been negative. Mother states that the child never does this kind of thing once they get to the hospital.*
>
> *Twice during the conversation and exam of the toddler, the mother changes her story. She says that the child had a seizure and then stopped breathing. When you try to get clarification, she gets very angry and demands to be transported to the hospital. You become concerned that her story does not sound the same each time she tells it.*
>
> *You transport the child and mother to the hospital and document your exact conversation with the mother on the encounter form. You pass along your concerns to the nurse and physician at the emergency department.*

▶ REVIEW QUESTIONS

1. Define the following terms: maltreatment, neglect, abuse, sexual abuse, and emotional abuse.

2. List the major types of child maltreatment.

3. For infants and toddlers, _____ continues to be a serious cause of mortality and morbidity.

4. List three examples of physical needs of an infant or child.

5. List three examples of emotional needs of an infant or child.

6. List three risk factors for physical abuse.

7. List six types of sexual abuse.

8. You are called to the home of a child who has been injured. The six-year-old girl is crying and states she was riding her brother's bicycle when she fell and hurt her "privates." You should immediately suspect sexual abuse. True or False?

9. The following items are indicative of child abuse.
   a. Multiple bruises in various stages of healing
   b. Burns to both feet with a specific line where the burn stops
   c. Any loss of hair
   d. a and b only

10. A three-month old baby who is unconscious after falling out of his crib should raise suspicion of child abuse. True or False?

11. Additional information may be added to the encounter form or trip sheet back at the station as soon as it is remembered. True or False?

▶ REFERENCES

DiScala, C. et al. (2000). Child abuse and unintentional injuries—a 10-year perspective. *Archives of Pediatrics and Adolescent Medicine, 154*(1).

National Center on Child Abuse and Neglect. (1996). *A coordinated response to child abuse and neglect: A basic manual.* Washington, DC: National Center on Child Abuse and Neglect.

National Pediatric Trauma Registry. (1996). *Children and adolescents with disability due to traumatic injury: A data book.* Boston, MA: Department of Physical Medicine and Rehabilitation, New England Medical Center.

Wong, D. (1999). *Whaley & Wong's nursing care of infants and children* (6th ed.). St. Louis, MO: Mosby-Year Book.

▶ BIBLIOGRAPHY

American Academy of Pediatrics, Section on Child Abuse and Neglect. (1998). *A guide to references and resources in child abuse and neglect.* (2d ed.). Elk Grove Village, IL: American Academy of Pediatrics.

American Academy of Pediatrics, Committee on Hospital Care and Committee on Child Abuse and Neglect. (1998). Medical necessity for the hospitalization of the abused and neglected child. *Pediatrics, 101* (4 pt 1).

Emergency Nurses Association. (1997). *Emergency nursing pediatric course.* Chicago, IL: Kay Graphics.

Laraque, D., Ravenell, J., & DiScala, C. (1995). Child abuse: What have we learned and where are we going? *Current Issues of Public Health, 1,* 122–130.

Levin, A., & Sheridan, M. (1995). *Munchausen syndrome by proxy: Issues in diagnosis and treatment.* New York: Lexington Books.

Limbos, M., & Berkowitz, C. (1998). Documentation of child physical abuse: How far have we come?" *Pediatrics, 102,* (1 pt 1), 53–58.

Monteleone, J. (1996). *Recognition of child abuse for the mandated reporter.* (2d ed.). St. Louis, MO: Mosby-Year Book.

Nashelesky, M., & Dix, J. (1995). The time interval between lethal infant shaking and onset of symptoms: A review of the shaken baby syndrome literature." *American Journal of Forensic Medical Pathology, 16,* 154–157.

National Association of Emergency Medical Technicians. (1998). *Prehospital trauma life support.* St. Louis, MO: Mosby-Year Book.

Sanders, M. (2000). *Mosby's paramedic textbook* (2nd ed.). St. Louis, MO: Mosby-Year Book.

U.S. Department of Health and Human Services. (1996). *The third national incidence study of child abuse and neglect.* Washington, DC: U.S. Government Printing Office

Wertz, E. (1997). Pediatric Emergencies. In B. Shade, et. al. (Eds.), *Mosby's EMT—intermediate textbook.* St. Louis, MO: Mosby-Year Book.

Chapter 13

Ethical and Legal Considerations

OBJECTIVES

Upon completion of this chapter, the student should be able to:

- Describe the child-parent-caregiver relationship.
- Discuss the ethical principles of beneficence, autonomy, and fidelity as they relate to prehospital personnel's obligation to children.
- Discuss the legal principles of consent and refusal as they relate to the conduct of prehospital personnel when dealing with a sick or injured child.
- Identify emancipated and mature minors.
- Describe the importance of medical control and documentation in dealing with ethical and legal principles.

KEY TERMS

advance directive
autonomy
beneficence
consent
ethics
fidelity
implied consent

law
living will
loco parentis
nonmaleficence
off-line or indirect medical control
on-line or direct medical control
policy

procedure
prospective medical control
protocol
retrospective medical control
self-determinism
standing orders
veracity

Case Scenario

You are called to the house of a six-year-old girl with end-stage brain cancer. You have been to her house on many occasions and know the child and the family. You are surprised to be called since you thought the child had a "do not resuscitate" order when she went home the last time from the hospital. When you arrive, the child is lying in a bed in the living room. Two adults are fighting over what to do for her. How do you handle this situation?

INTRODUCTION

Ethics and law provide the framework for guiding the obligations and conduct of prehospital personnel when providing care to their patients. **Ethics** deals with the rightness or wrongness of an individual's obligations to himself or herself and to others in society. **Law** provides the rules of human conduct that are accepted by society. It is important for prehospital personnel to realize that what is lawful may conflict with what is ethical and vice versa. For example, abortion may be legal; but there remains the question for many people as to whether it is ethical.

When prehospital providers are summoned to the scene of a sick or injured adult, they are not only confronted with the physical and emotional needs of the patient, but also with a wide range of ethical and legal dilemmas that can make decision making difficult. When children become patients, ethical and legal dilemmas may make decision making even more difficult because of the lack of a uniform outlook on the evolving position of children within our society. In order to resolve some of the ethical and legal dilemmas confronting the provider when dealing with children, it is important to understand the fundamentals of ethical thought and recognize the legal principles derived from them.

DEFINITIONS

Several terms are commonly used to describe pediatric ethical and legal situations. **Beneficence** is the duty to do good or promote the welfare of a child. **Nonmaleficence** is the duty not to harm or burden the child. **Autonomy** is the ability to make one's own decisions. With pediatric patients, parents or legal guardians have the autonomy to make decisions for their children, including those concerning medical treatment. **Self-determinism** is deciding or determining what is best for oneself. **Veracity** is the duty to tell the truth. **Fidelity** is the duty to keep one's promise or word.

THE CHILD-PARENT-PROVIDER RELATIONSHIP

When a child is involved as a patient, a relationship develops between the child and the health care provider as well as between the parents and the provider. This connection is called the *child-parent-provider relationship* (Figure 13-1).

Under common law, children were found to be incapable of making legally binding decisions based on their inability to understand all possible consequences. Thus, common law provided parents with the right to make decisions for their children, including those concerning medical treatment (i.e., autonomy). As a general rule, courts will not challenge this right unless

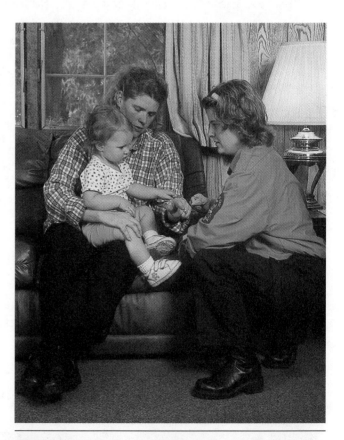

FIGURE 13-1 The child-parent-provider relationship develops when a child is the patient.

interference is in the best interest of the child (i.e., beneficence).

A patient-provider relationship is developed when a health care provider, including prehospital personnel, performs an act that may be construed as administering care. This act may be as simple as a health care provider introducing herself to a prospective patient. For a long time, the patient-provider relationship has been one-sided with the physician, especially, being the only active participant in the decision-making process.

This relationship has changed. The decisions made by physicians and other health care providers regarding what care to administer to sick or injured adult patients have become more complicated due to the ethical principles of patient autonomy and self-determinism. What this has done is change the role of patients in the decision-making process. Today, the patient-provider relationship is a collaborative relationship.

However, with children as patients, the decisions made by providers concerning the care to administer become even more complicated. At odds are the rights of children versus the rights of their parents; the rights of the parents versus the duty of the providers to the sick or injured child; and the interests of the decision-makers and those of the state (Chapter 14—Dealing with Families and Caregivers). Also at odds are the ethical principles of beneficence/nonmaleficence and autonomy/self-determinism.

CONSENT

Consent is the legal agreement of a patient to accept medical intervention. Central to the ethical principles of autonomy and self-determinism, consent allows a patient to choose, whenever possible, what he or she wants regarding medical care. Historically, patients have been given the right to consent upon reaching the legal age of majority. In most states that age is defined as 18 years of age. If the patient was younger, the ability to accept medical intervention was up to the parent or legal guardian. However, all state jurisdictions have recognized exceptions to the general rule of consent for patients under the age of 18. These are minors in an emergency, emancipated minors, mature minors, and certain state statutes allowing minors to consent to specified medical treatments.

Children in an Emergency

The courts have always been willing to utilize an **implied consent** theory when dealing with children in an emergency. This implied consent theory states that if

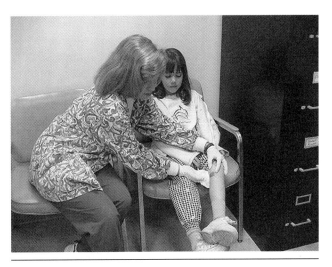

FIGURE 13-2 A child injured at school may be treated through *implied consent* if the parent or legal guardian cannot be contacted.

a child is involved in a medical emergency and the providers are unable to reach the parents, consent for treatment of the child is assumed because the parents would want what is best for their child (Figure 13-2). However, what constitutes an emergency? The courts have said that an emergency exists when immediate treatment is necessary to either save the child's life or alleviate pain and suffering. The important word in the definition of an emergency is "immediate." Any condition that does not require immediate intervention is not granted an exception to the general rule of consent.

The provider that gives care without the appropriate consent of the parents has the burden to prove that an emergency actually existed. Therefore, documentation of the existence of an emergency and the probability that a delay would have adversely affected the health of the child is important.

Emancipated Minors

The law recognizes the emancipated minor as an exception to the general rule of consent. Factors considered by the courts in determining emancipation vary. However, a child is usually considered emancipated if any one of the following conditions exist:

• The child lives apart from his or her parents.
• The child is financially self-supporting.
• The child is married.
• The child is pregnant.
• The child is in the military service.

The concept of emancipation also includes college students, even though they are financially supported by their parents, and minor parents who are unmarried. It is not necessary for a provider to have documentation from a minor proving emancipation. All the provider needs is for the minor to provide representation as being emancipated (e.g., the minor tells the prehospital provider that she is married).

Mature Minors

Developed under common law, this rule allows minors who can understand the nature and consequences of the medical treatment offered to consent to treatment. In general, the mature minor rule states that a minor may consent to treatment if:

- He or she is 14 years of age or older.
- The treatment is for the benefit of the minor only.
- The minor has the perceived ability to understand the nature and risks of the proposed treatment.
- The proposed treatment is described as minor or not serious.

The mature minor rule places the obligation on the provider to determine whether a minor is of necessary age and maturity to provide consent for his or her medical treatment. Factors that may assist the caregiver in making the decision to apply the mature minor rule are:

- Age
- Ability
- Experience
- Educational background and maturity as determined by the minor's behavior

It is important for prehospital personnel to contact medical control when trying to establish the maturity of a minor. Physicians are the only providers capable by law of determining the maturity of a minor.

Certain State Statutes

The final exception to the general rule of consent is the statutory and common laws that allow minors to consent to certain types of medical treatment. These medical treatments include treatment for venereal disease, alcohol and drug abuse, pregnancy, and psychiatric conditions. Public policy concerns about the spread of disease and providing incentives for a minor to seek medical care have provided the backbone for many of the statutes.

Exploring the Web

- Search your state Emergency Medical Services (EMS) or Department of Health Web site. Identify the state statutes affecting consent. What medical treatments are minors allowed to consent to by state law?

Special Situations

Children are often at school, a child care center, camp, or at a babysitter's house when they become sick or injured (Figure 13-3). In these situations, many parents sign a blanket consent form whereby the school, child care center, and other sites where children spend their time stand in *loco parentis,* in place of the parents, and may consent for routine medical care. If a form has not been signed, parents retain the right to decide the routine medical care the child should receive. This situation means every effort should be made to contact at least one parent before initiating treatment. In an emergency, a child of any age may be treated without permission of the parents. It is important to remember, however, the definition of an emergency as discussed previously.

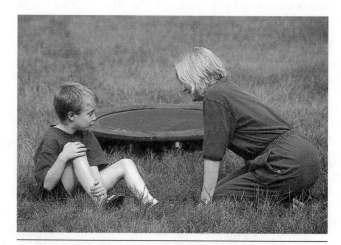

FIGURE 13-3 Consent may be given for treatment of a child who is hurt at a child care center by the director in *loco parentis,* in place of the parents, for routine medical care.

REFUSAL OF TREATMENT

Situations may arise in which refusal of treatment occurs by the child, parents, or legal guardians. The same ethical and resultant legal principles discussed previously should be kept in mind.

Refusal by a Child

Unless the child is an emancipated minor, a mature minor, or is covered by one of the treatment statutes, the child is not legally allowed to refuse consent for medical treatment. If a provider is confronted with this type of situation, every attempt should be made to contact the parents or legal guardians as well as consult with medical control and law enforcement.

Refusal by a Parent or Legal Guardian

Refusal of treatment by a parent or legal guardian may occur as the result of religious beliefs or parental marital conflict. The First Amendment right of religious freedom does not include the right to deny children access to medical care. Parents are allowed to make decisions for their children but cannot deny treatment in which that denial could result in harmful effects to their child.

If an emergency exists, prehospital providers should do what is best for the child. It may help to have law enforcement on the scene while you are explaining to the parents that treatment under an emergency is a medical obligation under the law. Their refusal may be reported to the local child protection agency depending on local protocol. If there is no emergency, the provider should respect the wishes of the parents. However, medical control consultation should be established in any of these situations. Whether parental refusal is accepted or not, good documentation is extremely important.

When parental marital conflict exists, the child may be caught between the parents. The parent who has legal custody holds the legal right to decide on the medical treatment rendered to the child. However, if the parent without legal custody is the only one available for a decision, it should be assumed that he or she has the authority to provide the necessary consent. Regardless of which situation the prehospital provider confronts, when an emergency exists, care should be administered under the obligation of beneficence and nonmaleficence. The provider will be viewed in a more positive light in the eyes of the courts if care is provided with the best interest of the child in mind.

WITHHOLDING OR PROVIDING MINIMAL TREATMENT

Several instances exist in which treatment may be withheld or only minimal treatment provided. The prehospital provider must be familiar with the policies and procedures in his or her state or local jurisdiction.

In the instance of a child with a chronic or life-threatening disease, the parents or legal guardians may be struggling with a decision to prolong life while knowing the child will have a high degree of burden and suffering. The parent or guardian may be trying to balance the burdens of the condition with the positive dimensions of providing quality to the child's life.

In other situations, the parent or guardian may have decided that enough is enough. They may want to alleviate their child's pain and suffering by not allowing certain life-sustaining treatments.

"Do Not Resuscitate" Orders

In children with end-stage disease processes, the family may have decided that certain procedures are not to be instituted to prolong the child's life. Some situations may allow for pharmacological therapy (i.e., pain control or suppression of premature ventricular contractions) but not intubation or cardiopulmonary resuscitation. "Do not resuscitate" or DNR orders are regulated differently from state to state, and the prehospital provider must know the laws applicable in his or her state.

Identification of the child with a DNR order is necessary. In Connecticut, for instance, a bracelet is worn by the child indicating that no cardiopulmonary resuscitation is to be performed "including chest compressions, defibrillation, or breathing or ventilation by any assistive or mechanical means including, but not limited to, mouth-to-mouth, mouth-to-mask, bag-valve mask, endotracheal tube, or ventilator for a particular patient." Prehospital providers document the presence of this bracelet and then treat (or do not treat) the child according to the directions in the DNR order.

In Maryland, the Maryland Institute for Emergency Medical Services Systems (MIEMSS) worked with the Board of Physician Quality Assurance and other key individuals in their state to develop a specific EMS/DNR Protocol (Bass & Alcorta, 1998). Dr. Robert Bass, Executive Director of MIEMSS, stated in the original introduction to legislation on July 1, 1995:

This protocol greatly expands access to palliative care and do not resuscitate orders within the State. More importantly, it enables EMS providers to honor patient wishes to the greatest extent possible, with dignity, humanity, and compassion.

In 1998, the Maryland legislation was updated to include a section for physicians outlining what medical conditions met the persistent vegetative state, end-stage condition, and terminal condition criteria as described in their Health Care Decisions Act (Bass & Alcorta, 1998). A program booklet also included guidelines for attorneys, federal facilities, and facilities outside of the state requesting to use the forms (Figure 13-4).

Federal Patient Self-Determination Act

The Patient Self-Determination Act was enacted as Sections 4206 and 4751 of the Omnibus Budget Reconciliation Act of 1990, P.L. 101-508 (1990). It became effective on December 1, 1991, and allows adults (i.e., those individuals greater than or equal to 18 years of age) admitted to a health care facility to accept or refuse

medical treatment. A competent adult can decide how to handle future health care issues through an **advance directive.** The advance directive can be a **living will** (written instructions authorizing the provision, withholding, or withdrawal of health care), the identification of a durable power of attorney (written appointment of an agent to make health care decisions for the patient), or an oral statement to a physician explaining instructions for health care or appointing an agent.

Unfortunately, legislation does not exist for those individuals under the age of 18. Many adolescents (i.e., children ages 12 to 17) may have the capacity to be part of the decision-making process but are not legally permitted to refuse lifesaving medical care. In some instances, the parent or guardian may want the emergency care provided yet the adolescent does not want the treatment. At this time, there is no legal protection to support the adolescent's rights. Prehospital providers are forced to respect the wishes of the child's parent or legal guardian.

Right to Die

The "right to die" is evident in three specific places:

- The right of self-determination (as previously discussed)
- The U.S. Constitution
- The doctrine of informed consent

The Fourteenth Amendment Due Process clause of the U.S. Constitution gives an American citizen the right to control what happens to his or her body (Romano, 1998). This "right to die" includes the right to refuse medical treatment.

The doctrine of informed consent includes action by prehospital personnel to disclose information to the patient (parent or legal guardian in the case of a child) about his or her medical condition. The provider in turn obtains the parent's or guardian's informed consent to treatment.

In some states, the parent or legal guardian may petition the courts to let the child die. How would this situation involve prehospital providers? Think about a child with a severe brain injury after a near-drowning event who has been in a persistent, vegetative state. The child has been kept alive for years by a feeding tube and ventilator. He is cared for at home with no hope of recovery. The parents may have received documentation from neurologists that the child will never recover. They obtain permission to disconnect the child's ventilator and then panic when he is struggling to breathe. EMS may be summoned to the house because of the parents' fear of watching the child suffer. Upon EMS arrival, there

MARYLAND
EMERGENCY MEDICAL SERVICES
DO NOT RESUSCITATE PROGRAM

Originally Issued 7/1/95
1st. Revision 4/1/96 (Update)
2nd. Revision 7/1/98

developed by the

Maryland Institute for Emergency Medical
Services Systems (MIEMSS)
653 West Pratt Street
Baltimore, Maryland 21201-1536
Office: (410) 706-4367 (4DNR)
FAX: (410) 706-4366

and the

Board of Physician Quality Assurance (BPQA)
P.O. Box 2571, 4201 Patterson Avenue
Baltimore, Maryland 21215-0095
(410) 764-4777

pursuant to

Subtitle 6, Health General Article, Annotated Code of Maryland
Sections 14-205, 14-303, and 14-305, Health Occupations Article, Annotated Code of Maryland (Expiring 12/31/98)
Section 13-508(a)(1), Education Article, Annotated Code of Maryland
and Section 13-516, Education Article, Annotated Code of Maryland (Effective 12/31/98)

FIGURE 13-4 Maryland's DNR program booklet.

may be a great deal of turmoil between family members regarding further treatment of the child even though they had previously agreed to turn off the ventilator.

ORGAN AND TISSUE DONATION

Organ and tissue donation is usually a subject that is discussed once the child is at the hospital. However, there may be instances in which family members or other caregivers ask about donation during the emergency phase of care if it appears that the child will die or have permanent brain damage. Have information available for the family or know where to refer the family for guidance.

 Exploring the Web

● Search the United Network for Organ Sharing (UNOS) Web site. What information is available related to organ donation and pediatric patients?

ROLES OF MEDICAL CONTROL AND DOCUMENTATION

Medical oversight and the proper recording of all incidents and treatment are crucial to the practice of prehospital care. Each concept is discussed below.

Medical Control

Medical control is an integral part of all activities associated with prehospital care. Physician oversight exists to determine that appropriate actions are taken during the care of infants, children, and adolescents. Consulting with medical control can provide the support necessary to make some, if not all, of the critical ethical and legal decisions when providing care to pediatric patients.

On-Line or Direct Medical Control

On-line or **direct medical control** occurs when there is communication between the prehospital provider and the physician over the telephone or radio. This method may be required at certain points in the treatment of pediatric patients due to the complexity of their care. Examples include:

● Administration of a narcotic to a child (e.g., rectal diazepam to a child in status epilepticus)
● Dealing with suspected child abuse (e.g., parents are arguing over permission to transport the child to the hospital)
● Confirmation of destination (e.g., burn center for a child with severe burns)
● Pronouncement of death permitted in some states (e.g., child found in crib with rigor mortis)

Off-Line or Indirect Medical Control

Off-line or **indirect medical control** can be prospective or retrospective. **Prospective medical control** includes developing specific treatment protocols and policies, requiring specific pediatric equipment at the basic life support and advanced life support levels, and requiring training and ongoing continuing education to perform certain pediatric skills.

Retrospective medical control provides accountability and enables the physician to ensure that appropriate care was rendered to the pediatric patient. Performance of the individual or system is compared to accepted standards of care as well as existing policies, procedures, and protocols. For example, if a problem is identified with the initiation of pediatric intubation, additional continuing education and clinical practice can be scheduled to enhance the prehospital provider's skill (Figure 13-5).

Policies, Procedures, and Protocols

A **policy** is defined as a principle that governs an activity. Employees or members of the ambulance service are

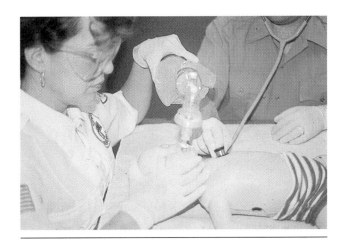

FIGURE 13-5 This paramedic practices bag-valve ventilation on an infant manequin.

expected to follow policies. A **procedure** is the actual sequence of steps to be followed by prehospital providers.

Standing orders are written documents that contain the rules, policies, procedures, regulations, and orders for patient care as related to specific clinical situations. They are developed collectively by a group of physicians involved in emergency and prehospital care. They are categorized by the condition and then outline the specific actions to be taken including any medications, dosages, routes of administration, and other specific procedures. **Protocol** is a written plan that specifically outlines the procedures to be followed for a particular condition and is sometimes used to mean standing orders.

Documentation

Thorough and accurate documentation of decisions made and care rendered is the best protection for prehospital personnel in a court of law. The statute of limitations for filing a lawsuit concerning medical care issues is two to three years. It is important to remember, however, that when children are involved as patients, this statute of limitations does not begin until the child reaches the age of majority, which is 18 in most states. Thus, prehospital personnel need to take the time to make sure their documentation is thorough and accurate since many years might pass before the incident is brought into a court of law.

SUMMARY

Children provide special challenges to prehospital personnel. Clinical expertise to provide good pediatric care and an understanding of ethical and legal principles are necessary to make appropriate decisions.

The status of children continues to evolve within society. Children have been given a greater ability to participate in the decisions concerning their medical care. There are 50 different jurisdictions within the United States. It is extremely important that providers receive current information regarding the laws within their specific jurisdictions.

Management of Case Scenario

Upon questioning the parents, you find out that the grandfather wants the child resuscitated because he cannot stand to see her struggling for breath. The mother produces a written DNR order that has been signed by the child's physician. In your state, you know that the DNR order is legal and recognized by the courts. Since the mother is the legal guardian and she produces a valid DNR order, you do not resuscitate the child.

You remain with the family until the child is no longer breathing. You then assess the child and run an electrocardiogram (EKG) strip which is flat-line. No heart sounds are heard. You contact medical control and confirm the child's death.

Since you have known this child and her family for almost a year, you begin to cry while you are comforting the mother. You continue to support the family while they contact the child's physician and the funeral home.

When you return to the station, you discuss the call with your partner. Your supervisor suggests a debriefing session to which you reluctantly agree. After the meeting, you feel more positive about your role in helping this family say goodbye to their child.

▌ REVIEW QUESTIONS

1. Define the following terms: ethics, law, consent, loco parentis, autonomy, and beneficence.

2. The patient-provider relationship is one of collaboration. True or False?

3. The term "self-determinism" means:
   a. The child can make his or her own decisions
   b. The parent can make decisions for the child
   c. The caregiver can make decisions for the child
   d. The EMT or paramedic can make decisions for the child

4. What is the age of majority in most states?

5. The courts have said that an emergency exists when immediate treatment is necessary to either save the child's life or alleviate pain and suffering. True or False?

6. A minor is considered emancipated when which of these conditions exists?

 a. Child is living apart from his or her parents

 b. Child is married

 c. Child is pregnant

 d. All of the above.

7. A *mature minor* is a child who is 18 years of age or older. True or False?

8. List three locations where a child may be in which *loco parentis* would be the consent for routine medical care.

9. The First Amendment right of religious freedom includes the right to deny children access to medical care. True or False?

 REFERENCES

Bass, R. R., & Alcorta, R. L. (1998). *Maryland Emergency Medical Services Do Not Resuscitate Program*. Baltimore, MD: Maryland Institute for Emergency Medical Services Systems (MIEMSS).

Omnibus Reconciliation Act (Patient Self-Determination Act [PSDA]), Title IV, Section 4206, h12456–h12457. (1990). *Congressional Record*, October 26, 1990.

Romano, J. (1998). *Legal rights of the catastrophically ill and injured: A family guide*. 2nd ed. Norristown, PA: Joseph L. Romano, Esq.

BIBLIOGRAPHY

American Academy of Pediatrics Committee on Bioethics. (1994). Guidelines for forgoing life-sustaining medical treatment. *Pediatrics*, 93(3), 532–536.

American Heart Association (2000). Guidelines for cardiopulmonary resuscitation and emergency cardiovascular care. *Journal of the American Heart Association* 120(8).

Americans with Disabilities Act of 1990. (1990). 42 USC 12101 *et seq.*

Jackson, P., & Vessey, J. (1996). *Primary care of the child with a chronic condition*. St. Louis, MO: Mosby-Year Book.

McCabe, M. A., Rushton, C. H., & Glover J. J. (1994). *Operational guidelines for involving adolescents in health care decisions*. Washington, DC: Children's National Medical Center.

National Association of EMS Physicians (1994). *Prehospital systems and medical oversight*. St. Louis, MO: Mosby-Year Book.

President's Commission for the Study of Ethical Problems in Medicine and Biomedical and Behavioral Research. (1983). *Deciding to forgo life-sustaining treatment*. Washington, DC: U.S. Government Printing Office

Shade, B., Rothenberg, M., Wertz, E., & Jones, S. (1997) *Mosby's emergency medical technician-intermediate textbook*. St. Louis, MO: Mosby-Year Book.

Wharton, R. H. (1994). Parental wishes regarding participation in critical health care planning for children with disabilities (abstract). *Pediatric Resuscitation*, 35:47A.

Wong, D. (1999). *Whaley & Wong's nursing care of infants and children* (6th ed.). St. Louis, MO: Mosby-Year Book.

Chapter 14

Interacting with Parents and Caregivers

OBJECTIVES

Upon completion of this chapter, the student should be able to:

- Define "family-centered care" and list three principles used to incorporate this concept into emergency care.

- List three types of relationships that caregivers may have with pediatric patients and describe each.

- Discuss examples of how to interact with the various categories of caregivers at an Emergency Medical Services (EMS) scene.

- Discuss the importance of addressing the emotional needs of parents and caregivers at the scene.

- Describe the importance of preparation to help avoid difficult circumstances with parents and caregivers when taking care of a child.

- List at least two strategies to use when delivering bad news to a parent, guardian, or other family member.

- List one unique situation involving a pediatric patient, and describe how to address the family members.

KEY TERMS

empowerment

enable

family-centered care

parent-professional partnership

Case Scenario

You are called to the scene for a girl hit by a car. Bystanders at the scene report that a 15-year-old female darted out of her house away from her parents after a heated argument. She was hit by a car while running across the street. The argument between the girl and her parents was over a boyfriend of which the parents did not approve.

Upon arrival, the boyfriend and parents are at the scene in addition to several neighbors. The patient is conscious enough to emphatically insist that the boyfriend, not her parents, is to accompany her during transportation to the hospital. What do you do?

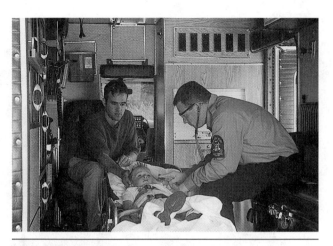

FIGURE 14-1 Families must be included in the care of ill and injured children.

INTRODUCTION

One of the least targeted subcategories in pediatric education is how to interact with the parents, guardians, siblings, caregivers, and other family members of children. Typical prehospital training teaches how to assess and treat the patient's airway, breathing, circulation, and other associated problems. How many emergency care classes include instruction for inclusion of a family member as part of the treatment team?

Just as there are higher emotional needs of a pediatric patient, there are higher emotional needs for the parents, caregivers, and other family members when a child is sick or injured. In addition, emergency care providers experience a higher level of emotion when attending to a pediatric patient no matter the chief complaint.

The intent of this chapter is to recognize that treating children does not happen in a vacuum. Pediatric patients offer situations and pressures that are not typical of the traditional "adult" patient treatment scenario. Health care providers in the prehospital setting need to:

1. Be aware of their own feelings and emotional needs concerning the treatment of ill or injured children.
2. Be ready to work in a more "family friendly" environment and focus on "family-centered care" (Figure 14-1).

FAMILY-CENTERED CARE

Family-centered care is an "approach to health care that offers a new way of thinking about relationships between families and health care providers," according to the Institute for Family-Centered Care (2000). It involves the philosophy that the family is the constant in the child's life (Wong, 1999). Health care providers will come and go as the child grows yet the family relationships, whatever they may be, remain the child's central core of caregivers.

First and foremost, families must be appreciated for what they are—families. In addition, children must be appreciated as children. They have an assortment of concerns, emotions, strengths, and aspirations beyond what they may need related to their illness or injury.

Major Components

There are two major components to family-centered care. The first one, **empowerment**, involves allowing the family to have or develop a sense of control over their own family lives. The respectful interaction between the EMS provider and the family helps the family feel appreciated and allows them to build on their strengths, actions, and abilities.

The second concept is to **enable** families. In other words, providers need to give families a chance to use their own skills and abilities. For instance, if the parent knows how to suction the child with a chronic respiratory disease, allow the parent to perform that skill and assist in the resuscitation. Whenever possible, help the family acquire new skills that may be necessary to meet the ongoing needs of their child. In the example above, perhaps another method of suctioning or a different way to irrigate the tracheostomy tube may save the parent time and accomplish the same goal.

Empowering and enabling the family can be fostered by **parent-professional partnerships**. Parents are respected for their contributions and have a right to be part of the decision-making process. Professionals use their medical expertise to care for the child while supporting and strengthening the family in their role of nurturing their child. This mutual relationship encourages teamwork and the sharing of various competencies. In addition, the family, in most instances, will be appreciative of the opportunity to be recognized as a valuable member of that team.

Traditionally, care has been rendered at the convenience of the provider. The provider decides when to move the child, the provider decides when to initiate transport, and the provider decides who rides where in the ambulance. Whenever possible, families should be offered choices:

- At the scene, can the parent remain with the child during painful or stressful procedures?
- Should the parent be at the child's side during cardiac arrest resuscitation?
- Should the parent assist during resuscitation?
- Should the parent be permitted to ride in the patient compartment on the way to the hospital?

Obviously, there will be times when the family is not capable of participating in their child's care. If the parent is outwardly traumatized by the illness or injury,

he or she cannot be a good support system to the child. Custody situations may present a challenge in that family members may be fighting with one another and not be capable of realistically tending to the specific needs of the child. Family members under the influence of drugs or alcohol are also not appropriate for support. Use good judgment as to whether the participation of the parent or family member will benefit or harm the child.

Remember, however, to err on the side of inclusion. While it may be much easier to cast the parent aside or have the parent ride in the front of the ambulance, do whatever is necessary to keep the parent and child together as much as possible. Take time to answer those few extra questions and provide those additional words of encouragement.

Key Principles

Surgeon General C. Everett Koop formulated eight specific elements of family-centered care in 1987 (Wallace, Biehl, MacQueen, & Blackman, 1997). In 1990, a ninth element was added. See Table 14-1 for the key principles of family-centered care (Wallace et al., 1997; Wong, 1999).

TABLE 14-1
Key Principles of Family-Centered Care

1. The family is the constant in the child's life while services provided to the child as well as the support personnel utilized within those services change. Incorporate this concept into policies and practices.

2. Family/professional collaboration should be facilitated at all levels of care—in the community, in the hospital, and in the home—to include:
   a. Care of an individual child
   b. Program development, implementation, and evaluation
   c. Policy formation

3. The racial, ethnic, cultural, spiritual, educational, geographic, and socioeconomic diversity of families must be honored at all times.

4. Each family has different methods of coping with their child's illness or injury. Recognize and respect those differences. Build on family strengths and individuality.

5. Family-to-family support and networking should be encouraged.

6. Each family has a right to complete and unbiased information about their child. Share this information with families on a continuing basis while being supportive to their needs and coping abilities.

(continues)

TABLE 14-1
(Continued)

---

7. Learn about the developmental needs of infants, children, adolescents, and their families. Understand and incorporate these concepts into the delivery of services.

8. Comprehensive programs and policies that meet the needs of families and provide emotional and financial support must be implemented.

9. Home, hospital, community service, and support systems must be flexible, accessible, culturally competent, comprehensive, and responsive to family-identified needs.

Adapted from Shelton, T. L., & Stepanek, J. S. (1994). *Family-centered care for children needing specialized health and developmental services*. Bethesda, MD: Association for the Care of Children's Health.

CAREGIVER RELATIONSHIPS

Just like patients, caregivers come in all shapes and sizes. When treating a child, a parent may not always be there as the caregiver. Children in school may have a teacher, principal, guidance counselor, or school nurse as their caregiver at the time of treatment. Other nonparent caregivers may be childcare workers, chaperones, babysitters, home health nurses, or guardians for children with special health care needs (Figure 14-2). These relationships can typically be classified in one of three ways: formal, informal, and emotional.

Formal Relationships

Formal relationships can be defined as a mother, father, step-parent, grandparent, legal guardian, or other direct

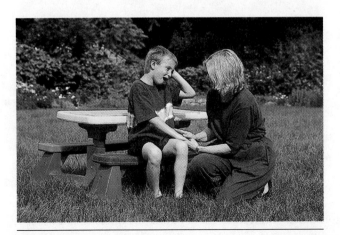

FIGURE 14-2 Caregivers may include the teacher, school nurse, or principal.

family member of the patient. These caregivers are typically capable of providing background related to the patient's history and are legally authorized to give treatment consents.

Informal Relationships

Children often refer to their parents' friends as "uncle" or "aunt." Sometimes an elderly neighbor is referred to as "grammy" or "pap." These are examples of *informal relationships*. A child may be very comfortable with these informal relatives. The prehospital provider, however, needs to clearly assess these relationships. While these individuals may be the caregivers at the actual time of treatment and take responsibility for the child, they may not have any legal authority to do so. Therefore, be careful with decisions they are making with regard to the patient until a formal relationship can be established. In addition, be aware of patient confidentiality issues.

The prehospital provider's best action is to clearly identify the person with the child. If there is no formal relationship to the patient, try to locate someone who can legally make decisions about the patient's care. If the child wishes and is comfortable with the informal relative at his or her side, feel free to use that person in an emotional support role.

Emotional Relationships

Most people do not want to see a child ill or injured and may have a difficult time with emotions tied to that child especially if there was a sudden event. Generally, the prehospital provider will be expected to "do something to help the child." While an adult at an emergency scene may have no formal or informal relationship to the child, this person may have an emotional relationship. Being a witness to the emergent event or possibly the cause of the event will provide a certain emotional tie to the patient. Legally, this person has no right to make decisions about the child's care nor does he or she have any right to know confidential information. Caregivers who have an emotional relationship with the child may sometimes be the most difficult relationship to handle while treating the patient.

INTERACTING WITH PARENTS AND CAREGIVERS AT THE SCENE

During a pediatric emergency, there may be multiple people at the scene of the accident or at the house of an ill child. It is important to prioritize care upon initial arrival.

The Informant

The prehospital provider's first priority is treating the patient. During that treatment, the prehospital provider will interact with all of the formal, informal, and emotional relationship caregivers at the scene. Try to determine fairly quickly who the individuals at the scene are and what type of relationship they have with the patient.

Most importantly, identify who at the scene, other than the patient, can act as the informant about the current situation. At certain ages, the child may be the most dependable informant. Whenever possible, identify a third party to add to or verify the child's history of events.

The informant is the most important person at the scene other than the patient. This person is someone who is intellectually and emotionally capable of relaying pertinent history about the child (Figure 14-3). Remember, while a parent at the scene may have the intellect to explain the child's pertinent medical history, he or she may not be emotionally capable of clearly and concisely sharing those details. The parent may not have the ability to cope with what is happening.

Ascertain the credibility and ability of the informant to provide the necessary data by asking the following questions:

- Is the informant a child, parent, or other caregiver?
- Is the informant focused on the questions being asked or simply speaking without providing clear answers?
- How willingly is the informant providing information?
- Does the informant provide consistent answers to repeated questions?

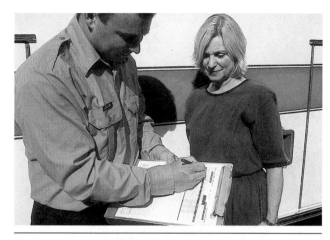

FIGURE 14-3 The informant is capable of providing you with pertinent, reliable information about the scene and the patient.

A reliable informant is the person who willingly gives consistent answers to the questions.

Other Caregivers at the Scene

The prehospital provider needs to determine which adults providing care at the scene need to know what information. Again, not everyone at the scene is legally entitled to know about the patient. While it may seem as if there is a moral or emotional obligation to provide specific information, remember that patient confidentiality laws prohibit disclosure.

It may be very difficult to withhold information from those people who have an informal or emotional relationship with the patient. As a matter of fact, it may be harder for them to understand than it is to explain. However, do not breach patient confidentiality! A passerby who has stopped to help will, no doubt, want to know about the patient's condition as treatment is provided at the scene. However, be very vague when sharing information at the scene or after an incident.

Using Caregivers to "Help"

Once it has been determined which parent or caregiver is the most competent to provide necessary information, look to this individual for assistance. Everyone may want to help, but orchestrate each person to help in very specific ways. Compare it to the old rule of having someone boil water when a baby is delivered. This activity puts that person to good use, gives the individual a sense of

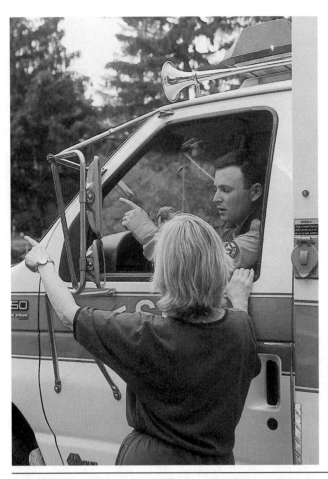
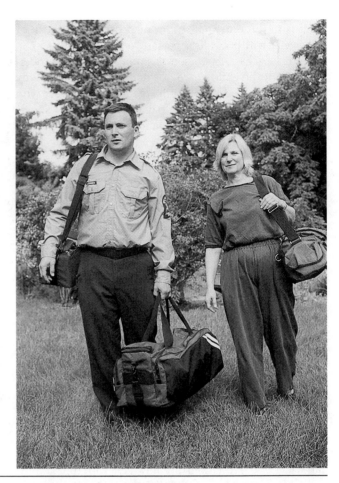

FIGURE 14-4 Caregivers can provide assistance in many ways in order to "help," such as giving directions and carrying equipment.

helping, and allows the mother to deliver the baby without added distraction. The informant can provide the necessary information, another properly assessed caregiver can assist in providing emotional support to the patient, and those individuals with an emotional relationship to the patient or situation can be asked to help with utility functions (e.g., carrying equipment, waiting for additional resources, or crowd control) as in Figure 14-4.

CAREGIVERS IN TRANSPORT

Once initial care has been given to the child, determine if any of the on-scene caregivers are appropriate to accompany the patient during transport. Unfortunately, the lines drawn at this point are not always clear. Certain caregivers may not want to be any more involved than they already are. At certain ages, a pediatric patient's close confidant or primary support person may not be a

parent or someone who might seem to be an "obvious" support person.

Even formal relationships may not be clearly defined at the scene. A formal relationship may exist between a patient and the father or mother. However, it could be that one of those parents has never cared for the patient until the particular incident that has made the child a patient. Rely on previously developed skills to

Exploring the Web

● Search the Web for information on dealing with parents of pediatric patients on the scene of an emergency. What useful tips and information can you find? Can you find any guidelines for transport of the pediatric patient and the caregivers?

determine who is the most reliable informant during your assessment. This person will in turn be the most appropriate formal relative to accompany the patient to the hospital and make treatment consent decisions. In some cases, it may be difficult to make this choice.

PATIENT NEEDS VERSUS CAREGIVER NEEDS

It is important to address the patient as well as the caregiver during the assessment and treatment phases. Remember that each group has specific needs.

Explanation of Process

Throughout this book you will see examples of specific needs of the pediatric patient. Follow the same guidelines for the caregivers' needs. A child will want to know what is going to happen next. He or she will want to know where the ambulance is going, how long it will take to get to there, what will happen during the transport, and what will happen at the hospital. The caregiver will want to know the same information. Whether the caregiver is a school nurse, teacher, parent, or temporary guardian, explain what will occur throughout the treatment and transport (Figure 14-5).

Provide information about ongoing treatment based on the caregiver's relationship to the patient. This interaction will help to keep the scene calm and, in turn, keep the child from becoming more anxious. Be sure to communicate in a way that does not offend the caregiver.

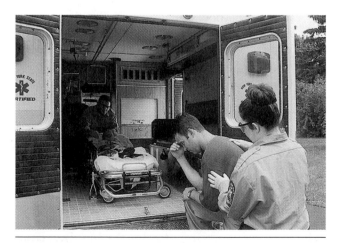

FIGURE 14-5 If the patient's condition permits, tell the patient and the caregivers what to expect during treatment and transport.

For example, a child who has been playing midget football sustains a back injury with associated loss of feeling below the waist. It may be necessary to explain to the team physician or athletic trainer on the field that the child should be transported to a particular hospital, preferably a pediatric trauma center, due to the suspected injury. Share the fact that spine injury studies are currently being conducted at that particular facility or that certain equipment and physician expertise are available 24 hours a day there.

For other health care professionals, be more explicit during the explanation. When speaking to someone without a medical background, use simpler terms such as, "We are going to take this child to ABC Hospital for some special x-rays."

Anxieties

Placing the child in the back of the ambulance causes a certain amount of fear, much of which is due to separation anxiety. Even if the child knows that someone familiar is going to ride in the front seat of the ambulance, there is a certain amount of anxiety about being all alone in the back.

The caregiver may have similar fears. Be aware that the family driving behind the ambulance or the family member sitting in the passenger seat may feel separation anxiety. When possible, reassure the patient and the caregiver during these anxious times. As previously discussed, practice family-centered care and allow the parent to ride in the patient compartment with his or her child. If current policy prohibits that option, lobby for a change in the policy to help with future situations.

Remember to use what is already known about treating pediatric patients in order to make them feel more at ease. For instance, infants and young toddlers should be held by their parents during your assessment whenever possible but NEVER during transport. Have the appropriate caregiver ride in the back compartment whenever possible to help decrease feelings of helplessness.

When assessing a school-aged patient, allow the child to touch some of the emergency medical services (EMS) equipment such as a stethoscope. While this action has a tendency to build a rapport with the patient and establish trust, it also builds rapport and decreases a certain amount of anxiety in the onlooking parent or caregiver.

Younger patients are also an age group in which anxiety in the patient and caregivers can be decreased simply by using familiar terms. When the patient is going to be physically separated from a family member, try to find some useful nicknames, phrases, or a special toy that may be unique between the two of them. This activity will help develop trust with the patient. The fact that a few extra minutes were taken to make this patient encounter a little more personal for "his or her child" will make the parent or caregiver less anxious about being separated from the child.

During a busy shift, it is the simple things that are most likely forgotten or overlooked. Imagine what one supportive statement would do for the patient. Imagine how hearing the prehospital provider express empathy would make the family feel.

As discussed above, if it would be beneficial for the child and the parent to be together, allow the parent to ride safely secured in the patient compartment. If the child is critically injured or ill, it may be more appropriate to have the parent ride in the front. Remember that each situation is different. Some parents are medically trained and may have had extensive experience caring for a child with a long-term or chronic condition. These parents may be the best resource even in the patient compartment. Be sure to work with the administrative team at the ambulance service to review the legal obligations before this situation arises.

Delivering Bad News

Delivering bad news to family members is one of the hardest tasks that a prehospital provider must do. If the child is found dead and treatment would be inappropriate, the family must be informed. If a resuscitation is attempted at the scene and then stopped, the focus changes to the grieving family.

The manner in which the news is delivered and the type of immediate support given will be remembered by the family for a long time. The family can be negatively affected from a psychological standpoint if caring and compassion are not used in this situation.

One difficulty for the provider is changing gears. During the resuscitation, prehospital providers are doing everything possible from a technical aspect to save the life of the child. They are concentrating on procedures and techniques and not on their feelings about the child in distress. Once the resuscitation ends, the providers now begin to experience their own feelings of loss and empathy for the family. They may become emotionally exhausted because their efforts were not successful, making it difficult to support and counsel the family.

The following tips were initially suggested by the American Heart Association at its conference in 1992 (American Heart Association, 1992). They are still valuable today and have been modified to apply to the pediatric patient.

1. **Designate a team leader.** Quickly decide who at the scene might be the most appropriate to deal with the death of a child.

2. **Collect information about the death.** Try to get as much information about the child, the family, and the circumstances surrounding the death. Review the events as they occurred, and document them on the written report. Include the child's medical history, the event (i.e., illness or injury), the relationship between the child and the people at the scene, and plans for disposition of the body. Per local protocol, involve law enforcement if there are any signs of a suspicious death.

3. **Locate a quiet area for discussion.** Move to an area away from the body and one that is safe from any hazards. Some family members may have an involuntary physical response such as walking, moving around, or banging fists against a wall in anger. Try to provide enough space for movement.

4. **Move to a position equal with the family.** Whenever possible, ask the family to sit down and sit down with them. Do not "tower" over the survivors when delivering bad news. If sitting is not possible, kneel down next to the parents, guardians, or primary caregivers if the parents are not at the scene.

5. **Use eye contact.** Look directly at the parents or guardians when speaking. Make some eye contact with other individuals in the room as appropriate.

6. **Use touch appropriately.** Some people do not like physical closeness even in times of emergency or emotional distress. If someone reaches out first or the individual is familiar, feel free to touch a hand, shoulder, or hug that person.

7. **Provide a brief summary of what happened.** Go over the events to make sure the family understands as much as possible about the death of their child. Allow as much time as necessary, and answer questions as much as possible. If there are extenuating factors about the death, involve law enforcement personnel as well.

8. **Use the actual words "death," "dead," or "has died."** Do not get caught up using other phrases such as "passed on," "moved to a better place," or "she is no longer with us." Be direct so that the family does not misunderstand anything.

9. **Be prepared for a reaction.** Family and friends may experience a variety of physical, mental, and behavioral reactions. If there were any conflicts in the family, it may be helpful to have a police officer available.

10. **Express your sympathy for the family.** It is not necessary to apologize for anything. "I'm sorry," may be interpreted to mean that something was done wrong which led to the child's death. Instead, say things like, "You have my (our) sin-

cerest sympathy," to convey your feelings. Many providers have cried with families when a child has died. Act in a manner that feels most comfortable and is appropriate for the circumstances.

11. **Find an immediate support person.** Do *not* leave a family member alone. Ask if there is a neighbor, close friend, someone from the local church, or other relative that can be called. If another call comes in, ask for support from the police department to stay with the family member until someone else is available.

12. **Allow the family to say goodbye.** Use the child's first name, and ask the family if they would like to say goodbye to him or her. In many instances, this activity helps the family realize that death has occurred. If there is still equipment in the child, let the family know before they view the body. Explain why it needs to stay in place.

13. **Review the plan for disposition of the body.** Let the family know what will happen next. Who will sign the death certificate? If the death is considered a coroner's case and needs legal intervention, let the family know. They will still need to make funeral arrangements and can work directly with law enforcement personnel. Know the policies and procedures for certification of death and disposition of the body before encountering a situation such as this one.

14. **Provide another opportunity for questions.** Ask again if the family has any additional questions. Provide simple answers as people in crisis may not be able to understand complicated information.

15. **DO NOT LIE!** Be honest at all times. This technique is critical in the event of a crime scene or when an autopsy is necessary. Tell the family that their child must be transported to the hospital or morgue for an autopsy to find out why he or she died. Explain that this information may prevent the same type of problems in other children.

16. **Provide information for follow-up.** Give the family a list of names that has been prepared ahead of time (e.g., social worker at the local hospital, (sudden infant death syndrome [SIDS]) support group, chaplain, or counselor). If time permits, offer to speak with the child's primary care physician to answer any questions.

UNIQUE SITUATIONS

Dealing with the emotions of parents and caregivers is never routine. Unique situations that may require a certain amount of finesse or nonroutine responses to identify responsible caregivers at a scene may include:

- *Certain religious beliefs.* Unfamiliar religious beliefs may not permit treatment of the child according to standard care practices (e.g., Jehovah's Witness in which the family does not want the child to receive blood or blood products).

- *Broken family scenarios or caregivers with personal agendas contrary to the child's well-being.* A child may be in the middle of a domestic dispute between his or her parents making it difficult to assess and treat the patient. A parent may be trying to harm or kill the child.

- *Caregivers under the influence of drugs or alcohol.* The child's caregiver may not be capable of making consent decisions for the treatment of the patient due to substance abuse.

These situations may require on-line consultation with a medical control physician or action of law enforcement personnel. In any event, the first priority still must be treatment of the patient according to what is standard for that particular illness or injury. Although attempting to control the emotions of caregivers in these situations may be difficult, always act in the best interest of the patient AND personal safety.

SUMMARY

Dealing with caregivers and parents of pediatric patients is an ongoing process. As the prehospital provider deals with the patient, consider the wide array of caregivers associated with that child. Those caregivers can have formal, informal, or emotional ties to the child. Each one of these subsets of caregivers has certain needs as treatment of the child progresses. Through ongoing questioning at the scene, identify an appropriate caregiver to provide patient information and support.

Parents and caregivers may have the same anxieties as the children being treated. The same things that

Exploring the Web

- Search the Web for information on death and grief. What information can you find that will enable you to better support the grieving family? What information can you find that will help you to cope with the loss of a patient?

make the patient comfortable with the prehospital provider will make the parents comfortable with what is being done to their child.

Be prepared to deliver bad news in the event of the death of a child. Review the techniques necessary, and develop guidelines before being faced with this type of encounter.

Some situations with caregivers are unique enough to require assistance from law enforcement personnel, medical control, or other appropriate support agencies such as regional children's agencies and health departments. In these events, maintain personal safety, protect the patient from further harm, and treat according to standard care procedures.

Management of Case Scenario

Your first priority is to immobilize the patient and perform a physical examination. Once you have ruled out any life-threatening injuries, complete the remainder of the examination.

You will need to intervene and advise the patient that her parents are the only individuals that can consent to her treatment and therefore, somehow, must accompany her, at least, to the hospital. In situations like these, you may have to intervene as a referee and help the patient determine an appropriate individual to accompany him or her during treatment and transport.

If the situation becomes volatile, request the assistance of law enforcement personnel. You may need to separate the patient from the boyfriend and family members arguing over her. The priority is to get the patient safely to the hospital for definite treatment. The police officers can address the other individuals.

▶ REVIEW QUESTIONS

1. Define the following terms:
   a. Advocacy
   b. Empowerment
   c. Enable
   d. Family-centered care
   e. Parent-professional partnership

2. List the two major components to family-centered care.

3. Parents have the right to be part of the decision-making process for their child. True or False?

4. To promote family-centered care, the prehospital provider should do all of the following except:
   a. Allow a family member to actively participate in the resuscitation whenever possible
   b. Take extra time to answer the family's questions
   c. Allow family members under the influence of drugs or alcohol to ride in the patient compartment
   d. None of the above

5. The family is the constant in the child's life. True or False?

6. The following is not an example of caregiver relationships.
   a. Formal
   b. Semiformal
   c. Informal
   d. Emotional

7. Who is a reliable informant?

8. Describe several instances in which other caregivers can "help" at the scene.

9. It is appropriate for a family member to hold an ill child in the back of the ambulance during transport to provide emotional support. True or False?

10. List three techniques to be followed when delivering bad news.

11. Broken family scenarios or caregivers with personal agendas contrary to the child's well-being should be involved in the child's care whenever possible. True or False?

▶ REFERENCES

American Heart Association. (1992). *National American Heart Association Conference*.

The Institute for Family-Centered Care Web site, www.familycenteredcare.org 4/6/00.

Wallace, H., Biehl, R., MacQueen, J., & Blackman, J. (1997). *Mosby's Resource Guide to Children with Disabilities and Chronic Illness*. St. Louis, MO: Mosby-Year Book.

Wong, D. (1999). *Whaley & Wong's nursing care of infants and children* (6th ed. St.). Louis, MO: Mosby-Year Book.

BIBLIOGRAPHY

Dunst, C., & Trivette, C. (1996). Empowerment, effective helpgiving practices and family-centered care. *Pediatric Nursing, 22*(4), 334–337.

Heller, R., & McKlindon, D. (1996). Families as "Faculty": Parents educating caregivers about family-centered care. *Pediatric Nursing, 22*(5), 428–431.

Vessey, J., & Jackson, P. (1996). *Primary care of the child with a chronic condition*. St. Louis, MO: Mosby-Year Book.

Wertz, E. (2001). Pediatric emergencies. In B. Shade, M. Rothenberg, E. Wertz, & S. Jones, (Eds.), *Mosby's EMT—intermediate textbook*. St. Louis, MO: Mosby-Year Book.

Collaboration with Other Health Care Professionals and Programs

OBJECTIVES

Upon completion of this chapter, the student will be able to:

● Identify health care professionals with whom prehospital personnel would collaborate on pediatric-related issues.

● Discuss the importance of multidisciplinary collaboration.

● Describe activities that invite multidisciplinary collaboration.

● Compare and contrast primary, secondary, and tertiary levels of prevention.

● Describe how prehospital personnel can participate in prevention activities.

● Identify community resources related to pediatric prehospital care.

KEY TERMS

coalition
coalition building
primary prevention

secondary prevention
tertiary prevention

Case Scenario

Prehospital providers from the local emergency medical services (EMS) agency notice an increase in the number of trauma calls for children with head injuries. These head injuries occurred in the local park that has a paved bicycle pathway for residents to enjoy. The head injuries were often minor, but transport to the local Emergency Department was necessary. All of the children transported were not wearing bicycle helmets, were of school age (6 to 12 years), and were accompanied by parents who also rode without helmets. There is a mandatory helmet law in this state for children under the age of 12 years. The bicycle pathway is well maintained, but it is hilly and is parallel to automotive traffic. The falls from the bicycles occurred when children panicked or became frightened by speeding cars or when the pathway was crowded with faster riders.

Personnel from the EMS agency wondered if there was a way to promote safe bicycling in their community. What steps would be necessary to initiate a program and reduce these head injuries?

INTRODUCTION

Prehospital providers are in a unique position to participate in collaborative efforts with health care professionals, community organizations, and governmental agencies on pediatric-related health issues. EMS organizations are community based and serve as the first entry point to the health care system. Prehospital providers already collaborate with hospital-based (e.g., medical physicians) and community-based (e.g., school nurses) health care professionals to deliver care at the individual patient level. They experience first-hand the devastating effects of illness and injury on children and can provide insight into the consequences of unsafe or unhealthy situations to community-based organizations, such as child care centers. Finally, prehospital providers can share their perspectives on pediatric EMS-related issues with governmental agencies and legislators and advocate for children's health and safety.

While these efforts appear daunting, they are readily achievable. The purpose of this chapter is to discuss the importance of participation in and collaboration with health care professionals, community organizations, and governmental agencies. Suggestions for how to get started in this process are outlined.

COLLABORATION WITH INDIVIDUAL HEALTH CARE PROFESSIONALS

Every day, prehospital providers collaborate with other health care professionals as they deliver patient care within their communities. Together, prehospital personnel and health care professionals identify and modify illness and injury risks, provide care for acute illness and injury, and assist in the treatment of chronic conditions. These health care professionals also play important roles in EMS education, system planning, evaluation, research, and/or provision of patient care (U.S. Department of Transportation, National Highway Traffic Safety Administration, 1996). Prehospital providers deliver care as part of, or in combination with, systematic approaches intended to improve the health care for their community. Table 15-1 lists health care professionals with whom prehospital providers would collaborate on a routine basis.

Collaboration with health care professionals promotes a seamless continuity of patient care. For example, children with special health care needs may attend the local elementary school (see Chapter 7—Children with Special Health Care Needs, and Chapter 8—Children with Special Health Care Needs Assisted by Technology). The school nurse, parents, physician, and prehospital providers should collaborate on a plan to treat the child should an emergency arise during school hours. Because parents know their children best, their suggestions are invaluable when creating such a plan.

Prehospital providers can enhance collaboration with other health care professionals by:

- Inviting school nurses, aides, home health nurses, and other community health professionals to their agency for a tour and description of the services they provide

- Inviting these professionals to an educational session on pediatric EMS

- Providing cardiopulmonary resuscitation training (CPR) or other continuing education to these health care providers

- Meeting with school nurses, principals, emergency physicians, and others to provide plans for emergency responses to the school setting

- Working with school nurses to plan emergency treatment and evacuation of children with special health care needs

- Requesting inclusion in debriefing episodes in which children were involved

- Working with emergency physicians and nurses on pediatric equipment requirements

- Teaching in standardized courses, such as Pediatric Advanced Life Support (PALS), pediatric trauma courses, or Pediatric Education for Prehospital Providers (PEPP)
- Creating or participating in any activities that would promote multidisciplinary collaboration

TABLE 15-1
Health Care and Other Professionals Who Collaborate with Prehospital Providers

Physicians
    Emergency medicine
    Pediatrician
    Sports medicine
    Family practice
    Trauma surgeons

Nurses
    Emergency
    School health
    Home health
    Public health

Nurse practitioners/physician assistants

Social workers

Child life specialists

Therapists
    Respiratory
    Occupational
    Physical
    Speech/language

Other providers
    Baby-sitters
    Lifeguards
    Child care providers

Other professionals
    Veterinarians
    Dentists
    Public safety (police, fire, and animal control)

- Getting involved or organizing EMS Week activities. Materials for EMS Week are available free from the American College of Emergency Physicians. A theme is selected each year, and EMS providers can become involved in promoting this theme through collaboration with other health care professionals.

Prehospital providers are the experts in out-of-hospital emergency care, and this information can be shared with school and home care nurses. In exchange, these nurses have expertise in child development and treatment of childhood illness and injury. Educating one another is important, as each discipline has an overlapping yet different body of knowledge. Prehospital providers should be proactive and contact local schools or community nurses and health aides to offer planning and guidance before it is needed. Planning ahead benefits the children and averts potential obstacles and problems (Figure 15-1).

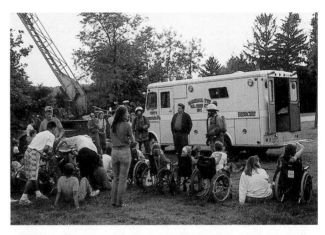

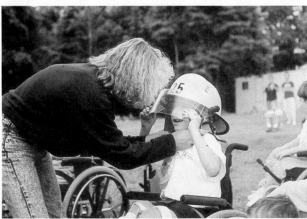

FIGURE 15-1 These prehospital providers demonstrate their equipment at a camp for children with spina bifida. Courtesy of Spina Bifida Association of Western Pennsylvania.

COLLABORATION WITH COMMUNITY AGENCIES

Prehospital providers maintain liaisons with public safety, social service, and other community agencies (U.S. Department of Transportation, National Highway Traffic Safety Administration, 1996). Table 15-2 describes community agencies and organizations with whom EMS providers would collaborate. Appendix D lists contact information of national organizations that may have branch chapters in the community. These agencies are known to promote children's health and safety and are potential partners with whom to collaborate.

Prehospital providers continue to expand their roles in public health by developing ongoing relationships with their community agencies. These providers are experts in knowing their community's emergency health and safety needs. For example, when responding

Exploring the Web

● Search the Web for kid-friendly agencies in your community. Make a list of the agencies that would be helpful in collaboration on pediatric health issues. Are there any programs in which you can get involved?

to an emergency call in the home setting, the scene is visually inspected for potential hazards. The home may have unsafe conditions, such as broken stairs, poor lighting, or other structural deficiencies. Poisons or matches may be readily available to young children. Traditionally, prehospital providers make note of these circumstances

---

TABLE 15-2
Community Agencies That Collaborate with Prehospital Providers

Youth groups
  Boys and Girls Clubs of America
  Boy Scouts and Girl Scouts of America

Religious-affiliated groups

Public safety agencies
  Police
  Fire

Child care centers

Medical explorers groups

Community organizations
  Kiwanis International
  Rotary International

Agencies for underserved populations
  Food banks
  Shelters
  Clinics

For-profit and not-for-profit health-related agencies
  American Cancer Society
  American Heart Association

American Red Cross
Epilepsy Foundation of America
National Safety Council
Safe Kids Coalition

Parent networks/helplines
  Parent-Teacher Associations/Organizations

Foster care/juvenile protective service agencies

Professional organizations
  American Academy of Pediatrics
  American College of Emergency Physicians
  American College of Surgeons
  Emergency Nurses Association
  National Association of EMS Educators
  National Association of EMS Physicians
  National Association of Emergency Medical
    Technicians
  National Association of Flight Paramedics
  National Flight Nurse Association
  National Registry of Emergency Medical
    Technicians

Tricks of the Trade

Among children ages 14 and under, 40 percent of deaths and 50 percent of nonfatal unintentional injuries occur in and around the home (Allen, 1997). These facts are why community-based prevention activities that involve various stakeholders are so important.

 Exploring the Web

● Search the Web for state and federal agencies that are promoting pediatric health issues. What type of programs exist? What type of programs could benefit from input from the EMS service?

and leave things as they are. In some communities, pre-hospital providers collaborate with community agencies in which they notify the agency of a family's needs, and assistance is offered. In this respect, prehospital providers give immediate care and play a significant role in preventing future injuries or illnesses.

Prehospital providers can initiate collaboration with community agencies by:

- Inviting community members to serve on the EMS agency's board of directors
- Inviting community organizations to the EMS agency to provide education on the organization's mission and purpose
- Contacting community organizations to set up potential pediatric health-related activities
- Joining a community agency
- Representing EMS on a community agency's board of directors

Community agencies are comprised of individuals that are members of that community—neighbors, friends, and family. These members use EMS agencies in their personal and professional lives. Prehospital providers should never miss out on an opportunity to represent emergency care or to collaborate on worthwhile projects that affect children's health!

COLLABORATION WITH GOVERNMENT AGENCIES

Prehospital providers already maintain liaisons with local and state health departments and other government agencies (U.S. Department of Transportation, National Highway Traffic Safety Administration, 1996). These governmental agencies generally have an understanding of the community's overall health. For example, EMS agencies may be required to submit their written reports to the state health department for analysis. These analyses should be available to the agency for its review. Such data can help prehospital providers in their collaboration with health care professionals, community organizations,

and government agencies to develop programs related to children's health and safety (Table 15-3).

Prehospital providers can collaborate with government agencies by:

- Inviting local legislators to the EMS agency for a tour and an education program on issues related to children's health

TABLE 15-3
Government Agencies That Collaborate with Prehospital Providers

Health departments
Local
State

National Safe Kids Coalition
Local level
State level
National level

Emergency Medical Services for Children (EMSC) Projects
Local
State
National

Other Agencies
Healthy Start grantees
Title V grantees
U.S. Consumer Product Safety Commission
U.S. Department of Transportation, National Highway Traffic Safety Administration
U.S. Maternal Child Health Bureau

- Sharing data with the local health department to develop prevention programs

- Inviting local and state EMS directors to the agency and sharing with them concerns and issues related to children's health

- Getting involved in the state's Emergency Medical Services for Children (EMSC) activities

- Working with the state EMS director to identify issues and solutions to pediatric health problems

- Serving on state-wide committees to advocate for children's health and safety

Government agencies are there to work for the community as well as the EMS agency! There is a lot of work to be done regarding children's health issues. By sharing resources, changes can be made to improve the health and well-being of children at the local level.

 Tricks of the Trade

Children in rural areas are more at risk for unintentional injury-related death as compared to urban areas because of the lack of organized trauma programs, prolonged response times, and decreased supply of medical personnel, equipment, and facilities for treatment. Collaborating with officials at the local and state levels, as well as hospital and community leaders, helps to focus on this issue and provides a basis for building the infrastructure needed for the proper care of children.

EMS PARTICIPATION IN PREVENTION ACTIVITIES

EMS agencies are active participants in prevention activities involving health care professionals, community organizations, and government agencies. While prevention is associated with an activity such as influenza immunization or smoke detector installation, prehospital providers contribute to pediatric injury and illness prevention in a number of ways.

There are three types of prevention activities. **Primary prevention** is an activity that prevents the development of an injury or disease among people who are well and are not ill or injured. **Secondary prevention** is an activity that identifies people who have an illness at an early stage in the illness' natural history during screening or early intervention (Gordis, 1996). **Tertiary prevention** is an activity that prevents complications

from an injury or illness. Tertiary prevention is what EMS providers employ when they initiate prehospital care, such as spinal immobilization to prevent the occurrence or worsening of a spinal cord injury. Table 15-4 lists examples of each prevention method.

Many EMS providers actively participate in prevention activities. For example, emergency medical technicians (EMTs) in New Mexico, through their state EMSC grant, educate children and families on injury prevention. These EMTs receive an eight-hour training session on how to become injury prevention advocates for children. From 1995 to 1997, 32 EMT Community Injury Prevention Projects were initiated by urban, nonurban, and Native American EMS systems. Included were programs on bicycle helmets, car seats, burn prevention, and playground safety (Stern, Olson, & Monahan, 1998).

In Rhode Island, EMS providers introduced Programa ALERTA, a pilot pediatric injury prevention program targeting Providence's Latino Community. Program components included church-based educational interventions, distribution of safety devices to participants, home safety visits, a concurrent Spanish language media campaign, and cultural sensitivity training for EMS providers (Gutman, Tyrrell, Smith, & Thompson, 1998).

In Pennsylvania, the Pennsylvania Chapter of the American Academy of Pediatrics used an EMSC grant to offer education to child care personnel. EMS providers were trained as evaluators and consultant/trainers. Child care sites were identified in two urban cities and one rural area of the state. Pre-education evaluations were done by the EMS team trained as evaluators. The EMS consultant/trainers then taught a first-aid training program to all of the child care providers at that site. Posteducation evaluations were done by additional EMS evaluators, and each child care site received a copy of *Risk Watch*™ to use for further training. Relationships were established with EMS providers in the child care centers' area so that future training, emergency preparation, and collaboration opportunities were enhanced.

Other activities include:

- Alameda County EMS conducted a project that demonstrated the efficacious and safe administration of immunizations to children (Pointer, Helander-Daugherty, & Kramm, 2000).

- Many EMS agencies sponsor a "Prom Promise" event, where a mock motor vehicle crash is enacted at the high school to illustrate the dangers of drinking and driving.

Finally, prehospital providers can collaborate with school health teachers to offer first aid and CPR training in the school setting through the Basic Emergency Life-Saving Skills (BELS) Framework (Maternal Child

TABLE 15-4
Examples of Prevention Activities

Level of Prevention	Description	Activity
Primary	Prevention of an injury or disease among people who are well and are not ill or injured	• Administering immunizations to children • Teaching children and parents how to use auto safety restraints • Teaching children and parents how to prevent burns, drownings, poisonings, and other childhood injuries • Teaching children and parents about the dangers of tobacco, drug, and alcohol use • Distributing bicycle helmets and instructing children and parents in their use • Assisting child care providers with fire safety, car seat use, playground safety, and other child-proofing activities • Collaborating with school officials on preparing for emergency responses • Teaching first aid and CPR classes to the community • Teaching safe babysitting training, lifeguard training, etc.
Secondary	Identification of people who have an illness at an early stage in the illness's natural history during screening or early intervention	• Conducting blood pressure, vision, height and weight, cholesterol, diabetes, and asthma screenings for children and adolescents • Conducting home safety audits • Conducting tobacco, drug, and alcohol cessation programs for adolescents • Assisting with criminal screening for child care providers • Assisting with mental health screening in adolescents • Identifying children at risk for abuse or neglect (e.g., immunization completion)
Tertiary	Prevention of complications from an injury or illness	• Initiating pediatric advanced life support interventions following a life-threatening illness • Initiating pediatric trauma life support interventions following a life-threatening injury

Health Bureau, 2000). This program is aimed at preparing school-aged children and adolescents to provide initial care during an emergency.

Prehospital providers can become involved in organizing and sponsoring childhood injury and illness prevention activities in their own communities by forming coalitions or alliances with child-friendly organizations. A **coalition** is a temporary alliance of distinct parties, persons, or states for joint action. **Coalition building** is "the ongoing process of cultivating and maintaining relationships with a diverse network of individuals

Exploring the Web

● Search the Web for prevention activities developed by EMS agencies in other states. Can you find programs that can serve as models for implementing programs in your state and local area?

and organizations who share a common set of principles and values" (Williams, 1997). Building relationships within the community is important to garner support and commitment for improving children's health and safety. These relationships will lead to an outcome-based coalition, in which the mutually developed project will have broad impact, long-term viability, and incomparable value (Williams, 1997). The benefits of outcome-based coalition building include (Williams, 1997):

- *Sharing of contacts and resources.* Building a relationship with one organization may prompt that organization to share its contacts with other community partners as well as its own resources. For example, an agency might share its mailing list with the EMS agency or EMS agency members to the local legislator. Another example is the owner of the sports equipment store who may be able to obtain bicycle helmets at a reduced cost for the EMS agency to distribute to the community during a bicycle rodeo.

- *Developing new products.* Organizations may help with developing new or improving upon existing products for distribution. These may include training curricula for child care providers or special reports to legislators.

- *Providing monetary and personnel resources.* Sharing costs is important when developing and marketing community programs. Financial costs may be offset by grants from local businesses or the health department. Personnel resources can be found in volunteers, such as nurses, retirees, or high school and college students who are willing to donate their time and energy in support of the project. Many middle and senior high schools have medical explorers clubs, in which students work with health-related agencies. An EMS agency could either sponsor or participate in these clubs, thereby involving students in the slated activities.

- *Establishing a policy agenda.* "Grassroots public policy is the process of local, state and national voters advocating for causes they believe will benefit their community" (Benson, 1997). Members of the coalition may have experience as child advocates and may offer advice on how to work with the local political system to affect changes in children's health and safety. Prehospital providers should make a concerted effort to know the local legislators by:
  - Inviting them to activities sponsored by the EMS agency
  - Submitting to the legislators recommended wording changes for bills to be introduced

- Establishing ties with the state health department, state EMS director, state EMS medical director, and governor's office
- Developing a legislative task force within the coalition (Benson, 1997)

Getting Started in Children's Health-Related Activities

Building relationships and coalitions within the community is the first step in enacting projects that affect children's health and safety. Suggestions for developing and implementing such projects are discussed below.

Identify Needs

Identify a health or safety need in the community. Review trip reports and talk with colleagues. Does there seem to be an increasing number of playground injuries at a certain school? Has the number of fire calls increased in the past year? Do there seem to be an increased number of improperly-restrained children injured in motor vehicle crashes? Discuss these findings with EMS colleagues. Do they agree that a need exists for safety education in one topic area (e.g., burn prevention, car safety, or playground safety) among community members? If so, follow up with the manager of the EMS agency, who may want to contact the state EMS agency or local health department to corroborate these findings.

Make Contacts

Contact community agencies that are interested in children's health, as listed in Appendix D. Search the Internet, go to the local library, or look in the telephone book under community resources to see if the community has local chapters of these organizations. If the community has a Safe Kids Coalition (the local health department is usually the lead or sponsoring agency), contact this group. They will have ideas for how to proceed to initiate targeted safety education in the community. For

 Tricks of the Trade

Unintentional injuries affect poor children more and result in more fatalities than in children with greater economic resources. For this reason, knowing one's community, its people, and its resources is important for targeting prevention and health-related activities.

example, many coalitions have trained car seat inspectors who can inspect car seats for damage and proper installation. Find out if the coalition is interested in working with the EMS agency in cosponsoring, with a car dealership, a car seat safety check event.

Another resource is the local health department. Health department officials are usually eager to work with the community to prevent illness and injury. They can supply excellent written materials, at no or minimal cost, for community-wide distribution. State representatives or senators may distribute health-related literature from their offices and may be contacted for copies of their pediatric health-related literature, which would be free of charge and carry the legislator's name and address.

Determine Your Approach

Identify the type of activity that would best meet the identified health need. Coalition members can help determine the best activity and then help with the planning and co-sponsoring. For example, the EMS agency may be stationed at the community's annual Fourth of July holiday celebration. While the ambulance is on-site for emergency care, the EMS crew can have literature available at the ambulance for summer safety, such as water safety, playground safety, pet safety, burn, and personal safety. The EMS crew can work with other community co-sponsors on additional activities for that day.

Another example is when the EMS agency co-sponsors a community day, in which various community agencies come together to share information about their services. During this time, the EMS agency and other community volunteers focus time on specific educational needs.

The EMS agency can also conduct home safety audits. Coalition members may want to join in these audits; or they may supply equipment, such as smoke detectors, flashlights, etc.

The range of activities that the EMS agency and the coalition undertake is as involved as the EMS agency wants it to be—from distribution of materials to teaching CPR classes to new parents. The coalition can decide where to conduct the event—at the EMS base, a church, a community recreation center, a school, etc. Many McDonald's restaurants employ an activities coordinator who is eager to work with the community to promote children's health. For any event, the most accessible location is selected to enhance attendance. Any activity, though, requires funding, which is the next step.

Acquiring Funding

Work with the coalition to secure financial assistance for the project. EMS agencies, as well as most community agencies, are not wealthy organizations. However, with each organization contributing resources, the financial burden is borne by all, making the activity more likely to be implemented.

Develop a budget to include every conceivable cost. Justify the costs. While funding agencies may pay for safety devices, such as gun trigger locks, they may not pay for overhead or salaries. The coalition members can then work together to find ways to meet these expenses.

A local hospital or trauma center may want to be involved. Many trauma centers are required to have outreach and prevention activities as part of their mission. The EMS manager can meet with the director of the Emergency Department, the trauma director, or another administrator to explain the program and to ask again for cosponsorship.

Other community agencies, such as local grocery store chains, pharmacies, health insurance plans, or organizations such as the Kiwanis may provide small grant awards to help with the project.

Building community partnerships and being good neighbors are crucial for EMS. Cosponsorships should be entertained and welcomed.

Promotion

Develop a media campaign to promote the activity. EMS agencies generally do not employ advertising agencies to market their organizations, but there are community organizations within the coalition who do have such resources available to them. Some simple, low cost strategies to consider include (Wise, 1997):

- Go to the local public library and review a copy of *The Gebbie Press All-in-One Directory* or the *News Media Yellow Pages*. These publications list all print and broadcast media by state and local areas. The library may have additional media resources to peruse.

- Contact the media in advance; don't wait until an issue arises or the day of the event to request media coverage. Instead, be proactive. Invite a reporter to the EMS agency to discuss children's safety issues. Supply the reporter with information about the EMS agency as well as the coalition.

- Advertise in all of the community's free and paid newspapers. Write a letter to the editor about the coalition or write a brief article about the coalition and its upcoming event.

- Have a local newspaper reporter come to the EMS agency to write an article about the upcoming event. This action will save advertising dollars, although advertising in the local newspaper is valuable as well.

- Write public service announcements (PSAs) for radio and television broadcast. Coalition members may have advertising or media personnel that could help with the writing and production of these advertisements.

- Invite a radio station to broadcast live from the event. This option should be explored as well.

Implementation and Evaluation

Hold the event and evaluate the outcome. While this is an event targeted for children's safety, there should be activities for both children and adults. Children's activities should include quiet and active play, such as a short video on burn safety followed by everyone practicing stop, drop, and roll. Teaching older children and parents CPR together also is a possibility.

Parent teaching includes active and passive learning, as well as the distribution of safety devices and literature.

After the event, write a brief summary of the day's activities. Describe the event and list its cosponsors. Include the number of people who attended, the approximate number of safety devices and/or literature distributed, and a general rating of the program's success. Decide how to do things differently for the next event.

Finally, review the trip reports in the coming months to see if the intervention had any impact at all on the targeted injury. Do not be discouraged if no changes are immediately noted. It takes time to change people's behaviors.

Be sure to write thank-you letters to the coalition and EMS colleagues for a job well done! Then, be ready to plan the next event!

 Tricks of the Trade

Children ages 4 and under are at greater risk of unintentional injury-related death and disability and account for almost half of the deaths under age 14. Including activities for parents to keep young children safe, as well as activities that parents and all children can participate in together, helps to get prevention education where it is needed most.

SUMMARY

Prehospital providers must collaborate with health care professionals, community organizations, and government agencies to optimize health in children and their families. Collaborating with health care professionals impacts on the health of individuals, while collaborating with community and government agencies impacts on the overall health of the community. Delivery of care through primary, secondary, and tertiary prevention improves the health of the community.

Prehospital providers must continue to expand their role into public health opportunities by developing ongoing relationships with community and government agencies. Participating in health-promotion activities, such as education and screening, reinforces EMS's role as a provider of community health. Through these endeavors, the health and safety of the community's children will be enhanced.

Management of Case Scenario

The EMS agency meets with the local police department, who report that a substantial number of traffic tickets are written for speeding drivers in this area. The police talk to parents about obeying the helmet law; but because the fine amounts to more money than buying a helmet, the officers are reluctant to penalize the parents.

The EMS agency and police agree to form a coalition with the local Safe Kids Coalition, local bicycle shop, local bicycling group, and local legislators to sponsor a bicycle rodeo at the park for children and families. They select a weekend, because this is a busy time for cyclists. The legislators' office contacts the media. The funds for the helmets and rodeo are secured through the police, EMS, bicycle shop, Safe Kids Coalition, and the local bicycling club. Together, they sponsor a rodeo, give away helmets, provide education on safe bicycling, and teach about safe driving in this area. Media coverage helped to gain attention to the event. A local grocery chain donated cold drinks for the participants, and the local trauma center and health department donated educational materials. Approximately 100 families attended the event.

The coalition was pleased with its work. All agencies received excellent media coverage and visibility to the parents and children. In addition, all agencies were able to promote themselves at the event. The local legislators were able to meet with their constituents. In the ensuing weeks, the police notice a decline in the number of speeding drivers and an increase in the number of helmets worn by the children. The EMS agency noted a slight decrease in the number of children transported for head injuries following bicycle crashes in this area. Together, over time, EMS agencies can make a difference in promoting the health and well-being of children in their communities.

REVIEW QUESTIONS

1. An EMS agency decides to offer CPR classes to children and their families. This action is an example of:

   a. Primary prevention

   b. Secondary prevention

   c. Tertiary prevention

   d. Quaternary prevention

2. All of the following are acceptable methods for identifying a health need in the community EXCEPT:

   a. Reviewing trip sheets

   b. Contacting local health department officials

   c. Asking members of a different community

   d. Meeting with other health care professionals

3. The first step in preparing a community-based health-related program is to:

   a. Contact the media

   b. Identify a health or safety need in the community

   c. Purchase items to give away, such as smoke detectors

   d. Post flyers at the local grocery stores

4. All of the following are benefits of coalition building EXCEPT:

   a. Sharing of contacts and resources

   b. Developing new products

   c. Having wealthy agencies pay for all of the costs

   d. Establishing a policy agenda

5. Which is an example of a government agency?

   a. The National Highway Traffic and Safety Administration

   b. An HMO

   c. The March of Dimes

   d. The American Heart Association

6. Give an example of a primary prevention activity. How would an EMS agency go about planning for such an activity?

7. Describe the importance of including local and state legislators in any community activity. How would such legislators be contacted and encouraged to participate?

8. Identify key individuals who provide health care to children in the community setting. How would an EMS agency initiate contact with these individuals to participate in planning and evaluating emergency care?

REFERENCES

*Allen, K. (1997). *Preventing childhood emergencies: A guide to developing effective injury prevention initiatives.* Washington, DC: Emergency Medical Services for Children National Resource Center.

*Benson, P. (1997). *EMSC's role in shaping policy: A practical guide to changing minds and saving lives.* Washington, DC: Emergency Medical Services for Children National Resource Center.

Gordis, L. (1996). *Epidemiology.* Philadelphia, PA: W.B. Saunders.

Gutman, D., Tyrrell, E., Smith, R. & Thompson, L. (1998). A church-based Spanish language intervention. *1998 National Congress on Childhood Emergencies.* Washington, DC: Emergency Medical Services for Children Project.

Maternal Child Health Bureau. (2000). *Basic emergency life-saving skills: The BELS Framework.* Washington, DC: Maternal Child Health Bureau.

Pointer, J., Helander-Daugherty, K., & Kramm, P. (2000). "Paramedics' administration of childhood immunizations: A first in California." Poster presentation. *National Association of EMS Physicians Annual Meeting,* Dana Point, CA, January 6–8, 2000.

Stern, A., Olson, L., & Monahan, C. (1998). Emergency medical technicians: Community advocates for injury prevention. *1998 National Congress on Childhood Emergencies.* Washington, DC: Emergency Medical Services for Children Project.

U.S. Department of Transportation, National Highway Traffic Safety Administration. (1996). *Emergency medical services agenda for the future.* Washington, DC: U.S. Department of Transportation, National Highway Traffic Safety Administration. DOT HS 808 441.

*Williams, K. (1997). *Reaching out: A guide to effective coalition building.* Washington, DC: Emergency Medical Services for Children National Resource Center.

*Wise, J. (1997). *Pounding the pavement: Getting the media to work for you.* Washington, DC: Emergency Medical Services for Children National Resource Center.

*Available at no charge from EMSC National Resource Center, 111 Michigan Avenue, NW, Washington, DC 20010. Phone: (202) 884-4927; fax: (301) 650-8045; email: info@emscnrc.com.

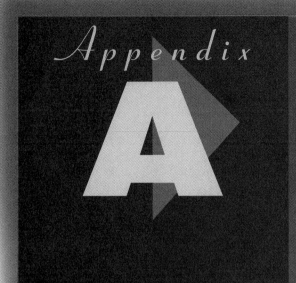

Appendix A
Commonly Used Pediatric Medications

Drug	Dose	Route/Comments
Activated charcoal	• Less than 1 year: 1–2 g/kg • Greater than 1 year: 25–50 g	NG tube or PO
Adenosine (Adenocard®)	• 0.1 mg/kg up to max of 12 mg • Give another 0.2 mg/kg if first dose not effective	Rapid IV/IO push Rapid flush to central circulation Monitor EKG during administration
Albuterol 0.5% (5 mg/mL solution for inhalation)	• <15 kg: 2.5–5.0 mg diluted in 3 mL of normal saline, nebulized • >15 kg: 5–10 mg diluted in 3 mL of normal saline; nebulized • May be repeated every 20 minutes × 3 doses or used continuously in critically ill patients	Aerosol inhalation
Amiodarone For pulseless VF/VT For perfusing tachycardias	• 5 mg/kg • Loading dose to 5 mg/kg	IV/IO via rapid bolus IV over 20 to 60 minutes
Atropine sulfate	• 0.02 mg/kg • minimum dose: 0.1 mg • maximum single dose: child—0.5 mg adolescents—1.0 mg may repeat once	IV, IO, or ET May cause tachycardia and pupil dilation
Benadryl	1 mg/kg up to max of 50 mg	IV, IO, or IM

(continues)

Drug	Dose	Route/Comments
Calcium Chloride 10% = 100 mg/mL	• 20 mg/kg up to max of 500 mg (0.2 mL/kg)	IV or IO slowly, preferably via central line Monitor EKG; may see bradycardia
Dextrose (25%) Newborn (10%) Child (25%) Adolescent (50%)	• 0.5–1.0 g/kg • 1–2 mL/kg • 2–4 mL/kg • 5–10 mL/kg	IV or IO slowly
Epinephrine *Note:* 1:10,000 = 0.1 mg/mL 1:1,000 = 1 mg/mL *Note:* Doses as high as 0.2 mg/kg of 1:1,000 may be effective.	• First dose: 0.01 mg/kg of 1:10,000 solution • Second dose: 0.1 mg/kg of 1:1,000 solution, repeat every 3–5 minutes • First dose: 0.1 mg/kg of 1:1,000 solution • Second dose: 0.1 mg/kg of 1:1,000 solution, repeat every 3–5 minutes • 0.01 mg/kg; may repeat every 20 minutes × 3 doses up to max dose of 0.3 mg for management of wheezing • 3–5 mg (3–5 mL) of 1:1,000 nebulized	IV or IO ET dose SQ Aerosol inhalation
Racemic epinephrine (2.25% solution for inhalation)	• 11.25 mg (0.5 mL) in 3 cc NS (for croup)	Aerosol inhalation
Glucagon	• If less than 10 kg: 0.1 mg/kg up to max of 1 mg • If greater than 10 kg: 1.0 mg/kg	IM, IV, or SQ
Furesomide (Lasix®)	• 1 mg/kg up to max of 40 mg	IV or IO
Xylocaine (Lidocaine®)	• 1 mg/kg	IV or IO rapid bolus
Midazolam (Versed®)	• 0.1 mg/kg	IM
Naloxone (Narcan®)	• 0.1 mg/kg	IV, IO, or ET
Sodium bicarbonate (8.4%) newborn (4.2%)	• 1 mEq/kg • 2 mEq/kg	IV or IO IV or IO slowly
Diazepam (Valium®)	• 0.1–0.3 mg/kg up to max of 5 mg • 0.5 mg/kg initial dose • 0.25 mg/kg for subsequent doses	IV or IO at maximum rate of 1 mg/min pushed over 5 minutes Rectal

American Heart Association (2000). Guidelines 2000 for cardiopulmonary resuscitation and emergency cardiovascular care. *Journal of the American Heart Association, 102*(8). I-307-319.

Abbreviations: ET, endotracheally; IM, intramuscularly; IO, intraosseous; IV, intravenously; NS, normal saline; SQ, subcutaneously.

NOTE: When giving medication via the ET tube, dilute medication with normal saline to produce a volume of 3–5 mL. Provide several positive pressure ventilations after medication administration.

Appendix B

Pediatric Skills Review

Note: It is assumed that all providers will wear protective equipment when performing these techniques. Gloves will be worn for every technique, and eye goggles and possibly a mask will be used for airway skills.

ASSESSMENT

Purpose

Assessment of the pediatric patient requires a different approach than when assessing adult patients.

Procedure

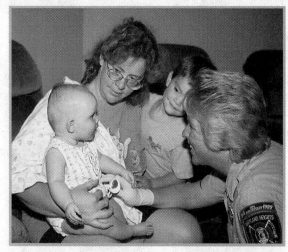

1. Infant patients should be assessed while being held by a parent or other familiar adult when possible.

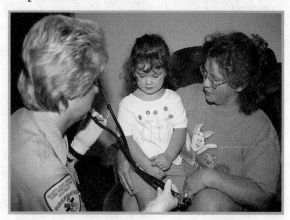

2. Toddler to preschool patients will need a familiar adult's reassurance and will need you to create a rapport with them. Talking to the patient at HIS or HER eye level is important.

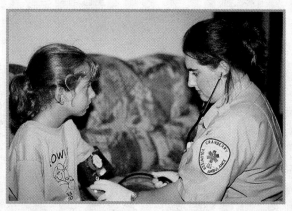

3. Elementary school-aged patients will need to relate to something "cool" or "neat" when time and patient condition permits.

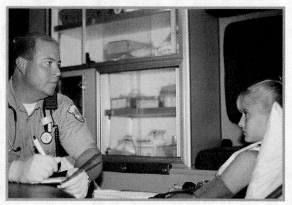

4. Preteen patients should be treated similarly to adults. Communicate in "real words," speak truthfully, and maintain patient privacy as much as possible.

BAG-VALVE-MASK VENTILATION

Purpose

Bag-valve-mask (BVM) ventilation is a critical skill when dealing with a pediatric patient in respiratory distress or failure. The key to performing this skill is to achieve an adequate seal on the child's face by using the appropriate equipment including a well-fitted mask and proper ventilation technique by the provider.

Procedure

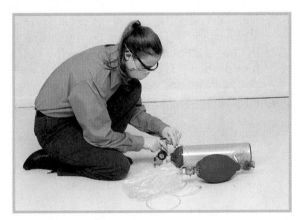

1. Assemble the following equipment: gloves (latex free whenever possible), a BVM device (at least 450 cc of volume), various pediatric oral airways, suction device with catheters, and an oxygen source.

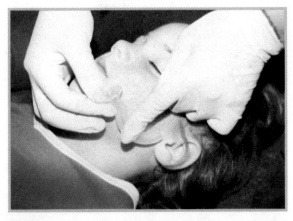

2. After determining that the child's ventilations need assistance, measure her for an oral airway. The airway should be from the corner of the mouth to the tip of the ear. Place the airway in the child's mouth. Make sure the airway is not too large for the child's mouth as it may cause injury or airway obstruction.

Note: NEVER insert an oral airway into any patient who is conscious or has a gag reflex present. A nasopharyngeal airway should be used for the patient with an active gag reflex or a child less than one year of age.

In addition, if the child has sustained facial trauma, using an oral or nasal airway can cause further injury as it may protrude into the brain. In that instance, use extreme caution or do not use the airway at all.

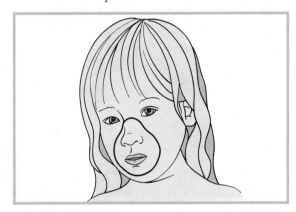

3. Select the proper size mask for the child. The mask should be transparent so that the provider can see the child's lips as well as note any emesis or fluids in or around the mouth. The mask should fit from the cleft in the chin to the bridge of the child's nose.

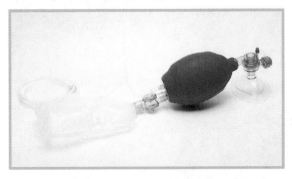

4. Select the proper resuscitation bag based on the size of the infant or child. A large bag is not appropriate for a small child and vice versa. The pediatric bag should be 450 to 750 cc while

an adult bag (1200 cc) can be used for adolescents and larger children. Some emergency services still use bags with a pop-off valve. If it is present, block the valve by holding one finger over it or *securely* taping it closed.

5. If trauma is suspected, maintain neutral, in-line stabilization of the head and neck and insert the oral airway using a jaw thrust maneuver. If no trauma is suspected, use the head-tilt/chin-lift maneuver to insert the airway. Even when trauma is not involved, do not hyperextend the neck as this action may cause airway obstruction.

6. Attach the BVM to an oxygen source and adjust the oxygen so that it flows at 15 liters/minute.

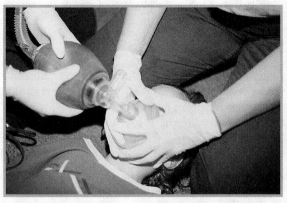

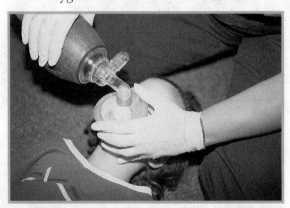

7. If only one rescuer is available, place the mask on the child's face. Obtain an airtight seal by using the C-clamp method. Do not push the mask into the face. Instead, pull the child's jaw into the mask without placing undue pressure on the soft tissue under the chin. Compress the bag with the dominant hand until the chest begins to rise.

8. If two rescuers are available, the first person holds the mask onto the face with two hands while keeping the airway open (as described above in no. 5). The second person compresses the bag with both hands. This method is preferred when it is difficult to get a good seal on the face with one person ventilating.

9. Observe the child for signs of gastric distention. If the transport will be long and endotracheal intubation is not available or has been unsuccessful, consider inserting an orogastric or nasogastric tube to decompress the stomach while continuing BVM ventilations.

ENDOTRACHEAL INTUBATION

Purpose

Endotracheal intubation is an optimal way to secure an airway yet may be complicated in the pediatric patient (as described in Chapter 4, Respiratory Emergencies). It provides a direct route to the lungs, an avenue for medication administration, and a way to decrease aspiration.

Procedure

Assemble the following equipment: gloves (latex free whenever possible), a BVM device (at least 450 cc of volume), various pediatric endotracheal tubes, pediatric laryngoscope with assorted blades, 10-cc syringe (if cuff on tube), a stylet (for older children), suction device with catheters, and an oxygen source. If a commercial carbon dioxide detector is available, plan to use it.

Select the appropriate size endotracheal tube. If using a tube size 6 mm or greater, inflate the cuff by using the 10-cc syringe filled with air. Make sure no leaks are present. Deflate the cuff, and leave the syringe attached. If a stylet will be used, insert it into the tube; and mold the tube into a "j" or "hockey stick" position.

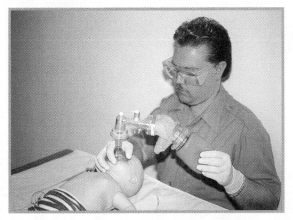

1. Select the laryngoscope and appropriate size blade. Assemble the equipment to ensure that the light is functioning on the blade.

   Position the child in the "sniffing" position as long as no trauma is suspected. If spinal immobilization is necessary, the second provider must maintain manual, in-line stabilization throughout the intubation attempt. Hyperventilate the child with the BVM before any attempts are made at intubation. Remove oropharyngeal airway if present.

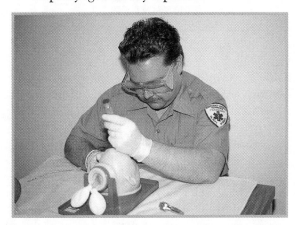

2. With the left hand, insert the laryngoscope blade into the mouth, sweeping the tongue to the left. If you are using a straight (Miller) blade, slide the blade along the tongue and lift the epiglottis out of the way. If you are using a curved blade (MacIntosh), slide the end of the blade into the vallecula, the space before the epiglottis. Lift the laryngoscope away from the child at a 45° angle, being careful not to use the child's teeth or gums as a fulcrum.

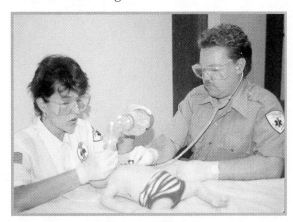

3. Once the larynx is visualized, insert the endotracheal tube through the cords. If in 15 seconds you are not able to see the cords, withdraw the laryngoscope and ventilate the child with the BVM.

Remove the laryngoscope from the child's mouth. Remove the mask from the BVM, and attach the end of the BVM device to the endotracheal tube. Hold the endotracheal tube in place until it is secured.

While the second provider ventilates, listen for breath sounds across the anterior chest and along the midaxillary line on each side. Listen over the abdomen for gastric sounds or gurgling.

Note: The provider who inserted the tube is responsible for verifying placement. If you put in the tube, make sure YOU listen for adequate breath sounds!

Signs of proper placement include: rise of chest on both sides, condensation in the tube, increase in heart rate (if the child was bradycardic), improvement in skin color (if the child was cyanotic), and improvement in the pulse oximetry reading.

If no breath sounds are heard or if distinct sounds are heard over the epigastrium (e.g., gurgling or a bubbling sound), remove the tube.

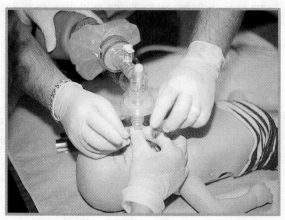

4. If using a tube size greater than 6 mm, inflate the cuff and then secure the tube using tape or a commercial device. Note the cm marking on the tube when wrapping the tape around it. Document this number in the written report.

Reassess the child periodically and after ANY movement. Be extremely careful to protect the tube when transferring the child to the stretcher, to the ambulance, or in the Emergency Department.

ASSISTING VENTILATIONS THROUGH A TRACHEOSTOMY TUBE

Purpose

Infants and children with tracheostomies may need suctioning if secretions or respiratory distress are present.

Procedure

Assemble the following equipment: gloves (latex-free whenever possible), a BVM device, and an oxygen source. Disconnect the mask from the BVM device. Make sure the reservoir bag is in place and that the device is connected to an oxygen source. Turn on the oxygen at 15 liters/minute and allow the reservoir bag to fill.

If an oxygen mask is present around the tracheostomy tube, remove it. If the child is on a ventilator, disconnect the ventilator tubing from the tracheostomy tube. Ask the parent or other caregiver to silence the alarm on the machine when it sounds.

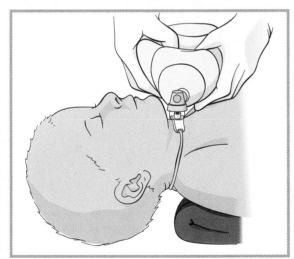

1. Connect the bag-valve device to the tracheostomy tube. If preparing for suction, hyperventilate the child for about 30 seconds.

If only assisting, give one ventilation every three to five seconds, depending on the size of the child. If the child is attempting to breathe, time your ventilations with the child's attempts. Use caution not to place undue pressure on the tracheostomy tube. In addition, try not to move the tube around too much so that you do not cause trauma to the stoma (opening) in the child's neck.

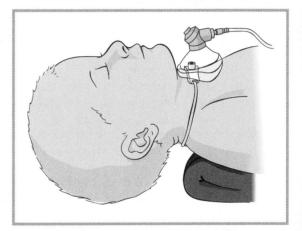

2. When finished, replace the oxygen mask or the ventilator tubing.

SUCTIONING A TRACHEOSTOMY TUBE

Purpose

There may be occasions in which the prehospital provider must suction a tracheostomy tube in an infant or child. If an obstruction is present, spontaneous respirations will be absent. In addition, it may be difficult or impossible to ventilate the child with a bag-valve device.

Procedure

Assemble the following equipment: a 3 or 5 cc syringe with normal saline (or commercial product filled with saline), a BVM device, a suction catheter, a suction device, and an oxygen source.

Consider a preassembled tracheostomy kit for quick access in an emergency situation if a child with a tracheostomy resides in the ambulance service area. Make sure various sizes of suction catheters are available to accommodate different sizes of tracheostomy tubes.

Disconnect the mask from the BVM device. Make sure the reservoir bag is in place and that the device is connected to an oxygen source. Turn on the oxygen at 15 liters/minute and allow the reservoir bag to fill.

Disconnect the ventilator. Ask the parent or other caregiver to silence the alarm on the machine when it sounds.

If secretions are thick, instill up to 1 cc of normal saline into the tracheostomy tube. Attempt to ventilate the tube with a bag-valve device to help loosen the secretions.

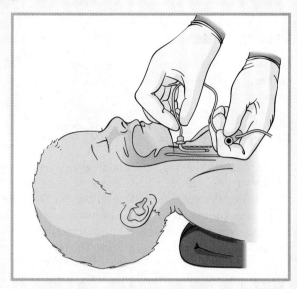

1. Insert the suction catheter into the tracheostomy tube WITHOUT using any suction. If you meet any resistance, do NOT force the catheter.

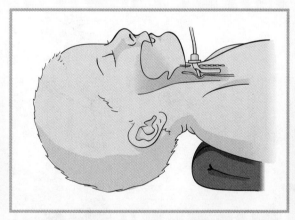

2. If the tracheostomy tube is fenestrated (has a hole in it), be careful that the suction catheter does not go through the hole into the tissue along the trachea. Pull back on the catheter and try again.

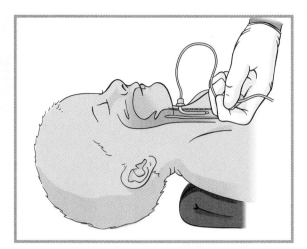 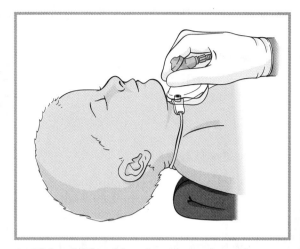

3. Cover the suction port, and slowly remove the catheter from the tube. Do not take more than ten seconds so that the child does not become hypoxic (or anoxic if there is a true obstruction). When using a portable suction machine, do not exceed 100 mm of pressure.

4. If the child is able to breathe on his or her own, provide blow-by oxygen at 10 liters/minute. If the child is on a ventilator, reconnect the ventilator and let the child breathe for about one minute. If the child was hypoxic for a period of time, connect the bag-valve device to the tracheostomy tube and hyperventilate with 100 percent oxygen (15 liters/minute).

CHANGING A TRACHEOSTOMY TUBE

Purpose

If the tracheostomy tube is obstructed or there are thick secretions, it may be necessary to change the tube.

Procedure

Assemble the following equipment: new tracheostomy tube, gloves (latex free whenever possible), BVM device, a 5 cc syringe, a vial of normal saline, cloth ties or another commercial device to secure the tube, a water-soluble lubricant, a suction catheter, a suction device, and an oxygen source.

Disconnect the mask from the bag-valve-mask device. Make sure the reservoir bag is in place and that the device is connected to an oxygen source. Turn on the oxygen at 15 liters/minute, and allow the reservoir bag to fill.

1. If present, inflate the cuff on the new tracheostomy tube to make sure it is adequate. Check for leaks in the cuff, and then deflate the cuff. Make sure the obturator is inside the tube.

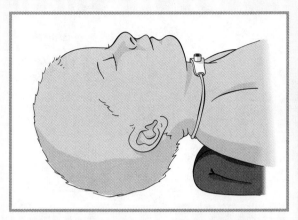

2. As long as no cervical trauma is suspected, place the child in a supine position with padding (e.g., rolled towel, pillowcase, or small blanket) under the shoulders. This action will hyperextend the child's neck.

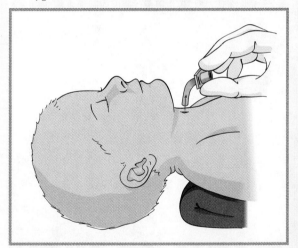

3. Untie the cloth ties or remove whatever other device is present that holds the tracheostomy tube in place. Deflate the cuff if present, and pull out the current tube. If there are a lot of secretions around the stoma in the child's neck, it may be necessary to suction the stoma.

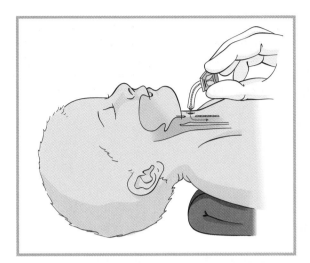

4. Insert the new tracheostomy tube (with obturator in place) into the stoma. It may be necessary to use a water-soluble lubricant to ease insertion of the new tube. If lubrication does not make the insertion easier, use a smaller tracheostomy tube.

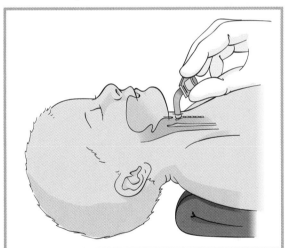

5. NEVER push the tube in against resistance. You may actually push the tube into the tissue and tracheal wall around the child's stoma. This *anterior dissection* may cause bleeding or subcutaneous air in the neck or upper chest.

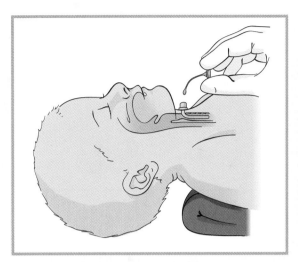

6. Remove the obturator, and inflate the cuff if it is present. Hold the tube in place, and ventilate the child a few times with the bag-valve device to insure correct placement. Listen to breath sounds, and observe for adequate chest rise bilaterally.

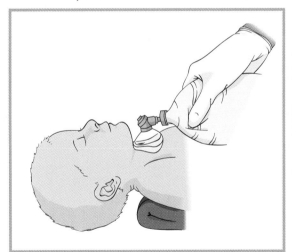

7. If bleeding or subcutaneous air is present, you cannot ventilate the child, or there is no chest rise when using the bag-valve device, suspect an anterior dissection. Remove the tube and control bleeding. Attach a small mask to the bag-valve device, and attempt to provide ventilation through the stoma. Rapidly transport the child to the nearest hospital.

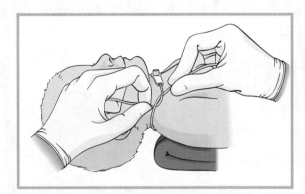

8. Secure the tube by using cloth ties or whatever commercial device is available. It may be necessary to suction the tube if secretions are present. Reattach an oxygen mask or ventilator tubing to the new tracheostomy tube.

PLACING AN ENDOTRACHEAL TUBE IN THE TRACHEAL STOMA

Purpose

If the tracheostomy tube has been dislodged and another appropriately sized tracheostomy tube is not available, an advanced life support provider may insert an endotracheal tube in the stoma to control the airway.

Procedure

Assemble the following equipment: several endotracheal tubes depending on the size of the child, gloves (latex free whenever possible), a BVM device, a 10-cc syringe if the tube has a cuff, a suction catheter, a suction device, and an oxygen source.

Disconnect the mask from the bag-valve-mask device. Make sure the reservoir bag is in place and that the device is connected to an oxygen source. Turn on the oxygen at 15 liters/minute and allow the reservoir bag to fill.

If present, inflate the cuff on the endotracheal tube to make sure it is adequate. Check for leaks in the cuff, and then deflate the cuff.

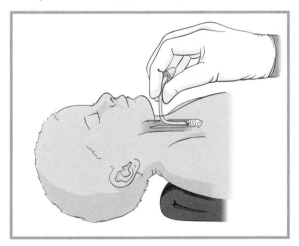

1. Insert the endotracheal tube into the stoma, and inflate the cuff if present. Be careful not to intubate the right mainstem bronchus. Hold the tube, and ventilate the child a few times with the bag-valve device to insure correct placement. Listen to breath sounds, and observe for adequate chest rise bilaterally.

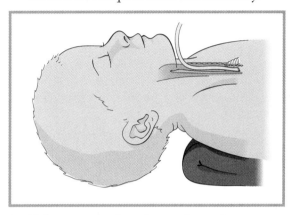

2. If there are no breath sounds or chest rise on the left side, deflate the cuff (if present) and pull the tube slightly back. Reassess breath sounds and chest rise. If ventilation is successful, reinflate the cuff. Secure the tube around the neck. It may be necessary to suction the tube if secretions are present. Ventilate the child manually or connect the ventilator tubing.

INTRAOSSEOUS INFUSION

Purpose

Intraosseous (IO) infusion is used to achieve vascular access when methods to establish a peripheral intravenous line have been unsuccessful. In addition, IO infusion may be used when peripheral access cannot be performed rapidly. Examples of situations in which IO infusion may be helpful include severe dehydration, circulatory failure, and cardiopulmonary resuscitation. IO infusion is performed by an advanced life support provider properly trained in the procedure. It is appropriate for children six years of age and younger.

Procedure

1. Assemble the following equipment: gloves, one IO needle or a Jamshidi needle, antiseptic wipes, one 10-cc syringe filled with normal saline, IV administration set, IV extension tubing, 500 cc or 1 liter of normal saline or lactated Ringer's, 30 cc syringe for boluses, material for a dressing, tape, and a pressure bag for rapid fluid boluses if necessary. Connect the IV bag and tubing and prime the IV line with whatever fluid will be used.

2. Slightly flex the child's knee. Have another provider hold the child's leg above and below the site to be used or secure it into position with tape and towels or a small blanket.

3. Identify landmarks on the child's leg. Palpate one to two fingerbreadths (1 or 2 cm) below the tibial tuberosity. This flat side of the bone is the preferred site. Make sure that the leg chosen is not injured or burned. The distal one-third of the femur may be used in newborns.

4. Prepare the needle, and cleanse the area with an antiseptic wipe. If a stylet is present in the needle to be used, ensure that it is appropriately aligned.

5. Insert the needle into the skin at an angle perpendicular to the bone.

6. Use a rotating motion to push the needle into the bone. A "pop" will be felt as the resistance is decreased once the needle pushes through the bone. Use caution not to push too hard causing the needle to protrude through the other side of the bone.

7. At this point, the needle should stand unsupported in the bone.

8. If a stylet was used, remove it at this time. Attach the prefilled 10 cc syringe, and aspirate to see if bone marrow comes back in the syringe. If no marrow is aspirated, inject 2 to 3 cc of saline.

9. If the fluid does not flow through the syringe or if any fluid goes into the surrounding tissue, discontinue infusion attempts. Remove the needle, and place a small dressing on the site. Attempt the procedure in the other leg if not injured or burned.

10. Secure the IV infusion set onto the hub of the needle, and attach the IV bag with administration set. Directly infuse the fluid through the IO site or give 20 cc boluses using the 30 cc syringe. If rapid infusion is necessary, use a pressure bag around the IV bag. Inflate it to approximately 300 torr.

11. Secure the needle and IO site with a dressing. Reassess the site frequently for swelling or oozing of fluid indicating possible infiltration. Also assess the dependent part of the leg for any signs of extravasation of fluid from the bone marrow. If either of these conditions occur, stop the infusion immediately.

ADMINISTERING MEDICATION THROUGH A VENOUS ACCESS DEVICE

Purpose

There may be occasions in which the prehospital provider may utilize an existing venous access device for intravenous fluid administration. This technique is performed by an advanced life support provider properly trained in the procedure.

Procedure for Peripherally Inserted Central Catheter or Hickman®/Broviac® Catheter:

Gather the necessary equipment: gloves, antiseptic wipes, IV administration set, IV fluid, 10 cc syringe filled with saline, 21- to 18-gauge needle (depending on the size of the lumen), and dressing material.

1. Uncap the end of the device (which may be called the lumen or port), and attach the IV line. Infuse whatever fluid is appropriate for the child's condition.

2. If a peripheral lock (also known as heparin lock or saline lock) is present at the end of the device, cleanse the end of the lock. Attach a regular needle to the end of the IV line, and insert it into the lock. Tape the connection so that it is secure, and tape the tubing to the child's chest. Infuse whatever fluid is appropriate for the child's condition. A 5 or 10 cc syringe may be used for flushing.

   Rapid fluid replacement is not recommended for this device because of the small lumen size.

Procedure for Implanted Port

Gather the necessary equipment: gloves, noncoring Huber needle, antiseptic wipes, IV administration set, IV fluid, 10 cc syringe filled with saline, and dressing material.

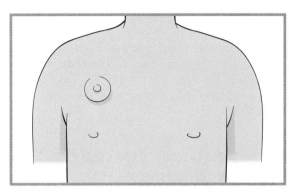

1. Identify the site of the implanted port. A small raised area should be palpable on the right side of the child's upper chest. Cleanse the overlying skin with an antiseptic. To prevent infection, ideally the site should be accessed using a sterile procedure. In the prehospital setting, sterile conditions are not usually available. Therefore, it is important to perform the procedure using the cleanest conditions possible.

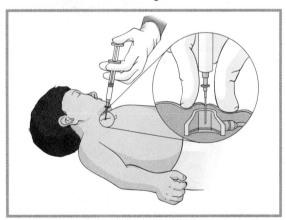

2. The diaphragm of the port is pierced on the top or side depending on the type of device implanted. Use ONLY a Huber needle. DO NOT use a regular needle as it will cause damage to the implanted port. Surgery will be required to replace the port if it is damaged. Infuse whatever fluid is appropriate for the child's condition. If a Huber needle is not available, do not attempt to use the implanted port.

Note: Remember that the child will feel pain as the needle is introduced through the skin into the port. Provide emotional support as necessary.

HELMET REMOVAL

Purpose

There are various types of helmets. Each one has a unique contour, face protection, and strapping devices. Helmets that cover the head all the way to the nape of the neck will need to be removed differently then those helmets that cover the upper portion of the head.

Procedure for Bicycle, Roller Blades, or Skateboard Helmets

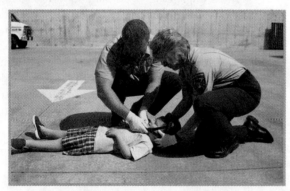

1. The provider at the head holds manual, in-line stabilization of the child's head and neck while the second provider loosens the chin strap.

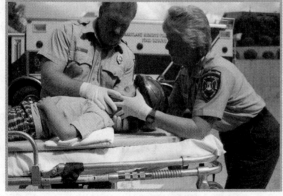

2. Frontal, in-line stabilization begins with provider 2 placing one hand in a position behind the head to support the head from dropping once the helmet is removed. Frontal in-line stabilization is complete when provider 2 places the other hand on the mandible and jaw to maintain side-to-side stability of the child's head.

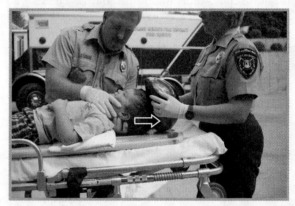

3. Provider 2 continues full stabilization of the head while provider 1 removes the helmet.

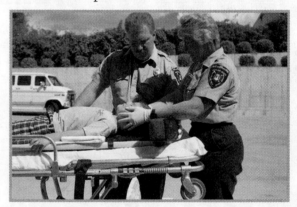

4. Once any helmet is removed, any voids left between the child's head and the long backboard need to be filled with towels, gauze wrap, or other appropriate material.

Procedure for Football or Equivalent Helmet with Face Mask

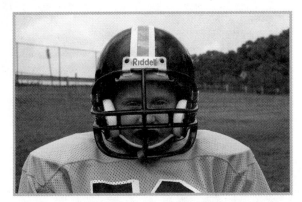

1. This type of helmet is designed to closely fit the child's head. The face mask protects the face from blunt injury. Notice the mouth guard in place.

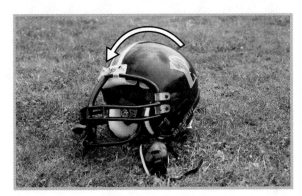

2. The helmet fits the contour of the child's head.

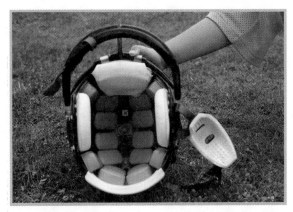

3. Extensive padding is present inside the helmet. This padding ensures that the helmet fits very snugly against the child's head so that no movement occurs inside the helmet.

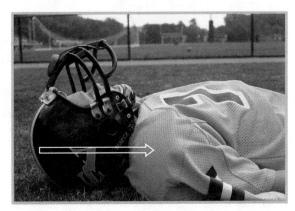

4. The helmet in conjunction with the shoulder pads keeps the child's spine in neutral alignment.

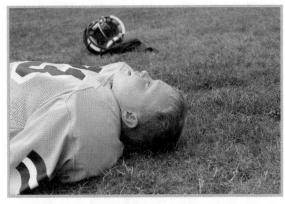

5. Notice the hyperextension of the child's cervical spine if only the helmet is removed. The shoulder pads continue to elevate his back.

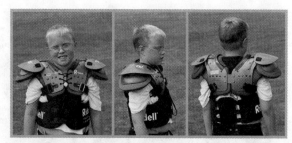

6. The shoulder pads are actually a unit of padding that extends down the torso along the front and back of the child. The child should be immobilized with the helmet and shoulder pads intact to protect the spine. Padding in the front may be untied to access the child's anterior chest. Removal of the padding and the helmet, however, will cause unnecessary manipulation of the child's head and neck.

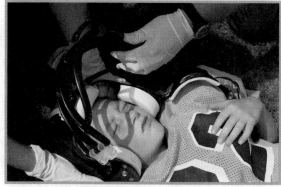

7. To gain appropriate access to the child's airway, the face plate should be removed. Special tools are available that cut through the plate itself. Once the face plate has been cut or QUICKLY disassembled, it should be moved out of the way.

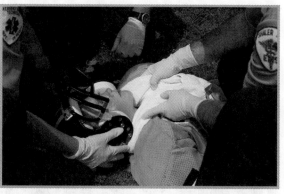

8. In most instances a cervical collar will not fit around the child's neck when the helmet and shoulder pads are in place. Attempt to immobilize the neck with a towel or blanket.

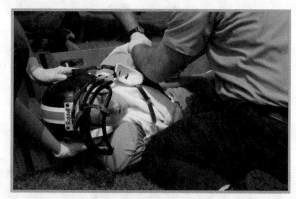

9. Roll the child as a unit onto the backboard with the equipment still in place. Secure the child's body first, and then secure the head and neck to complete immobilization.

HINTS FOR ADMINISTERING IV TREATMENT TO PEDIATRIC PATIENTS

Age Group	Ideal Site	Preparation of Child
Infant	Scalp vein, foot, or hand	Allow family member to hold patient and provide tactile and verbal reassurance.
Toddler	Hand, arm, or foot (use less dominant limb whenever possible)	Give simple, concrete explanation. Talk to child immediately before procedure. This age group has limited attention span.
Preschool	Hand or forearm (use less dominant limb whenever possible)	Explain procedure right before taking action. Demonstrate skill on toy or doll when possible.
Elementary school age	Hand or forearm (use less dominant limb whenever possible)	Let patient assist in preparing equipment for IV insertion (e.g., tearing open adhesive strips or tape). Tell the child it is OK to cry because needles sometimes hurt.
Adolescent	Hand or forearm (use less dominant limb whenever possible)	Approach discussion at adult level. Explain necessity of IV therapy and discuss equipment in adult terms.

SPINAL IMMOBILIZATION TECHNIQUES

Pedi-Pak Application

Purpose

This device is designed to safely restrain a pediatric patient up to 40 pounds on the stretcher.

Procedure

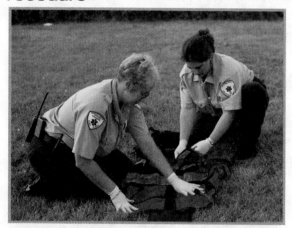

1. Unroll the device and separate the straps.

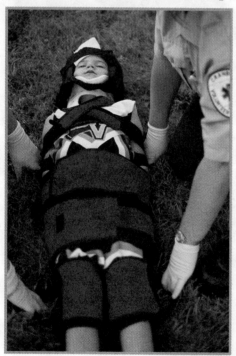

2. Logroll the child and place her on the center of the Pedi-Pak. Secure the straps across the chest, over the shoulders, around the abdomen,

and around the legs. Make sure they are snug but not too tight so as to restrict the child's breathing efforts. Secure the pieces around the head last.

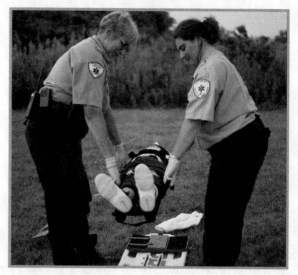

3. Lift the child, and place her on the long backboard.

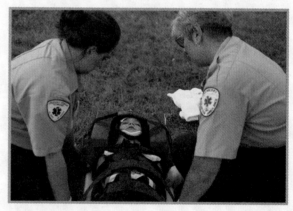

4. Once on the long backboard, secure the torso and then place a head immobilization device along the sides of the head for extra support.

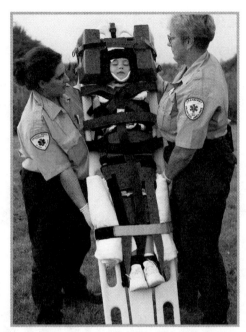

5. Extra padding may be needed along the side of the legs or arms to prevent side-to-side movement in the event that the backboard is tilted (if the child begins to vomit). The feet should also be secured so that the child does not slide down on the board.

Rigid Cervical Collar

Purpose

This device is used to immobilize the head and neck. It should fit the child without causing any hyperextension of the head. If the collar available is too large for the pediatric patient, DO NOT USE IT.

Procedure

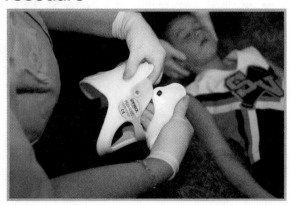

1. Maintain manual, in-line stabilization of the child's head and neck (provider #1 in background). Remove the cervical collar from its package (provider #2 in foreground).

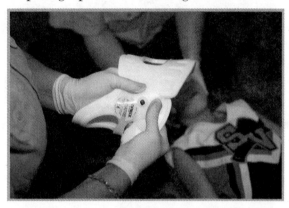

2. Complete assembly if necessary. With the collar shown, secure the chin portion of the collar.

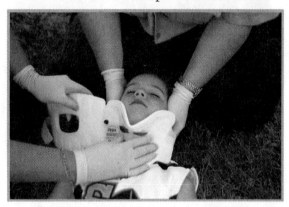

3. Make sure the collar fits the child. Briefly place the front of the collar under the child's chin to make sure it fits. Remove the collar.

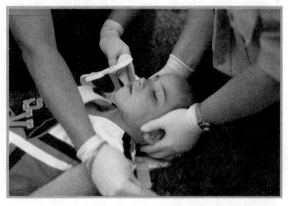

4. Slide the back of the collar behind the child's neck.

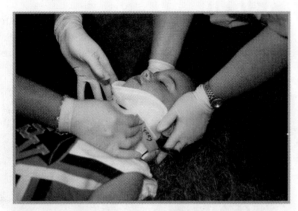

5. Secure the front of the collar under the child's chin, and wrap the back of the collar around the child's neck. Secure the Velcro strap just tight enough to keep the collar in place.

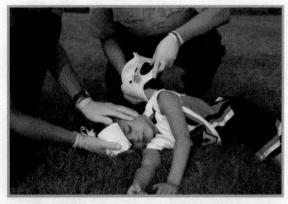

6. Not all pediatric patients will be found supine. For those children that are found prone or on their side, the first provider holds manual, in-line stabilization.

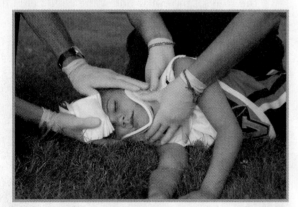

7. The second provider applies a rigid cervical collar before the child is moved.

Backboarding

Purpose

This device is designed to safely immobilize a patient in the usual anatomical position. Pediatric patients may need additional padding depending on their size.

Procedure

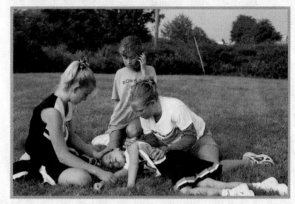

1. When a child is injured, there will usually be other people around. Siblings and/or friends of the child may also be present.

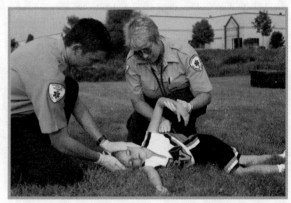

2. Provider 1 maintains manual, in-line stabilization of the child's head and neck while provider 2 completes the assessment. As each step is completed, explain what is happening to the child in language she will understand.

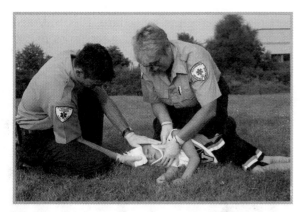

3. Provider 2 applies an appropriately-sized rigid cervical collar on the child as previously described.

4. Provider 2 prepares the backboard for use and assesses the child's extremities for injuries. Without complicating or worsening any injury, provider 2 places the child's arms along the side of the body in preparation for a log roll. The size of the child will determine the number of people needed to assist in logrolling the child onto the backboard. Use bystanders if necessary as long as they are calm enough to help.

Note: Do NOT roll the child on an injured extremity!

5. EMS providers at the child's side put their knees against the child so as to create a pivot point on which to logroll her. Firmly grip the side of the child opposite of where the knees are placed. Do not be tempted to grip the child's clothing or belt loops. Instead, grasp the child's body through her clothing.

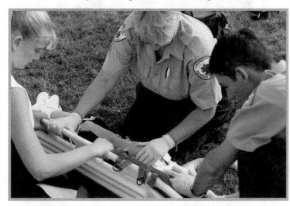

6. As a team, initiated with some kind of verbal command from the provider at the head, logroll the child as a unit onto her side. Have another

provider or bystander slide the backboard underneath the child as close to the child as possible. Use this time to check the posterior of the child for additional injuries.

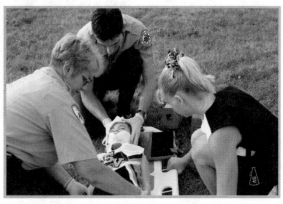

7. Lower the child onto the board. If she is not properly centered on the backboard, adjust her position.

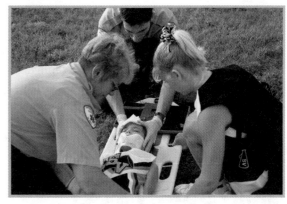

8. To adjust the child's position, provider 1 maintains manual, in-line stabilization of the head and neck. Upon verbal command of the provider at the head, the entire team moves the child down on the backboard (or up if the child is too low) in a diagonal motion toward centering the child.

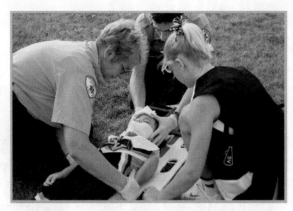

9. Provider 1 continues to maintain manual, in-line stabilization of the child's head and neck. Upon verbal command of the provider at the head, the entire team moves the child up on the backboard (or down as necessary) in a diagonal motion to a center position.

Straps should be used to secure the child to the backboard.

DO NOT: Place straps over the child's neck.

Place straps too tightly on child which may restrict chest or abdominal movement by tightening.

Place padding or some type of filling between child and the point where the strap connects to the backboard. This will keep the child from sliding underneath the straps during extrication and transport.

Child Safety Seat Immobilization

Purpose

A child safety seat can be used to immobilize a pediatric patient under 40 pounds if:

1. The infant's or child's condition warrants (no unstable or potentially life-threatening injuries)
2. The child safety seat is not cracked or broken
3. The child safety seat is an approved restraining device

Be aware that this procedure is controversial at the present time. Several organizations have recommended against using the safety seat to immobilize the infant or child after a crash. However, there has not been any research or substantial evidence to sup-

port discontinuing the procedure. It is still recommended by the American College of Surgeons' Committee on Trauma as appropriate immobilization for pediatric patients.

Procedure

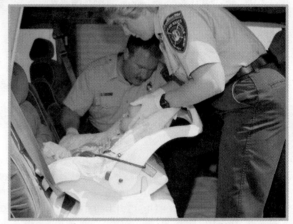

1. Provide manual in-line stabilization of the infant's head and neck while she is in the safety seat. Inspect the safety seat and the child or infant. As long as the patient's condition permits it and there is no obvious damage to the seat, immobilize the child or infant in the seat.

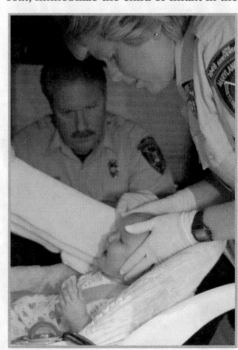

2. Apply a rigid cervical collar to an older child. If the patient is an infant, use padding around the

neck if an appropriately-sized rigid cervical collar is not available. DO NOT use a collar that is too big as it will cause hyperextension of the infant's neck leading to airway obstruction or further aggravation of a possible cervical injury.

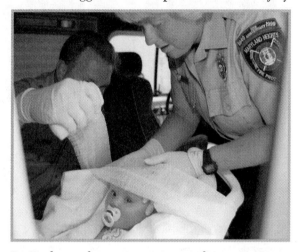

3. Pack towels, gauze wrap, or other appropriate material snugly around the patient's body and head to prevent any side-to-side movement. Wrap gauze around the forehead and back of the seat so that the child or infant cannot move forward. DO NOT place any tape or similar sticky substance against the patient's forehead or hair. If tape must be used, first place the sticky side of two long pieces together. Once the head has been appropriately secured, the first provider may discontinue manual stabilization.

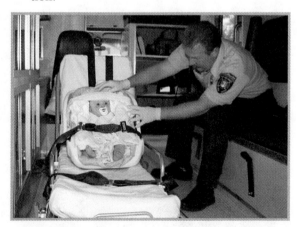

4. Properly secure the seat to the stretcher for transport. For infants, make sure that the seat is facing the rear doors of the vehicle.

Moving a Pediatric Patient from a Child Safety Seat to Another Full-Spine Immobilization Device

Purpose

The infant or child may need to be moved to another full-spine immobilization device because:

1. The patient has become unstable
2. Further examination is required, usually once the patient reaches the hospital
3. The staff at the receiving Emergency Department may feel uncomfortable with moving the patient and request your assistance

A short backboard, long backboard, or vacuum mattress may be used. A pedi-pak is used in the following procedure.

Procedure

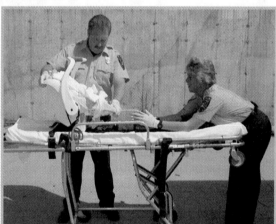

1. Place the entire safety seat on the device. The first provider stands at one end of the stretcher. The second provider gently moves the back of the seat to a lying position. The patient is now supine in the seat.

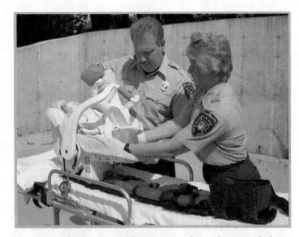

2. Provider 1 provides manual, in-line stabilization of the infant's head.

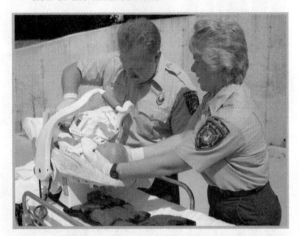

3. Provider 2 removes all padding and releases any straps.

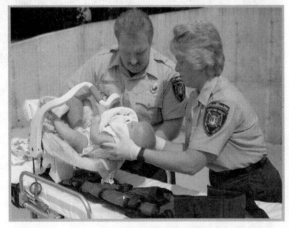

4. Provider 1 continues manual, in-line stabilization while provider 2 gently slides the infant or child out of the seat and onto the backboard (pedi-pak). This transfer should occur as one

movement with the provider at the infant's head directing the move. DO NOT PULL THE CHILD OUT BY HER HEAD AND/OR NECK!

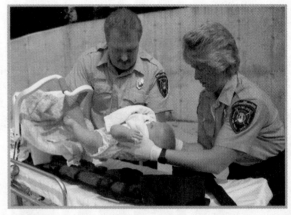

5. Depending on the size of the infant or child, support of the back may be required.

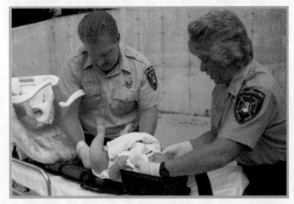

6. Adjust the child's position on the backboard or in the pedi-pak.

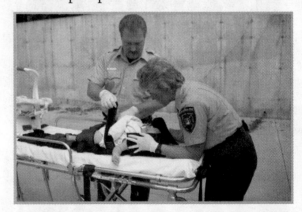

7. Secure the infant or child to the long backboard (or pedi-pak) for transport if the patient is not at the hospital.

Transferring a Child from a Wheelchair or Special Stroller to a Long Backboard

Procedure

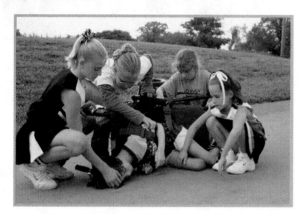

1. Children with special health care needs who use wheelchairs or specialized strollers can be injured while in these devices.

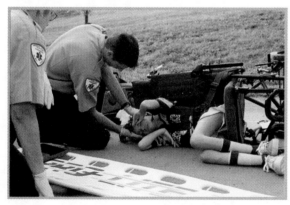

2. Once the need for immobilization has been identified, provide manual, in-line stabilization of the child's head and neck.

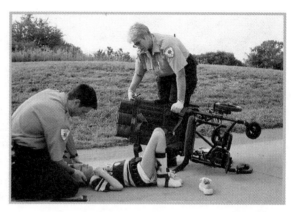

3. Provider 1 continues to provide stabilization. Provider 2 removes any straps from around the child, and moves the wheelchair or special stroller out from under the child. After briefly examining the back, place the child in a supine position. This child also has braces (ankle-foot orthoses or AFOs) on her lower extremities. If no injuries are found in those areas, leave the AFOs or similar devices in place.

Note: Try not to cut any straps or other devices securing the child to the chair or stroller. This equipment is *very* expensive and may not be easily replaced. Use good judgment. *ONLY* use scissors if the child has a life-threatening injury and cannot be easily removed from the equipment.

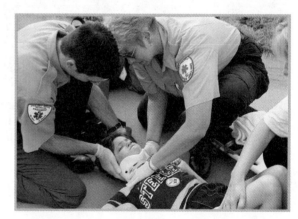

4. Provider 1 continues manual, in-line cervical stabilization while provider 2 applies a rigid cervical collar. Explain what is being done in terms that the child, family, or other caregivers will understand. Ask questions about the child's disabilities and modify your treatment as appropriate.

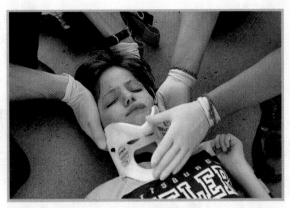

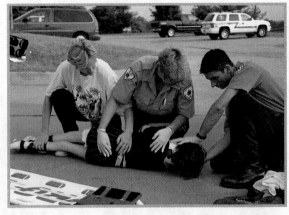

5. Make sure the collar is secure around the child's neck. Several explanations may be necessary during the procedure as the child may not understand what is happening. The young girl used in this example was nonverbal and had the understanding of a 12-month-old child (even though she was 13 years old). She needed frequent verbal reassurance during the simulation.

REMEMBER to provide frequent emotional support to the child, parent, and /or caregiver throughout the process.

7. Logroll the child up onto her side upon verbal command from the person at the head. The remainder of the procedure is the same.

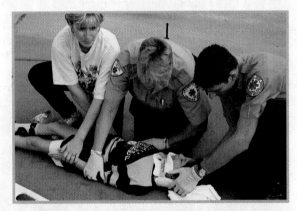

6. Prepare the child for logrolling. Use a parent or other caregiver for assistance as available. In this photograph, the child's aunt assists with the procedure.

ADMINISTERING RECTAL DIAZEPAM GEL (DIASTAT®)

Purpose

Rectal diazepam gel (Diastat®) can be administered to a child in status epilepticus. This rapid intervention may stop or reduce the seizure activity, leading to an improvement in the child's outcome.

Procedure

1. Place the child on his or her side while protecting the head.

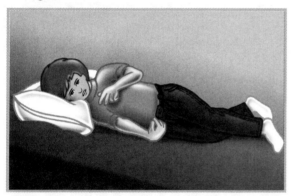

2. Determine what dosage is necessary. Diastat® comes in six unit doses.

Pediatric pack	1.	2.5 mg
	2.	5 mg
Universal pack		10 mg
Adult pack	3.	15 mg
	4.	20 mg

Note: Each Twin Pack contains two Diastat Quick-Dose™ rectal delivery systems, two packets of lubricating jelly, and administration instructions.

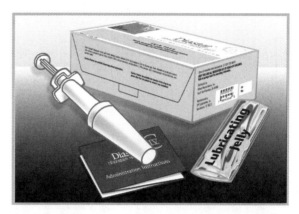

3. Select the syringe from the items contained in the box.

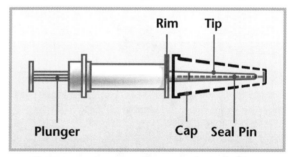

4. Push up with thumb and pull to remove protective cover from syringe.

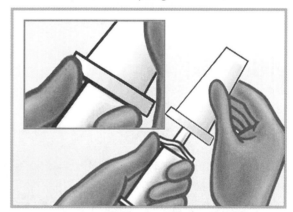

5. Lubricate rectal tip with lubricating jelly.

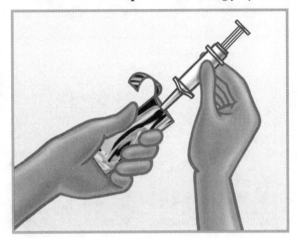

6. Turn child on side facing you.

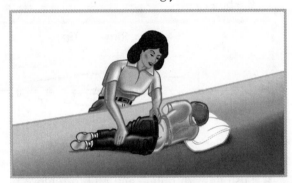

7. Bend the upper leg forward to expose the rectum. If the child is wearing a diaper, ask the parent or caregiver to help you move the diaper to expose the rectum.

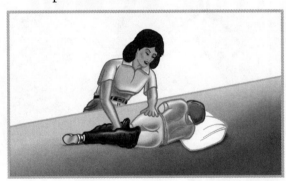

8. Separate buttocks to expose the rectum.

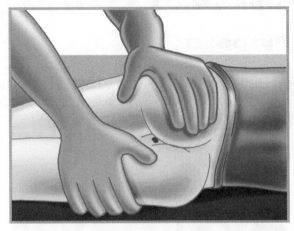

9. Gently insert the syringe tip into the rectum. The rim should be snug against the rectal opening.

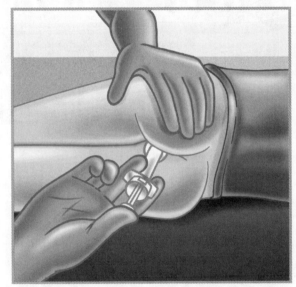

10. Slowly count to three while gently pushing the plunger in until it stops.

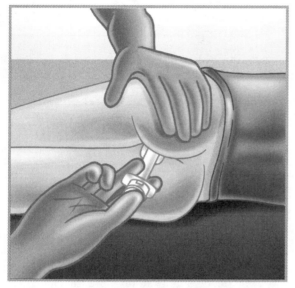

11. Slowly count to three before removing the syringe from the rectum.

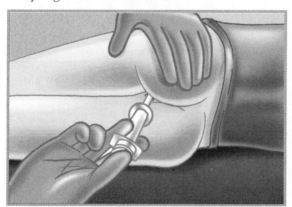

12. Slowly count to three while holding the buttocks together to prevent leakage.

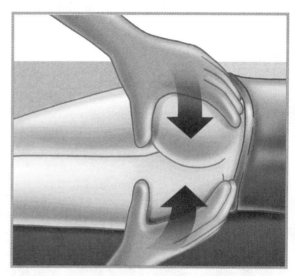

13. Once Diastat® has been given, keep the child on his or her side facing you. Note the time the medication was given, and continue to observe the child.

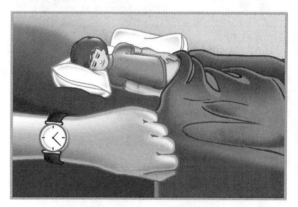

Illustrations reprinted with permission © Elan Pharmaceuticals.

TRANSPORTING SKILLS

Purpose

Taking care of a pediatric patient IS different than taking care of an adult. This difference includes the "typical" activity in the patient compartment of the transporting vehicle. Be aware of what you say and what you do.

Procedure

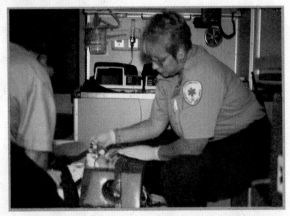

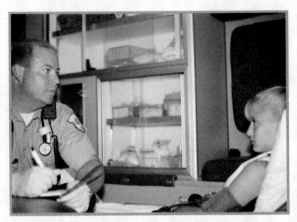

1. Try to always sit in full vision of the child. Make radio or cellular communications from the bench seat when possible. Try not to go behind the patient and out of his or her view.

2. When possible, let the patient's parent or a familiar adult ride along in the patient compartment of your transporting vehicle. Place the adult in an area that does not impede your path to equipment during transport, and secure him or her in a safety belt.

3. Take time to talk to the patient during transport. Do not get caught up with writing your report, talking to your partner, or sorting through EMS equipment. Pediatric patients will need your attention more than an adult.

4. Speak in the patient's terms of understanding. Most will not understand what a "hematoma" is as compared to a "boo-boo" or "black-and-blue-mark." If you do not routinely interact with children, you will need to make a concerted effort to do so.

Appendix C ▶ Guidelines for Pediatric Disability Awareness

1. Do not use the term "handicap" or "handicapped." The more appropriate term is "disability" or "disabled."

2. **Use "person first" language. In fact, license plates in many states now have the abbreviation "PD" instead of "HP." PD refers to a person with a disability instead of HP, which referred to a handicapped person. Use "child with diabetes" instead of a diabetic child or just diabetic. Do not say "epileptic" when referring to a child with epilepsy or a seizure disorder. The person is mentioned before the condition, and reference to the person should always be included.**

3. Use positive terms whenever possible. For instance, a wheelchair actually enables a child to have increased mobility. Therefore, that child is not "wheelchair bound" or "confined to a wheelchair." Do not use "suffers from," "invalid," or "inflicted with" to described the child. Do not use "fits" when referring to a seizure or "mongoloid" when referring to a child with Down syndrome.

4. Avoid the "N" word. "Normal" should be replaced with "typically developing" or "child without a disability."

5. Emphasize how children are alike instead of pointing out their differences.

6. Be sensitive to the family's coping skills. When a child with a disability is a family member, there is stress on the entire family. Allow the parents to vent if necessary, and try to provide resources for assistance whenever possible. Do not be surprised if they are not all that concerned about an emergency—they may have had to deal with the same situation multiple times. Encourage positive interaction with brothers and sisters when they are present.

7. Encourage "parent-professional" partnerships as much as possible. Parents are an integral part of their children's lives, especially when that child has a disability. Treat them as valued team members. Use them as a resource for medical information, how to communicate with their child, what makes their child uncomfortable (e.g., loud siren), and general physical and emotional comfort measures to use.

8. Do not be judgmental. Some parents may not be well educated or may not be as actively involved in their child's care. The degree of parent and sibling involvement may vary from family to family. While it is appropriate to report legitimate suspicions of child abuse, do not assume the child is being harmed because of his or her disability. For instance, the child with attention deficit hyperactivity disorder (ADHD) may require restraint during an emotional and/or physical outburst. This action by the parent or other family member may be entirely appropriate for the situation.

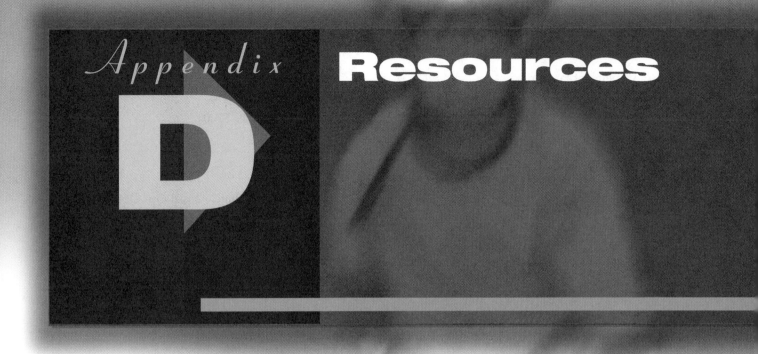

Appendix

D

Resources

Federal Sites

Centers for Disease Control and Prevention
1600 Clifton Road
Atlanta, GA 303333
1-800-311-3435
www.cdc.gov

Emergency Medical Services for Children
EMSC National Resource Center
111 Michigan Avenue, NW
Washington, DC 20010-2970
202/884-4927
Fax: 301-650-8045
www.ems-c.org

Forum on Child and Family Statistics for America's
Children
www.childstats.gov

Health Resources and Services Administration (HRSA)
Maternal and Child Health Bureau
See the web site for the address of the bureau in your
region.
www.mchb.hrsa.gov

National Center for Health Statistics
U. S. Department of Health and Human Services
Centers for Disease Control and Prevention
National Center for Health Statistics
Division of Data Services
Hyattsville, MD 20782-2003
301-458-4636
www.cdc.gov/nchs

National Highway and Traffic Safety Administration
(NHTSA)
400 Seventh Street, SW
Washington, DC 20590
1-800-424-9153
www.nhtsa.dot.gov

U.S. Consumer Product Safety Commission
4330 East West Highway
Washington, DC 20814
1-800-638-2772 → Consumer hotline: Call toll-free to
obtain product safety information, report unsafe products, and obtain other agency information.
www.cpsc.gov

U.S. Department of Health and Human Services
200 Independence Avenue, SW
Washington, DC 20201
1-877-696-6775
www.dhhs.gov

U.S. National Library of Medicine (National Institutes
of Health)
8600 Rockville Pike
Bethesda, MD 20894
1-888-346-3656
Public Information Office: 1-888-FIND-NLM
www.nlm.nih.gov

Organizations

American Academy of Pediatrics
141 Northwest Point Boulevard
Elk Grove Village, IL 60007-1098
1-800-433-9016
847-434-4000
Fax: 847-434-8000
www.aap.org

American College of Emergency Physicians
1125 Executive Circle
Irving, TX 75038-2522
1-800-798-1822
www.acep.org

American College of Surgeons
1155 16th Street NW
Washington DC 20036
(202) 872-4600
(800) 227-5558
www.acs.org

Safety

Bicycle Helmet Safety Institute
4611 Seventh Street South
Arlington, VA 22204-1419
703-486-0100
Fax: 703-486-0576
www.helmets.org

Children's Safety Network
CSN National Injury and Violence Prevention
Resource Center
National Center for Education in Maternal and Child
Health
2000 15th Street North, Suite 701
Arlington, VA 22201-2617
703-524-7802
Fax: 703-524-9335

CSN National Injury and Violence Prevention
Resource Center
Education Development Center, Inc.
55 Chapel Street
Newton, MA 02458
617-969-7101, ext. 2207
Fax: 617-244-3436

CSN Adolescent Violence Prevention Resource Center
55 Chapel Street
Newton, MA 02458
617-969-7100 ext 2374
Fax: 617-244-3436

CSN Rural Injury Prevention Resource Center
National Farm Medicine Center
Marshfield Clinic
1000 North Oak Avenue
Marshfield, WI 54449-5790
715-389-4999
888-924-7233
Fax: 715-389-4996

CSN Injury Data Technical Assistance Center
California Center for Childhood Injury Prevention
Graduate School of Public Health
Maternal and Child Health Division
San Diego State University
6505 Alvarado Road, Suite 208
San Diego, CA 92120
619-594-3691
Fax: 619-594-1995

National SAFE KIDS Campaign
1301 Pennsylvania Avenue, NW
Suite 1000
Washington, DC 20004-1707
202-662-0600
Fax: 202-393-0272
www.safekids.org

National Safety Council
1121 Spring Lake Drive
Itasca, IL 60143-3201
1-800-621-7615
630-285-1121
Fax: 630-285-1315
www.nsc.org

Burns

American Burn Association
625 North Michigan Avenue
Suite 1530
Chicago, IL 60611
1-800-548-2875
312-642-9260
Fax: 312-642-9130
www.ameriburn.org

Shriner's Burn Institutes
International Shriner's Headquarters
2900 Rocky Point Drive
Tampa, FL 33607-1460
813-281-0300
www.shrinershq.org

Child Abuse

American Association for Protecting Children
American Humane Association
63 Inverness Drive East
Englewood, CO 80112
1-800-227-5242 (outside Colorado)
1-800-227-4645
303-792-9900
www.americanhumane.org

C. Henry Kempe National Center for the Prevention
and Treatment of Child Abuse and Neglect
1205 Oneida Street
Denver, CO 80220
303-321-3963

Emergency Child Abuse Hotline
Childhelp USA
1150 Connecticut Avenue NW
Washington, DC 20036
1-800-422-4453 or 1-800-4-A-CHILD

National Clearinghouse on Child Abuse and Neglect
Information
330 C Street SW
Washington, DC 20447
703-385-7565 or 800-FYI-3366
Fax: 703-385-3206
www.calib.com/nccanch

National Committee for Prevention of Child Abuse
332 South Michigan Avenue Suite 1600
Chicago, IL 60604-4357
312-663-3520

National Resource Center on Child Sexual Abuse
107 Lincoln Street
Huntsville, AL 35801
1-800-543-7006

Parents Anonymous, Inc
675 W. Foothill Boulevard, Suite 220
Claremont, CA 91711
909-621-6184
Fax: 909-625-6304
http://parentsanonymous-nah.org

Parents United International, Inc.
P.O. Box 952
San Jose, CA 95108
408-453-7616

Family-Centered Care

Association for the Care of Children's Health
19 Mantua Road
Mt. Royal, NJ 08061
609-224-1742
Fax: 609-423-3420
www.acch.org

Institute for Family-Centered Care
7900 Wisconsin Avenue Suite 405
Bethesda, MD 20814
301-652-0281
Fax: 301-652-0186
E-mail: info@familycenteredcare.org
www.familycenteredcare.org

Project Copernicus
2911 East Biddle Street
Baltimore, MD 21213
410-550-9700
Recognizing Family-Centered Care and other publications are available from this organization.

National Center for Infants, Toddlers, and Families
15th Street NW
Washington, DC 20005-1013
202-638-1144
Equals in This Partnership, a free pamphlet, and other
information about parent-professional partnerships are
available from this organization.

Sites for Information Regarding Children with Special Health Care Needs (CSHCN)

For information on the Emergency Information Form
(EIF) for Children with Special Health Care Needs:

www.pediatrics.org/cgi/content/full/106/4/e53
www.acep.org/library/index.cfm/id/7
www.acep.org/policy/po400267.html

Administration for Children and Families
370 L'Enfant Promenade, SW
Washington, DC 20447
www.acrf.dhhs.org

Archives of Pediatric and Adolescent Medicine
American Medical Association Headquarters
515 North State Street
Chicago, IL 60610
312-464-5000
Obtain and review articles from journals.
http://archpedi.ama-assn.org

Latex Allergies
www.latexallergyhelp.com
www.latex.org

Cancer

American Brain Tumor Association
2720 River Road
Des Plaines, IL 60018
847-827-9910
Fax: 847-827-9918
Patients: 1-800-886-2282
www.abta.org

American Cancer Society
1599 Clifton Road, NE
Atlanta, GA 30329
1-800-ACS-2345
www.cancer.org

Candlelighters Childhood Cancer Foundation
3910 Warner Street
Kensington, MD 20895
1-800-366-2223
www.candlelighters.org

Children's Hospice International
2202 Mt. Vernon Avenue
Suite 3C
Alexandria, VA 22301
703-684-0330
Fax: 703-684-0226
1-800-2-4-CHILD
www.chionline.org

National Brain Tumor Foundation
414 13th Street Suite 700
Oakland, CA 94612-2603
510-839-9777
Fax: 510-839-9779
1-800-934-CURE (2873)
www.braintumor.org

National Cancer Institute
Building 31 Room 10A03
31 Center Drive MSC 2580
Bethesda, MD 20892-2580
301-435-3848
1-800-4-CANCER
www.cancernet.nci.hih.gov

National Hospice and Palliative Care Organization
1700 Diagonal Road Suite 300
Alexandria, VA 22314
703-837-1500
www.nho.org

Physical Disabilities
Cleft Lip/Palate

Birth Defect Research for Children, Inc.
930 Woodcock Road Suite 225
Orlando, FL 32803
407-895-0802
www.birthdefects.org

Cleft Palate Foundation and American Cleft Palate-Craniofacial Association
104 South Estes Drive Suite 204
Chapel Hill, NC 27514
919-933-9044
Fax: 919-933-9604
1-800-24-CLEFT (parent hotline)
www.cleftline.org (old site was www.cleft.com)
E-mail: cleftline@aol.com

March of Dimes
March of Dimes Birth Defects Foundation
1275 Mamaroneck Avenue
White Plains, NY 10605
888-MODIMES (663-4637)
www.modimes.org

Congenital Heart Disease

American Heart Association
National Center
7272 Greenville Avenue
Dallas, TX 75231
1-800-AHA-USA1
www.americanheart.org

Hearing Impairment

Alexander Graham Bell Association for the Deaf and
Hard of Hearing
3417 Volta Place NW
Washington DC 20007-2778
(202) 337-5220 Voice and TTY
(202) 337-8314 Fax
www.agbell.org

Canadian Hearing Society
271 Spadina Road
Toronto, ON M5R 2V3
(416) 964-9595 Voice
(416) 964-0023 TTY
(416) 928-2525 Fax
www.chs.ca

Muscular Dystrophy

Muscular Dystrophy Association—USA
National Headquarters
3300 East Sunrise Drive
Tucson, AZ 85718
1-800-572-1717
www.mdausa.org

Spina Bifida

Hydrocephalus Association
870 Market Street Suite 705
San Francisco, CA 94102
415/732-7040
Fax: 415/732-7044
E-mail: hydroassoc@aol.com
www.hydroassoc.org

Spina Bifida Association of America
4950 MacArthur Boulevard, NW
Suite 250
Washington, DC 20007-4226
1-800-621-3141
202/944-3285
Fax: 202/944-3295
www.sbaa.org

National Easter Seal Society
230 West Monroe Street
Suite 1800
Chicago, IL 60606
312/726-6200 (voice)
312/726-4258 (TDD)
312/726-1494 (fax)
1-800-221-6827
E-mail: info@easter-seals.org
www.easter-seals.org

Blindness

American Foundation for the Blind
11 Penn Plaza, Suite 300
New York, NY 10001
Phone: (212) 502-7600
E-mail: afbinfo@afb.net
www.afb.org

Division for the Blind and Handicapped
National Library Service for the Blind and Physically
Handicapped
Library of Congress
Washington, DC 20542
Telephone (202) 707-5100
Fax (202) 707-0712
TDD (202) 707-0744
E-mail: nls@loc.gov
www.loc.gov/nls

Helen Keller National Center
111 Middle Neck Road
Sands Point, NY 11050
(516) 944-8900 (Voice)
(516) 944-8637 (TTY)
Fax: (516) 944-7302
www.helenkeller.org

The Lighthouse, Inc.
New York City Headquarters
111 East 59 Street
New York, NY 10022-1202
(212) 821-9200
(800) 829-0500
Fax: (212) 821-9707
TTY: (212) 821-9713
www.lighthouse.org

Cystic Fibrosis

The Cystic Fibrosis Foundation
6931 Arlington Road
Bethesda, MD 20814
(301) 951-4422 or
(800) FIGHT CF (344-4823)
Fax: (301) 951-6378
E-mail: info@cff.org
www.cff.org

Epilepsy

Epilepsy Foundation of America
4351 Garden City Drive
Landover, MD 20785
(800) 332-1000
(301) 459-3700
www.efa.org

Hemophilia

National Hemophilia Foundation
116 West 32nd Street, 11th Floor
New York, NY 10001
Phone: (212) 328-3700
Fax: (212) 328-3777
HANDI Phone: (800) 42-HANDI
HANDI Fax: (212) 328-3799
www.infonhf.org

HIV/AIDS

Elizabeth Glaser Pediatric AIDS Foundation
2950 31 Street #125
Santa Monica, CA 90405
310/314-1459
310-314-1469 (fax)
E-mail: info@pedAIDS.org
www.pedAIDS.org

National Pediatric & Family HIV Resource Center
University of Medicine & Dentistry of New Jersey
30 Bergen Street ADMC #4
Newark, NJ 07103
973-972-0410
1-800-362-0071
Fax: 973-972-0399
www.pedhivaids.org

The Kids AIDS Site
720 Olive Way Suite 1800
Seattle, WA 98101
E-mail: comments@theKidsAIDSsite.com
www.theKidsAIDSsite.com

Organ Donation

American Association of Kidney Patients
100 S. Ashley Drive Suite 280
Tampa, FL 33602
(800) 749-2257
Fax (800) 223-0001
E-mail: aakpnat@aol.com
www.aakp.org

United Network for Organ Sharing (UNOS)
1100 Boulders Parkway
Suite 500
P.O. Box 13770
Richmond, VA 23225-8770
1-888-TXINFO1
www.unos.org

Mental Retardation

American Association on Mental Retardation
444 North Capitol Street, NW
Suite 846
Washington, DC 20001-1512
202/387-1968
800/424-3688
Fax: 202/387-2193
www.aamr.org

Association for Retarded Citizens of the United States
National Headquarters Office
1010 Wayne Avenue Suite 650
Silver Spring, MD 20910
301-565-3842
Fax: 301-565-5342
E-mail: Info@thearc.org
www.thearc.org

Governmental Affairs Office
1730 K Street, NW
Suite 1212
Washington, DC 20006
202-785-3388
Fax: 202-467-4179
GAOinfo@thearc.org

Autism Society of America
7910 Woodmont Avenue Suite 300
Bethesda, MD 20814-3015
1-800-3AUTISM Ext. 150
Fax: 301-657-0869
www.autism-society.org

The Council for Exceptional Children
1920 Association Drive
Reston, VA 20191-1589
1-800-CEC-SPED
703-620-3660
TTY (text only) 703-264-9446
Fax: 703-264-9494
www.cec.sped.org

National Down Syndrome Congress
7000 Peachtree—Dunwoody Road NE
Lake Ridge 400 Office Park
Building #5, Suite 100
Atlanta, GA 30328
800-232-NDSC
770-604-9500
www.ndsccenter.org

National Down Syndrome Society
National Down Syndrome Society
666 Broadway
New York, NY 10012
NDSS Phone: 212-460-9330 or 800-221-4602
NDSS Fax: 212-979-2873
www.ndss.org

National Fragile X Foundation
P.O. Box 190488
San Francisco, CA 94119
1-800-688-8765
510-763-6030
Fax: 510-763-6223
E-mail: natlfx@sprintmail.com
www.nfxf.org

Special Olympics, Inc.
1325 G Street, NW
Suite 500
Washington, DC 20005-3104
E-mail: jobsso@aol.com
www.specialolympics.org

Youth Groups

Americorps
Corporation for National Service
1201 New York Avenue NW
Washington, DC 20525
202-606-5000
www.cns.gov/americorps/index.html

Association of Junior Leagues International
132 West 31st Street
New York, NY 1001-3406
212-951-8300
Fax: 212-481-7196
www.ajl.org

Benevolent and Protective Order of the Elks
2750 N. Lakeview Avenue
Chicago, IL 60614-189
312-477-2750

Boy Scouts of America
www.bsa.scouting.org

Boys and Girls Clubs of America
1230 W. Peachtree Street, NW
Atlanta, GA 30309
404-815-5700

Circle K International
3636 Woodview Terrace
Indianapolis, IN 46268-1168
1800-KIWANIS
317-875-8755
Fax: 317-879-0204
www.circlek.org

Four H
7100 Connecticut Avenue NW
Chevy Chase, MD 20815
301-961-2820

Future Farmers of America
5632 Mt. Vernon Memorial Highway
Box 15160
Alexandria, VA 22309-0160
703-360-3600

Future Homemakers of America
1910 Association Drive
Reston, VA 22091-1584
703-476-4900

General Federation of Women's Clubs
1734 N. Street NW
Washington, DC 20036-2990
202-347-3168
Fax: 202-835-0246
www.gfwc.org

Girl Scouts of America
420 Fifth Avenue
New York, NY 10018-2798
800-478-7248
www.gsusa.org

Jaycees
PO Box 7
Tulsa, OK 741002-0007
800-529-2337
918-584-2481

Key Club International
3636 Woodview Trace
Indianapolis, IN 46268-3196
800-KIWANIS
317-875-8755 ext. 247
Fax: 317-879-0204

Kiwanis International
363 Woodview Trace
Indianapolis, IN 46268-3196
800-KIWANIS
317-879-0204
www.kiwanis.com

Lions Club International
300 22nd Street
Oak Brook, IL 60521
630-571-5466

Loyal Order of Moose
Moose International
Mooseheart, IL 60539
630-859-2000

National Exchange Club
3050 Central Avenue
Toledo, OH 43606-1700
800-924-2643

National Parent Teacher Association (PTA)
330 N. Wabash Avenue
Suite 2100
Chicago, IL 60611
312-670-6782
800-307-4782
Fax: 312-670-6783
www.pta.org

Optimist International
4494 Lindell Boulevard
St. Louis, MO 63108
314-371-6000
800-500-8130
www.optimist.org

Points of Light Foundation
1400 Street NW
Suite 800
Washington, DC 20005
800-59LIGHT
202-720-8000
Fax: 202-729-8100
www.pointsoflight.org

Rotary International
One Roatary Center
1560 Sherman Avenue
Evanston, IL 60201
847-866-3402
Fax: 847-866-3178

Young Men's Christian Association (YMCA)
101 N. Wacker Drive
Chicago, IL 60606
312-977-0031
Fax: 312-977-9063
www.ymcausa.org

Youth Volunteer Corps of America
6310 Lammar Avenue
Suite 125
Overland Park, KS 66202-4247
913-432-YVCA
Fax: 913-432-3313
www.yvca.org

Young Women's Christian Association (YWCA)
Empire State Building
350 Fifth Avenue, Suite 301
New York, NY 10118
212-273-7800
Fax: 212-465-2281
www.ywca.org

Glossary

absence seizure Seizure that produces some change in the patient's level of consciousness

abuse To physically or verbally attack or injure

acquired amputation The loss of a limb or part of a limb by accident or intentional surgery

acquired immunodeficiency syndrome (AIDS) A disease that involves a defect in cell-mediated immunity and is manifested by various opportunistic infections

acrocyanosis A bluish discoloration of only the hands and feet; present in most newborns for the first few minutes following birth; caused by a combination of a cool delivery environment and initially decreased blood flow to the extremities; not due to a lack of oxygen and does not require treatment

activated charcoal Indicated antidote for most ingested poisons; not used with any decrease in level of consciousness or for ingestion of alcohol, heavy metal, or caustics

adenosine Trade name Adenocard®; used to treat supraventricular tachycardia (SVT); causes a transient atrioventricular block that interrupts the re-entry circuit causing SVT

adolescent From 12 to 18 years of age

advance directive Living will, identification of a durable power of attorney, or oral statement to the physician explaining instructions for health care or appointing an agent

air embolism Blockage of a blood vessel with air

air leak syndrome Ball-valve effect that occurs from overinflation and rupture of alveoli as meconium is pulled into the lower airways

alopecia Loss of hair

alternating current (AC) Electrical current that reverses direction

amiodarone Antidysrhythmic used for a wide range of atrial and ventricular dysrhythmias; prolongs QT interval and QRS duration

amputation The loss of part of a limb or an entire limb

anaphylactic shock Shock precipitated by a severe allergic reaction

anaplastic A change in the structure or orientation of cells

ankle-foot orthoses (AFO) Braces that can help an individual walk

antidote Drug or other substance that counteracts a specific poison

antiretroviral drugs Drugs that prevent reproduction of new virus particles and slow the growth of HIV

Apgar scoring Standardized method for rating the condition of a newborn at one and five minutes following birth; involves five parameters: appearance or skin color, pulse or heart rate, grimace or irritability, activity or muscle tone, and respirations

Arnold-Chiari malformation (ACM) The child's cerebellum, medulla, pons, and fourth ventricle herniate down through an enlarged foramen magnum

asystole Lack of both cardiac output and electrical activity

ataxic breathing Breathing pattern due to a lesion in the medullary respiratory center; characterized by a series of inspirations and expirations

ataxic A type of cerebral palsy characterized by a wide-based gait

atelectasis Collapse of lung tissue preventing the exchange of carbon dioxide and oxygen

athetosis Slow, writhing movements of the extremities

Atlantoaxial instability Neck pain and weakness caused by the instability of the first two cervical vertebrae; usually occurs in children with Down syndrome

atropine Parasympathetic blocker that accelerates the sinus or atrial pacemaker and increases atrioventricular conduction

attention deficit disorder without hyperactivity (ADD-H)   Deficits to attention span with no hyperactivity

attention deficit hyperactivity disorder (ADHD)   A persistent pattern of inattention and/or hyperactivity-impulsivity that is more frequent and severe than is typically observed in individuals at a comparable level of development (American Psychiatric Association)

aura   Period of time right before a seizure begins

autism   A complex disorder that is usually detected within the first 30 months of life; it is characteristic of deficiency of social interaction, impaired communication, and a limited range of play interests and activities

autonomy   The right of parents to make decisions for their children, including those concerning medical treatment

battered child syndrome   Clinical condition in young children that results from serious physical abuse usually at the hand of a parent or foster parent

beneficence   The duty to do good or promote the welfare of the child

bradycardia   Heart rate less than 60 beats/minute

bradydysrhythmia   Dysrhythmia resulting from a slow heart rate

bronchiolitis   Acute viral infection of the lower respiratory tract that occurs primarily in infants under 1 year of age; characterized by respiratory distress, inflammation and obstruction of the bronchioles and expiratory wheezes

bronchoconstriction   The narrowing of the bronchi/bronchioles resulting in restricted air flow

bronchopulmonary dysplasia (BPD)   Chronic lung disease that occurs in the lungs of premature infants treated with positive-pressure ventilation and oxygen for respiratory distress syndrome

bronchorrhea   Discharge of fluid in the bronchi

Broselow system   Equipment system that allows quick identification of proper size of equipment and medication dosages for pediatric patients; uses a color-coded, length-based tape

cancer   A neoplasm characterized by the uncontrolled growth of anaplastic cells that tend to invade surrounding tissue and metastasize to distant body sites (Anderson, 1994)

capnograph   Device to monitor end-tidal carbon dioxide

carbonaceous   Containing carbon

carboxyhemoglobin   Red blood cell carrying carbon monoxide instead of oxygen

cardiac contusion   Bruising of the heart muscle

cardiac output   Volume of blood pumped by the heart in one minute

cardiogenic shock   Shock precipitated by the failure of the heart to pump adequate blood to maintain perfusion

cellulitis   Acute infection of the skin

central cyanosis   The bluish color that involves the entire body, including the mucous membranes; due to a decreased level of oxygen in the blood; may be present even when respirations and heart rate are adequate; occurs when there is adequate oxygen to maintain the heart rate but not enough to fully oxygenate the newborn

central neurogenic hyperventilation   Pattern of breathing with rapid and regular ventilations at approximately 25 per minute; the increasing regularity indicates an increasing depth of coma

cerebral palsy (CP)   A nonprogressive disorder of movement and posture caused by some injury to the brain during early development

cerebrospinal fluid (CSF)   The fluid surrounding the brain and spinal cord

Cheyne-Stokes respirations   Respiratory pattern with periods of shallow, slow breathing increasing to rapid, deep breathing, then returning to shallow, slow breathing followed by a short period of apnea; commonly associated with increased intracranial pressure

child maltreatment   Broadly describes intentional physical and emotional abuse or neglect of children as well as sexual abuse of children

children with special health care needs (CSHCN)   Children who have or are at increased risk for a chronic physical, developmental, or emotional condition and who also require health and related services of a type or amount beyond that required by children generally (McPherson, 1998)

circumoral cyanosis   A bluish discoloration around the mouth

clean intermittent catheterization (CIC)   The ability of a child to self-catheterize to relieve the bladder

cleft lip   A congenital anomaly resulting in one or more openings in the upper lip

cleft palate   A congenital anomaly resulting in an opening in the midline of the roof of the mouth

coalition   A temporary alliance of distinct parties, persons, or states for joint action

coalition building   The ongoing process of cultivating and maintaining relationships with a diverse network of individuals and organizations who share a common set of principles and values (Williams, 1997)

cochlear implant   A surgically placed device that converts sounds to electrical impulses and sends them to the auditory nerve

cognitive impairment   A general term that refers to any type of alteration in cognitive processes

cognitive   The mental processes of comprehension, judgment, memory, and reasoning

colostomy   A surgically created opening that brings a portion of the small or large intestine to the surface of the abdomen

compartment syndrome   Occurs with circumferential burns; swelling of the burn creates pressure or a "tourniquet" effect on the underlying structures and bones and will eventually constrict blood supply if not treated; will lead to loss of the limb if proper circulation is not restored

conduction   The transfer of heat from a warmer to cooler surface

congenital amputation   A limb or part of a limb of a fetus that does not develop completely while in utero

congenital heart disease (CHD)   The presence of any structural or functional defect of the heart or great vessels that is present at birth

congenital   Present at birth

congestive heart failure   The result of a cardiac defect that causes an increase in volume or workload of the ventricles

consent   The legal agreement of a patient to accept medical intervention

continuous positive airway pressure (CPAP)   A device that fits closely over the mouth and nose to provide constant airway pressure upon inhalation and exhalation

continuous quality improvement (CQI)   Process used to improve upon deficiencies identified by quality assurance activities

contractures   The condition of a joint characterized by flexion and fixation that is caused by the shortening of the muscles or by the loss of skin elasticity

convection   The transfer of heat away from the body by air movement

convulsive seizure   Seizure that involves some motor activity (e.g., tonic-clonic)

cricothyroidotomy   Emergency incision between the cricoid and thyroid membranes

croup   Acute viral infection of the upper and lower respiratory tract that occurs primarily in infants and young children up to 3 years of age; characterized by varying degrees of respiratory distress, hoarseness; fever, harsh "seal bark" cough, and inspiratory stridor; also known as laryngotracheobronchitis

cyanosis   Blue discoloration of the skin, nail beds, and mucous membranes as a result of inadequate oxygen concentration

cystic fibrosis (CF)   A condition in which the exocrine or mucus-producing gland does not function properly

deaf   Inability to hear

dehydration   Acute loss of body fluids resulting from either increased fluid loss or decreased fluid intake

dermatitis   Inflammation of the skin

diabetes mellitus (DM)   Chronic, systemic disease characterized by a disorder in the production of insulin

diabetic ketoacidosis (DKA)   Buildup of ketones due to metabolism of fat instead of glucose

diaphoresis   Profuse sweating

diazepam   Also known as Valium®; controlled drug (i.e., narcotic); benzodiazepine sedative and tranquilizer; used to treat anxiety, nervous tension, muscle spasm, and as an anticonvulsant

diplegia   A type of cerebral palsy involving the trunk and all extremities with the legs being the most involved

direct current (DC)   Electrical current that flows only in one direction and is relatively constant

dislodgement   Movement of a tube from its correct position

distributive shock   Shock that is precipitated by profound vasodilatation

Down syndrome (DS)   A congenital condition with varying degrees of mental retardation and other physical characteristics; also called trisomy 21

drowning   Death that occurs within 24 hours resulting from asphyxia during submersion

dry drowning   Death caused from respiratory obstruction and asphyxia due to prolonged laryngospasm; also known as drowning without aspiration

ductus arteriosus   The vascular channel in the fetus that joins the pulmonary artery directly to the descending aorta; usually closes after birth

dyskinetic   A type of cerebral palsy characterized by abnormal involuntary movements

dysphagia   Difficulty swallowing

early intervention   A federally funded program that provides early education for children with delays or disabilities or those at risk for disabilities

ethics   The rightness or wrongness of an individual's obligations to himself or herself and to others in society

Emergency Department Approved for Pediatrics (EDAP)   Facility where minimum pediatric staffing, equipment, and supplies are available for initial stabilization of pediatric patients

Emergency Medical Services for Children (EMSC)   National program with the goal of ensuring that children receive the same high-quality emergency medical care that is provided to adults in the EMS system; initiated in the mid-1980s with federal legislation and funding

emotional abuse   Any activity that attempts to destroy or significantly impair a child's self-esteem or competence

emphysema   Overinflation and destructive changes in alveolar walls causing a loss of lung elasticity and decreased gases

empowerment   Involves allowing the family to have or develop a sense of control over their own family lives

enable   Give families a chance to use their own skills and abilities

encephalocele   The formation of a fluid-filled sac on the back of the neck resulting from the brain and meninges herniating through a defect in the skull

entrance wound   Site where electricity first strikes the body (e.g., necrotic area on hand from touching a high-tension wire or on top of the head from a lightning strike)

epicardial   Pertaining to the outside layer of the heart

epiglottitis   Acute bacterial infection resulting in inflammation and swelling of the epiglottis; characterized by fever, sore throat, and stridor

epilepsy   Chronic seizure disorder; two or more seizures that are not provoked by any obvious cause

epinephrine   Drug that increases myocardial contractility and heart rate (beta effects) and increases vasoconstriction (alpha effects); increases perfusion and enhances oxygen delivery to the heart muscle and brain

escharotomy   Surgical incision into necrotic tissue of burn to expand the tissue and decrease ischemia from a circumferential burn

evaporation   Occurs as low humidity in the air converts water to vapor, thereby drawing heat from the core

exit wound   Site where electricity leaves the body (e.g., necrotic area on foot)

exudate   Pus or serum

family-centered care   An approach to health care that offers a new way of thinking about relationships between families and health care providers; it involves the philosophy that the family is the constant in the child's life

fasciotomy   Incision of the muscle sheath in an extremity; performed when an escharotomy is not successful in restoring distal circulation

febrile seizure   Seizure that results from rapid rise in body temperature; occurs primarily in children under the age of six years

fenestrations   Holes along the length of a tracheostomy tube so air can move up through the larynx and mouth upon exhalation

fidelity   The duty to keep one's promise or word

flail chest   Instability of the chest due to multiple rib fractures

fontanelle   Space between the bones of an infant's skull

foramen ovale   The opening in the septum between the right and left atria in the fetal heart; provides a bypass for blood that would otherwise flow to the fetal lungs; usually closes after birth

foreign body aspiration   Inhalation of a foreign body into either the upper or lower airways

fragile X syndrome   A condition that causes cognitive impairment that can range form mild learning disabilities to severe mental retardation

frenulum   The tissue between the upper lip and gum

fungal infection   An irritation of the stoma site due to leakage of gastric contents

gastrostomy   A surgically created stoma whereby the stomach is brought to the level of the skin

generalized seizure   Abnormal electrical activity spreads throughout the entire brain resulting in some motor activity or some change in the patient's level of consciousness

granulation   Growth of extra tissue around a stoma

hard of hearing   Decreased ability to hear; requires use of a hearing aid

hearing impairment   Reduction in the ear's responsiveness to loudness and pitch

hemiplegia   A type of cerebral palsy involving only one side of the body; this is the most common type

hemophilia   A group of hereditary bleeding disorders

hemoptysis   Coughing up blood

hemothorax   The collection of blood in the pleural space

human immunodeficiency virus (HIV)   The virus that causes AIDS

hyaline membrane disease Respiratory dysfunction that occurs in preterm infants as a result of their lungs not being mature upon birth; also known as *respiratory distress syndrome*

hydrocephaly An accumulation of cerebral spinal fluid in the ventricles of the brain

hyperbilirubinemia A high concentration of bilirubin in the blood stream

hypercarbia Increased carbon dioxide in the blood

hypercyanotic The occurrence of acute cyanosis and rapid, shallow respiration as a result of the heart's inability to meet an increased need for oxygen

hyperkalemia Increased serum potassium

hyperleukocytosis A peripheral white blood cell count that becomes greater than 100,000 cells/mm

hypertonia Increased muscle tone

hypertonic Solution that causes cells to shrink

hypoglycemia Low blood sugar

hypoperfusion Decreased perfusion

hypothermia Abnormal body temperature below 95°F

hypotonic Solution that causes cells to swell

hypovolemic shock Shock that is precipitated by blood or body fluid loss

hypoxemia Decreased oxygen concentration in the blood

hypoxia Decreased oxygen concentration at the cellular level

idiopathic No identifiable cause

ileostomy A surgically created opening that brings a portion of the small or large intestine to the surface of the abdomen

immunosuppression Drugs that are given to lessen the body's response to a foreign body

implied consent If the child is involved in a medical emergency, treatment of the child is assumed based on the theory that the parents would want what is best for their child

infant From one month to one year of age

intracranial pressure (ICP) A buildup of fluids and pressure in the brain

intractable Not easily managed

intraosseous Within the bone

Isolette™ A self-contained incubator unit that allows for the control of heat, humidity, and oxygen; used to transport premature and low-birth-weight neonates

jejunostomy tube A tube that is inserted temporarily through which nutritional supplements or medications can be pumped

jejunum Small intestine

ketogenic diet A diet high in fat, low in carbohydrates, and low in protein

ketones By-product of fat metabolism

Kussmaul respirations Hyperventilation characteristic of acidosis

laryngospasm Spasm of the larynx

law The rules of human conduct that are accepted by society

lead Part of the pacemaker that includes the insulated wire that conducts the impulses between the heart and the pulse generator

least restrictive environment (LRE) Children with disabilities are allowed to attend schools along with children without disabilities

lidocaine Trade name Xylocaine®; drug used for ventricular dysrhythmias; raises threshold for ventricular fibrillation and suppresses ventricular ectopy

living will Written instructions authorizing the provision, withholding, or withdrawal of health care

loco parentis In place of parents

lumen Opening in various tubes

mammalian diving reflex A reflex induced by cold water on the face and forehead that results in apnea, bradycardia, and shunting of blood to the heart and brain leading to a lowering of metabolic needs

meconium The newborn's first bowel movement; normally occurs after birth; may occur in utero as a response to distress

meninges The three membranes enclosing the brain and spinal cord—the dura mater, the pia mater, and the arachnoid mater

meningitis Inflammation of the meninges; may result from viral or bacterial infection; characterized by headache; photophobia, nausea and vomiting; altered mental status in bacterial; seizures may occur

meningocele The formation caused by a saclike cyst filled with meninges and cerebral spinal fluid

meningococcemia Disease that occurs when the *N. meningitides* bacteria spreads to the bloodstream

meningomyelocele A neural tube defect similar to spina bifida in which the protective sheath also contains meninges, spinal fluid, and a portion of the spinal cord with nerves; also called *myleomeningocele*

mental retardation   A mental difficulty or deficiency of subaverage intellectual functioning, deficits in adaptive behavior, and onset before 18 years of age (American Association of Mental Retardation)

midazolam   Trade name Versed®; parenteral central nervous system depressant; used for conscious sedation and preoperative sedation

multilumen   A catheter with more than one lumen

Munchausen syndrome by proxy   A rare type of child abuse in which one person (usually the parent) fabricates or induces illness in another person (ususally the child)

muscular dystrophy   A genetic muscle disorder resulting in muscle degeneration and weakening that is progressive and disabling

myelomeningocele   A neural tube defect similar to spina bifida in which the protective sheath also contains meninges, spinal fluid, and a portion of the spinal cord with nerves; also called *meningomyelocele*

nasogastric tube   A tube that is inserted temporarily through which nutritional supplements or medications can be pumped; inserted through the nose and ends in the stomach

nasojejunal tube   A tube that is inserted temporarily through which nutritional supplements or medications can be pumped; inserted through the nose and ends in the jejunum or small intestine

negative-pressure ventilation   Use of a hard shell or body suit to create a vacuum or negative pressure to inflate the lungs

neglect   A condition that exists when a parent or guardian fails to provide minimal physical and emotional care for the child

neoplasm   An abnormal growth of new tissue that can be either noncancerous or cancerous

neural tube   The tube that becomes the brain, spinal cord, and other neural tissue of the central nervous system

neurogenic shock   Shock precipitated by the loss of vasomotor tone below the level of a spinal injury

neurogenic   Originating in the nervous system

neuropathic   Inflammation of degeneration of the peripheral nerves

nonmaleficence   Duty not to harm or burden the child

obturator   A rigid guide inside tracheostomy tubes to help with insertion; it is removed after the tube is inserted; similar to a stylet

offline or indirect medical control   Can be prospective or retrospective (see **prospective medical control** and **retrospective medical control**)

on-line or direct medical control   Communication between the prehospital provider and the physician over the telephone or radio

open pneumothorax   A sucking chest wound that results in a collapsed lung

opisthotonic   A characteristic of cerebral palsy; exaggerated arching of the back

orogastric tube   A tube that is inserted temporarily through which nutritional supplements or medications can be pumped; inserted through the mouth and ends in the stomach

orojejunal tube   A tube that is inserted temporarily through which nutritional supplements or medications can be pumped; inserted through the mouth and ends in the jejunum or small intestine

orthostatic hypotension   Decrease in blood pressure with a change in position

osteogenic sarcoma   Bone cancer; also known as *osteosarcoma*

osteosarcoma   Bone cancer; also known as *osteogenic sarcoma*

otitis media   Inner ear infection

paradoxical respirations   The movement of the chest when a flail chest is present; the flail segment moves inward on inspiration and outward on exhalation, opposite of the rest of the ribs

paraplegia   A type of cerebral palsy involving only the legs

parent-professional partnership   A collaborative relationship in which parents are respected for their contributions and have a right to be part of the decision-making process; professionals use their medical expertise to care for the child while supporting and strengthening the family in their role of nurturing their child

partial seizure   One particular area of the brain is affected by abnormal electrical discharges; causes specific symptoms

patent foramen ovale   An opening in the atrial septum that does not close after birth

Pediatric Critical Care Center (PCCC)   Tertiary facility designed to provide a higher level of care (i.e., definitive care) than an EDAP; has pediatric intensive care unit (PICU) as well as pediatric and trauma care specialists

percutaneous endoscopic gastrostomy (PEG) or button   Low profile gastrostomy tube at skin level

pericardial tamponade   Accumulation of blood in the space between the heart and the pericardium

pericardiocentesis   Aspiration of the fluid from the pericardial space by use of a needle

peritonitis   Inflammation of the peritoneum causing severe abdominal pain

persistent pulmonary hypertension   Pulmonary arterial vasoconstriction from decreased ability to deliver oxygen to the alveoli; causes blood to be shunted through the still open foramen ovale and ductus arteriosus, resulting in severe hypoxemia

petechiae   Round, purple spot due to intradermal or submucosal hemorrhage

phantom limb pain   Complaint of pain in a limb that has been amputated; is believed to be the result of the disruption of nerve endings

photophobia   Abnormal sensitivity to light; especially in the eyes

physical abuse   Any physical injury that is deliberately inflicted on a child

policy   Principle that governs an activity; employees or members of the ambulance service are expected to follow policies

polycythemia   An increase in number of red blood cells

polydipsia   Increased thirst

polyphagia   Increased hunger

polyuria   Increased urination

positive-pressure ventilation   Use of positive pressure to inflate the lungs; the tidal volume is related to the pressure setting

postictal   Period of time right after the seizure is over

premature newborn   A baby born before 37 weeks gestation and weighing 5.5 pounds or less

preschooler   From three to six years of age

primary injury   Injury to the brain that occurs due to the injuring force

primary prevention   An activity that prevents the development of an injury or disease among people who are well and are not ill or injured

primary transport   Transport of patient to local facility for initial stabilization

procedure   Actual sequence of steps to be followed by prehospital providers

prospective medical control   Developing specific treatment protocols and policies, requiring specific pediatric equipment at the basic life support and advanced life support levels, and requiring training and ongoing continuing education to perform certain pediatric skills

prosthesis   The artificial replacement of a part of the body

protocol   Written plan that specifically outlines the procedures to be followed for a particular condition; sometimes used to mean standing orders

pulse generator   Part of the pacemaker that contains the electronic circuitry and the battery

pulse pressure   Difference between systolic and diastolic blood pressure

pulseless electrical activity (PEA)   electrical activity of the heart remains organized yet there is a lack of, or severely compromised, cardiac output resulting in the loss of central pulses

quadriplegia   A type of cerebral palsy with equal involvement of the arms, legs, head, and trunk

quality assurance (QA)   Organized system of tracking specific indicators to ensure that the quality of the system is maintained

radiation   Involves electromagnetic waves; warmer surfaces radiate heat to cooler areas with no physical contact occurring

reactive airway disease (RAD) or asthma   Increased responsiveness of the tracheobronchial tree to various stimuli, resulting in bronchoconstriction; asthma

respiratory distress syndrome   Respiratory dysfunction that occurs in preterm infants as a result of their lungs not being mature upon birth; also known as *hyaline membrane disease*

respiratory failure   clinical state of inadequate carbon dioxide elimination or inadequate oxygen in the blood

respiratory syncytial virus (RSV)   Single-strand virus that is a common cause of acute bronchiolitis, bronchopneumonia, and the common cold in young children

retinopathy of prematurity   Retinal damage that occurs in premature infants

retractions   Drawing backward

retrolental fibroplasia   Retinal detachment and blindness; complication of oxygen toxicity in the newborn

retrospective medical control   Provides accountability and enables the physician to assure that appropriate care was rendered to the pediatric patient

salicylism   Aspirin overdose

school-aged   From 6 to 12 years of age

scissoring   A characteristic of cerebral palsy; the legs are in a crossed position with stiff knees, hips, and ankles

secondary injury   Injury to the brain that occurs as a result of problems due to other organ system injuries

secondary prevention   An activity that identifies people who have an illness at an early stage in the illness' natural history during screening or early intervention (Gordis, 1996)

secondary transport   Transport of patient from local facility to tertiary center for definitive care

seizure   Disturbance in the electrical activity of the brain

self-determinism   Deciding or determining what is best for oneself

sepsis   Spread of infection from its initial site to the bloodstream initiating a systemic response that adversely affects blood flow to the vital organs

septic shock   Shock usually precipitated by an overwhelming systemic bacterial infection

sexual abuse   The use, persuasion, or coercion of any child to engage in sexually explicit conduct (or any simulation of such conduct) for producing any visual depiction of such conduct, or rape, molestation, prostitution, or incest with children

shaken baby syndrome   A condition that occurs when babies are shaken violently; obvious signs and symptoms may not be evident

shock   Inadequate tissue perfusion

shunt   A special catheter surgically inserted from the brain to either the chest or abdomen

sickle cell anemia   Most common form of sickle cell disease

sickle cell crisis   Acute, episodic condition that occurs in children with sickle cell anemia

sickle cell disease   Genetically determined disorder of the hemoglobin structure within red blood cells

simple pneumothorax   A collection of air in the pleural space that causes the lung to collapse

sinus tachycardia   Not considered a true dysrhythmia, occurs as the result of fever, anxiety or compensatory mechanism for a decrease in cardiac output

spina bifida   A neural tube defect that develops during the first 28 days of pregnancy; the spinal cord is encased in a protective sheath of bone in the meninges

standing orders   Written documents that contain rules, policies, procedures, regulations, and orders for patient care as related to specific clinical situations

Starling's law   Law stating that the force of the heart's contraction is determined primarily by the length of the muscle fibers in the wall

startle reflex   Uncontrollable stiffening of the body and flexion of the extremities that follows any stimulus for which there is usually no adaptation, such as a sudden noise, flash of light, or touching of a person

status asthmaticus   Acute, severe, prolonged asthma attack

status epilepticus   Continuous seizure lasting for more than 30 minutes or a series of seizures from which the child does not regain consciousness

stoma   A surgically created opening; an opening from the gastrointestinal or urinary tract to the outside of the body

strabismus   Misalignment of the eyes

stridor   Crowing sound heart on inspiration; caused by partial airway obstruction

stroke volume   The amount of blood pumped with each ventricular contraction

stump   The end of an amputated limb

subglottic   Below the glottis

subluxation   Partial or complete dislocation

sudden infant death syndrome (SIDS)   Sudden death of an infant or young child that is unexpected by history and in which an autopsy fails to reveal an adequate cause of death; also called "crib death"

superior vena cava syndrome   The compression of mediastinal structures that causes airway compromise and possible respiratory failure

supraventricular tachycardia (SVT)   Heart rate greater than 240 beats/minute in infants and greater than 180 beats/minute in children

syrup of ipecac   Used to induce vomiting

tachydysrhythmia   Dysrhythmia resulting from a rapid heart rate

tachypnea   Persistent, rapid respiratory rate

temperature demarcation   Line where cool skin ends and warm skin begins

tension pneumothorax   An accumulation of air pressure in the lungs that causes a shift in the mediastinum that compromises venous return and decreases cardiac output

teratogens   A substance, agent, or process that interferes with normal prenatal development

tertiary prevention   An activity that prevents complications from an injury or illness

toddler   From one to three years of age

tracheostomy   A surgical opening in the trachea on the front of the neck to aid in breathing

transplant   To transfer an organ from one person to another or from one body part to another

transtracheal jet insufflation Ventilation through the catheter used for cricothyroidotomy

transvenous Insertion into a vein

tripod position Sitting upright, leaning forward with arms down and extended

trisomy 21 A congenital condition with varying degrees of mental retardation and other physical characteristics; also called *Down syndrome*

urostomy A surgically created opening that brings a portion of the urinary tract to the surface of the abdomen

vagus nerve stimulator (VNS) A device that used to treat epilepsy; often referred to as the pacemaker of the brain

ventilation-perfusion mismatch Inability to adequately exchange oxygen and carbon dioxide

ventricular fibrillation (VF) Dysrhythmia characterized by rapid, disorganized depolarization of the ventricles of the myocardium; rare in children

ventricular tachycardia (VT) Dysrhythmia with at least three consecutive ventricular complexes at a rate of more than 100 beats/minute

ventricular-septal defect (VSD) Opening or defect in the heart wall (septum) between the left and right ventricles

ventriculoatrial shunt (VA shunt) A type of shunt that starts in the ventricle of the brain and ends in the right atrium of the heart

ventriculoperitoneal shunt (VP shunt) A type of shunt that starts in the ventricle of the brain and ends in the peritoneum

veracity Duty to tell the truth

verapamil Trade name Calan® or Isoptin®; calcium-channel blocker that acts to slow conduction in the atrioventricular junction

vesicostomy The creation of a stoma that brings the anterior wall of the bladder to the abdominal wall

visual impairment Varying degrees of sight ranging from complete loss of sight to blurred vision

wet drowning Death from asphyxia as well as changes caused by fluid aspiration while submerged; also known as drowning with aspiration

Index